Introduction

Dear readers.

The writer of this book is not a medical doctor, but a real physicist. This book is aimed to be easily understandable book for ordinary people, and also for medical doctors, nurses, students and researchers.

The population of the World is increasing at a very high rate, and especially the population in cities is increasing tremendously. This means, that the food intake and physical activity has also changed a lot. In older times people made a lot of physical work, they had a lot of sports activity and the food was simple but healthy. Obesity was very rare among people.

Nowadays hypertension, high cholesterol levels and obesity are extremely common all around the World. There exist over billion people with hypertension in the World, and there are hundreds of millions of people with high cholesterol levels and excessive body fat and obesity. Also diabetes has increased greatly, all around the World, also in the developing countries.

Non-natural medicines for both hypertension and hypercholesterolemia are used too often, without trying first to take care of these diseases with healthy food, more physical exercise, reducing weight, and reducing fat, sugar, alcohol, smoking etc.

It seems to be, that the education given to patients by doctors and nurses is not sufficient, partly because even they do not know, which natural methods should be used to lower high blood pressure and high cholesterol values.

There exist hundreds of foodstuffs, medicinal plants, animal products and physical methods, which can be used easily and with little money to decrease high blood pressure and high cholesterol values. This books explains only about 250 of those methods.

The book is based strictly on modern scientific research, and each research reference can be looked at the reference list, at the end of the book. Totally there are over 1400 research references in this book.

In reality there exist hundreds of medicinal plants all over the World, which are used in folk medicine to decrease high blood pressure or cholesterol. Only a small amount of these have been scientifically verified. But all the made research have shown, that the folk medicinal claims and uses have been right and they work. This is not astonishing, because the use of these medicinal plants is based on empirical experience, during several hundreds and even thousands of years.

Stig Froberg   07/2012, Naantali, Finland

Index

General

Some common shortnotes

p-value: This figure exists again and again in the text, when there is a comparison between the test group and control or placebo group, using statistical mathematical methods. The difference in measured value is statistically significant between the test group and placebo group, if $p < 0.05$, ie. If p-value is less than 0.05.

The difference in measured value is more significant, the less the p-value is, between the groups. For example, if $p < 0.001$, the difference in the measured value between test group and placebo group is much more, than if $p < 0.05$. For example, if $p < 0.01$, there is only 1% probability, that the difference in measured value between the groups did happen by accident. If $p < 0.05$, there is only 5% probability, that the difference in the measured value between the groups did happen by accident.

TC = Total cholesterol.

TG = Triglycerides.

LDL-cholesterol = "Bad" low density cholesterol.

HDL = "Good" high density cholesterol.

VLDL = "Very bad" very low density cholesterol.

SBP = Systolic blood pressure or the pressure in veins, when heart is contracting. This is always higher than DBP.

DBP = Diastolic blood pressure or the pressure in veins, when heart is relaxing.

Renin = Enzyme, which is made by the kidneys, and which regulates the blood pressure.

Angiotensinogen = Compound, which is made in liver, and which is converted by Renin to a compound called Angiotensin I.

ACE = Angiotensin Converting Enzyme = Enzyme, which acts as a catalytics by converting Angiotensin I to Angiotensin II. Angiotensin II contracts the blood vessels and causes high blood pressure. Many commercial medicines against hypertension work by inhibiting this ACE enzyme.

ET-1 = Endothelin-1 = a protein in human body, which strongly contracts blood vessels.

NO = Nitrogen Oxide. NO is made from the amino acid L-Arginine in food. It is a strong vasodilator, and decreases high blood pressure.

eNOS = Enzyme, which stimulates the NO synthesis from L-Arginine.

Aldosterone = Hormone, which increases blood pressure.

Hypertension

Hypertension or high blood pressure is a chronic disease, in which the blood pressure of arteries is elevated from the normal values. For this reason, the heart has to make more work to pump blood through the blood vessels. There are 2 different blood pressure values: Systolic (SBP) blood pressure and Diastolic (DBP) blood pressure. SBP is the blood pressure measured, when heart is contracting. DBP is the blood pressure, when heart is relaxing. The unit of blood pressure is mmHg. The English clergyman Stephen Hales was the first to measure human blood pressure in 1733.

The normal Systolic blood pressure is in the range betweem 90 – 140 mmHg, and the normal Diastolic blood pressure is in the range between 60 – 90 mmHg. The World Health Organization defines hypertension as SBP over 140 mmHg and DBP over 90 mmHg or shortly 140/90 mmHg.

At the moment, there are over 1000 million hypertensive people in the World. Hypertension varies among different cultures. In Poland about 70%, in USA 30% and in India 5% of population are hypertensive, whereas among the Yanomami Indians in Venezuela, hypertension is nonexisting, with 0% of hypertensives among population!

Most of hypertensives have so called primary hypertension, where the exact reason for hypertension is not known. The rest have so called secondary hypertension, where the reason to hypertension is know to be disease of heart, liver, kidney or arteries.

Hypertension is a strong cardiovascular risk factor, and it can cause stroke, heart attacks, peripheral arterial disease or chronic kidney disease, and finally death. The most common symptoms are headache, altered vision, tinnitus etc. Blood pressure increases normally due to aging.

Hypertension is mostly a lifestyle disease. The most important factors, which cause high blood pressure are excess salt, excess saturated fat, excess daily calories, excess alcohol intake, stress, obesity, infrequent exercise, excess sugar and fructose, smoking, too much coffee etc.

Angiotensin is a hormone, which cause the blood vessels to constrict, and cause hypertension. Angiotensin stimulates the hormone Aldosterone, which also causes hypertension. Angiotensin was first isolated late 1930s.

Liver produces a compound called Angiotensinogen. The enzyme Renin from Kidney acts on Angiotensinogen, and converts it to Angiotensin I. Angiotensin I is converted to Angiotensin II through the enzyme ACE (Angiotensin-Converting Enzyme). Angiotensin II causes hypertension.

Part of medicines used against hypertension inhibit ACE.

Other compounds, which constrict blood vessels and cause hypertension, are Endothelin-1 (ET-1), which is a protein. It is induced by hypoxia, oxidised LDL-cholesterol, pro-inflammatory cytokines etc.

Cholesterol

Cholesterol is an organic compound, which exists in almost all living cells. Most of Cholesterol synthesis happens in liver. The molecular mass of cholesterol is 386.65 g/mol, and its chemical formula is $C_{27}H_{46}O$.

Cholesterol is an important compound for the manufacture of bile acids, vitamin D and many hormones, especially the sex hormones Testosterone, Estrogen, Progesterone, DHEA etc. Other hormones manufactured from Cholesterol are Aldosterone and Cortisol.

However, high levels of Cholesterol in blood increases significantly the risk of cardiovascular disease, heart attack and stroke.

The average synthesis of Cholesterol in human body is about 1000 mg daily and the total Cholesterol body content is about 35 grams. The dietary intake of Cholesterol varies between 200 – 1000 mg per day. The food sources with highest Cholesterol content are eggs, liver, meat, cheese and butter.

The critical enzyme in Cholesterol synthesis is HMG-CoA (3-Hydroxy-3-Methylglutaryl CoA Reductase). Many Cholesterol medicines, such as Statins, inhibit this enzyme.

Cholesterol is insoluble to water. It is transported in the circulatory system with Lipoproteins, which are complex particles, composed of proteins and lipids. There are several types of Lipoproteins, for example Very-Low-Density Lipoprotein (VLDL), Low-Density Lipoprotein (LDL) and High-Density Lipoprotein (HDL). The more lipid and the less protein a Lipoprotein has, the less dense it is.

When the blood Cholesterol content is very high, a part of LDL-cholesterol is oxidized and taken up by macrophages, which become engorged and form foam cells. These cells are trapped in the walls of blood vessels, and form artherosclerotic plaque, and sooner or later block the blood vessels. These plaques cause heart attacks, stroke, high blood pressure and death.

But HDL-cholesterol transports cholesterol back to liver, in a process known as reverse Cholesterol transport. For this reason HDL-cholesterol is called "Good" Cholesterol, whereas VLDL-cholesterol and LDL-cholesterol are called "Bad" cholesterol. Total cholesterol is the sum of VLDL-cholesterol, LDL-cholesterol and HDL-cholesterol.

This means, that total cholesterol is not the most important risk factor for plaque formation, but the ratio Non-HDL-cholesterol/HDL-cholesterol, or in fact the ratio of Oxidized Non-HDL-cholesterol/HDL-cholesterol is the most important risk factor for plaque formation.

When cholesterol is measured in laboratory, the units are normally given either in millimoles/Liter (mmol/L) or milligrams/deciLiter (mg/dL).

Typical limits given for high cholesterol levels are 5.2 mmol/L or 200 mg/L for total cholesterol (TC) and 1.8 mmol/L – 2.6 mmol/L or 70 mg/dL – 100 mg/dL for LDL-cholesterol.

For treatment of hypercholesterolemia, the primary treatment is strict diet, exercise and excess body weight reduction.

The secondary treatment is medicinal, by synthetic medicinal compounds, normally by different Statin compounds. These are Atorvastatin, Fluvastatin, Pitavastatin, Pravastatin and Simvastatin. But Statins have serious complications. They strongly increase the risk of impotence, and reduce serum Testosterone levels strongly (Corona et.al. 2010; Rivzi et.al. 2002; Bruckert et.al. 1996). Other symptoms are muscle cramps. Statins decrease strongly Ubiquinone Q10, which is extremely important to every living cell, in producing energy.

Statins are nowadays used far more than they should, and for example in females, there are no scientific proof to show, that they decrease the risk of cardiovascular deaths.

Triglycerides

Triglycerides are esters, composed of Glycerol molecule together with 3 fatty acid molecules. There are many kinds of triglycerides, depending on the amount of Carbon atoms and the amount of unsaturated double bonds between the Carbon atoms. Triglycerides have a general short name TG.

Triglycerides are the main components of vegetable and animal fats. In human triglycerides are the mechanism to store unused energy. The triglyceride content of blood correlates strongly with the amount of carbohydrates in daily food.

Triglycerides are the main component of the VLDL-cholesterol, and the calorific content of triglycerides, 9 kcal/gram, is 2 times higher than the calorific content of proteins and carbohydrates.

In humans, the high blood triglycerides content represents a significant risk factor for cardiovascular disease. Diets, which contain large amounts of carbohydrates, increase triglyceride levels. Especially obese persons have very often very high triglyceride levels. Also frequent alcohol drinking will increase triglyceride levels. Physical exercise, fish oil and L-Carnitine are natural methods to decrease high triglyceride levels.

Triglycerides can be measured in laboratory, and the units are normally given as mg/dL (milligrams/deciLiter) or mmol/L (millimoles/Liter).. The normal levels are lower than 200 mg/dL or 2.25 mmol/L (American Heart Association).

Practical advice to lower high blood pressure and high cholesterol levels

Before we show over 250 different hypotensive and high cholesterol lowering foodstuffs, diets, nutrients and physical methods, we give here some practical advice to lower high blood pressure, high cholesterol or both. With this knowledge, each person can easily make a suitable diet and exercise program, to naturally lower both high blood pressure, high cholesterol levels, high triglyceride levels and high body weight.

Here is one detailed list of different possibilities.

Exercise
- At least 3 – 5 times weekly, 45 minutes – 1.5 hours of aerobic exercise, such as walking, Nordic walking, running, swimming, bicycling, ice skating, squash, tennis, ice hockey, football, basket ball, volley ball, roller skating, roller skiing, cross country skiing, weight lifting, water polo, ping-pong, badminton etc.

Coffee
Stop drinking Coffee, or replace it at least partly by the following teas
- Green tea
- Pu-Erh tea
- Mate tea
- Rooibos tea
- Cacao (Without sugar)
- Du-Zhong tea (Eucommia Ulmoides)
- Hibiscus tea
- Chrysanthemum tea
- Luobuma tea (Apocynum Venetum)
- You can also make a mixture of these teas

Alcohol
- Reduce alcohol consumption to 30 grams daily
- Replace lager beer with dark beer
- Replace lager beer and strong alcohol drinks with red wine, 2 – 3 dl daily

Meat
- Replace meat by chicken, turkey and fat fish (Rainbow Trout, Salmon, Trout, Atlantic Herring, Cod, Anchovies, Mackerel, Tuna, Bonito, Haddock, European Sprat, Halibut etc.)

Sugar
- Replace sugar by Honey, preferably with dark Honey

Butter and cream
- Replace butter and cream by margarine and vegetable oils (Virgin Olive oil, Sesame oil, Flaxseed oil, Amaranth oil, Rice bran oil, Groundnut oil)

Food and salad oils
Use the following vegetable oils
- Virgin Olive oil
- Sesame oil
- Rice bran oil
- Amaranth oil
- Groundnut oil
- Pumpkin oil

Nuts
Use daily the following nuts
- Almonds
- Walnuts
- Groundnuts (Non-salted)
- Pecan nuts
- Pistachio nuts

Milk products
Use daily a lot of fermented, fat free or low fat milk products with different lactic acid bacteria such as Lactobacillus Casei, Lactobacillus Bulgaricus, Lactobacillus Acidophilus etc.
- Youghurt
- Sour milk

Soymilk
- Replace milk totally or partially by soymilk
- It can be drank as such or put instead of milk to different foods

Berries
Eat a lot of the following berries
- Black Chokeberry
- Blueberry
- Red grapes
- Black raisins, Corinthian raisins
- Goji berries (Lycium Barbarum)
- Amla, Indian Gooseberry (Emblica Officinalis)
- Raspberries
- Mulberries
- Schisandra berry (Schisandra Chinensis)
- Seabuckthorn berry
- Rose hips (Also dried flour)
- Barberry

Fruits
Eat daily at least 2 – 3 fruits from the following list
- Water melon
- Apple
- Bergamot
- Clementine

- Mandarin
- Red grapefruit
- Lemon
- Guava
- Papaya
- Banana
- Passion fruit (Use also the skins, grind into flour and drink or put to different foods)
- Persimmon
- Kiwi
- Avocado
- Prunes and fresh black Plums
- Pomegranate
- Tamarind
- Pitahaya fruit

Vegetable roots
Eat a lof of the following
- Dark or red potatoes (Kongo, Inca Red, Shetland Black etc.)
- Sweet potatoes
- Carrots
- Purple Carrots
- Red beets
- Celery
- Maca (Lepidium Sativum)
- Chinese Bellflower

Vegetables
Eat daily a lot of vegetables from the following list
- Tomato
- Red cabbage
- Purslane
- Peppermint
- Garlic
- Red onions
- Parsley
- Dill
- Olives (Black and green)
- Fresh Ginger
- Fresh Galangal root
- Caigua
- Ashitaba (Angelica Keiskei)
- Celery (Stalks and leaves)
- Spearmint
- Chives
- Shallot
- Chinese Chives
- Welsh Onion

- Ramsons
- Society Garlic (Tulbaghia Violacea)
- Broccoli
- Kale
- Artichoke
- Eggplant
- Bottle Gourd
- Nettle (Also dried and freezed)
- Okra
- Indian Cress
- Amaranth leaves
- Wax Gourd
- Egyptian Luffa
- Pumpkin (Cucurbita Pepo)
- Asparagus
- Chayote

Sprouts
Eat the following sprouts
- Mung bean sprouts
- Alfalfa sprouts
- Fenugreek sprouts
- Azuki bean sprouts
- Black soybean sprouts
- Soybean sprouts
- Pintobean sprouts
- Red Kidney bean sprouts
- Quinoa sprouts
- Buckwehat sprouts
- Tartary Buckwheat sprouts
- Broad bean sprouts
- Broccoli sprouts
- Brown rice sprouts
- Sesame seed sprouts

Mushrooms
Eat a lot of mushrooms from the following list
- Shiitake
- White Button mushroom, fresh or dried
- Reishi
- Maitake
- Himematsutake
- Oyster mushroom
- Jew's ear
- King Boleto (Boletus Edulis)

Beans and peas
Eat a lot of the following beans and peas
- Soybeans
- Black soybeans
- Pinto beans
- Azuki beans
- Red Kidney beans
- Chickpeas
- Broad beans

Grains
Eat a lot of the following grain products, in different forms (Bread, Muesli, Gruel, French bread, baked rolls, Cookies, Sprouts etc.)

- Whole grain barley
- Whole grain oat
- Red rice
- Brown rice
- Black rice
- Purple Corn
- Black sesame
- Buckwheat
- Tartary Buckwheat
- Quinoa
- Proso Millet
- Foxtail Millet
- Amaranth seeds

Bran and germs
Use daily a lot of bran and germs in youghurt, bread etc.
- Rice bran
- Oat bran
- Barley bran
- Rye bran
- Wheat germs
- Sugar beet bran

Grass flour
Eat the following grass flours
- Wheat grass
- Barley grass

Sweeties
- Replace all sweeties by dark Chocolate
- Do not eat liquorice (It increases blood pressure)

Algae
Eat the following algae
- Wakame
- Chlorella
- Spirulina
- Kelp

Salt
- Reduce strongly the use of salt. Normally and during winter, the need for daily salt is only 1 – 2 grams. The Yanomami Indians in Venezuela get only 0.2 grams of salt from their daily diet, and they have the lowest blood pressure values in the whole World.
- Replace salt by spices and spice mixtures, which can easily be made by yourself.

Oil capsules
Use the following oils in capsule form
- Fish oil (EPA + DHA)
- Evening Primrose oil (GLA = Gamma-Linolenic Acid)
- CLA (=Conjugated Linolenic Acid)

Spices
Use a lot of spices and their mixtures from the following list
- Garlic
- Red Onion
- Ginger
- Parsley
- Dill
- Basil
- Curry
- Cinnamon
- Black Pepper
- Long Pepper (Piper Longum)
- Capers
- Cloves
- Coriander
- Rosmarin
- Chili
- Timjam
- Guinean pepper (Xylopia Aethiopica)
- Chives
- Fennel
- Nutmeg
- Caraway seeds
- Jeera
- Black Cumin
- Ajwain
- Cumin seeds
- Saffron

- Lemon Balm
- Lemon Grass
- Sage
- Pineapple Sage (Salvia Elegans)
- Cardamom
- Ketchup, Crushed Tomato, Tomato Puree
- Mustard

Cheese
Use fatfree Cottage Cheese

Diets
The following diets are excellent, they reduce obesity, high blood pressure, high cholesterol, high triglyceride values and high blood sugar
- Ketogenic diet
- Protein diet, hypocaloric
- Vegetarian diet
- Lactovegetarian diet
- Stone age diet
- Mediterranian diet
- Okinawa diet

Learn slow breathing techniques and Yoga Pranayama slow breathing exercises and a few Yoga relaxing Asanas.

Learn Shiatshu or learn electric Acupuncture stimulation technigues (Against high blood pressure).

Obesity
If you have very much overweight, drop it by exercise and diet. This will strongly decrease your blood pressure, total cholesterol, LDL-cholesterol, VLDL-cholesterol and triglycerides.

Mentality
If you are on strict diet and exercise program 6 days a week, it does not matter anything, if you at the weekend eat whatever fatty food, pizza etc., and drink alcohol, beer etc. It is a very good idea to have one "Do whatever you want" day in a week. It does not increase your blood pressure or cholesterol values.

Calcium, Magnesium, Potassium
- Increase your daily Calcium by 800 – 1200 mg
- Increase your daily Magnesium by 350 – 700 mg
- Increase your daily Potassium by 1000 – 2000 mg

Protein
The following are very good protein sources
- Fat free Soy protein flour
- Whey protein

You can add these into whatever foods or drinks or juice.

Dietary supplements

The following dietary supplements are very good against high blood pressure, high cholesterol levels, high triglyceride levels and high Homocysteine levels

- Pangamic acid
- Pantethine
- Ubiquinone Q10
- N-Acetyl-L-Cysteine (NAC)
- Lipoic acid
- Biotin
- Chromium Picolinate
- Folic acid
- Ferulic acid
- Chlorogenic acid
- Quercetin
- Apigenin
- Luteolin
- Soy Lecithin
- Rutin
- Carob flour
- Lycopene
- Propolis
- Royal Jelly
- Melatonin
- Vitamin D
- L-Carnitine
- Acetyl-L-Carnitine
- Apocynin
- Astaxanthin
- Berberine
- Genistein
- Glucuronic acid
- Grape seed extract (GSE)
- Pycnogenol
- Resveratrol
- C-vitamin (At least 1 gram daily)
- Tocotrienols
- Ellagic acid
- Stevioside
- Dioscorin

Vinegar

- Use a lot of Vinegar in food, either Apple Vinegar or Vinegar from Black Rice (Kurosu in Japanese)
- Drink daily the following: 2 dl water + 1 teaspoon Vinegar + 1 teaspoon dark Honey. Mix well and drink.

14

Fruit juices
Drink everyday 2 – 5 dl 100% fresh fruit juice
- Red Grapefruit juice
- Orange juice
- Pomegranate juice
- Red Grape juice (For example BIOTTA)
- Passion fruit juice
- Self made from the fruits or berries mentioned earlier, or a mixture of them.

Vegetable juices
Make fresh vegetable juices from the following
- Carrots (Self made or BIOTTA etc.)
- Celery juice (Self made or BIOTTA etc.)
- Red beet juice (Self made or BIOTTA etc.)

The following seeds can be eaten as such or added to bread and other food
- Flaxseed
- Black Cumin
- Fenugreek
- Garden Cress
- Black sesame
- Pumpkin (Cucurbita Pepo)
- Radish (Raphanus Sativus)

The following herbs are very valuable
- White Horehound
- Tienchi Ginseng
- Ginseng
- Ginkgo Biloba
- Sweet Violet
- Valerian
- Roman Chamomile
- Scrambling Gynura
- Brahmi
- Yarrow
- St John's Wort
- Tulsi, Holy Basil
- Motherwort
- Puncture wine (Tribulus Terrestris)
- Olive leaves
- Hawthorn (Leaves, fruits, flowers)
- Lime leaves
- Milk Thistle, seed
- Corn Silk
- Veldt Grape (Cissus Quadrangularis)
- Mistle
- Black currant leaves

- Japanese Honeysuckle, flower buds
- African Mango (Irvinga Gabonensis)
- Stevia (Stevia Rebaudiana)
- Arjuna (Terminalia Arjuna)
- Bahera (Terminalia Bellerica)
- Haritaki (Terminalia Chebula)
- Aloe Vera
- Avocado seed
- Red clover
- False Daisy, Eclipta (Eclipta Alba)

The following amino acids are very valuable
- GABA
- L-Arginine
- L-Serine
- L-Citrulline
- HMB
- L-Carnosine
- Taurine
- L-Tryptophan
- BCAA amino acids (Leucine, Isoleucine, Valine)

Water fast or fresh juice fast lowers extremely efficiently high blood pressure and body weight.

Avoid cholesterol in food
- Reduce the use of eggs
- Avoid using egg yolks
- Avoid using animal liver products
- You can eat egg whites as much as you wish, they do not contain cholesterol at all.
- Avoid fatty meat
- Avoid fatty cheese

Do not eat the following food, which contain a lot of fat, salt, calories and carbohydrates
- Pizza
- Hamburgers
- French fries
- Chips
- Sausages
- Fatty cheese
- Fatty milk
- Butter
- Cream
- Mayonnaise
- Convenience food
- Wheat flour
- Macaroni
- White bread

Acetyl-L-Carnitine

Acetyl-L-Carnitine is a natural, vitamin related compound found in human body, which has many physiological properties. In animal experiments, it slows the aging process, just like Lipoic acid.

Acetyl-L-Carnitine has
  – Blood pressure lowering properties

When 32 volunteers were given 2.0 grams Acetyl-L-Carnitine daily, for 24 months, systolic blood pressure decreased by average 7.95 mmHg (137.4 mmHg → 129.45 mmHg; $p < 0.001$), compared to the control group (Ruggenenti et.al. 2009).

When 36 volunteers were given Lipoic acid 400 mg and Acetyl-L-Carnitine 1.0 grams daily, for 8 weeks, systolic blood pressure decreased by 9.0 mmHg (145.0 mmHg → 136.0 mmHg; $p = 0.003$), compared to the control group (McMackin et.al. 2007). This was a doubble blind experiment.

In old (22 weeks) rats, Acetyl-L-Carnitine given 100 mg/kg daily, decreased triglycerides by 25.5% ($p < 0.01$) and total cholesterol by 20.8% ($p < 0.01$), compared to the control group (Tanaka et.al. 2004).

Acupuncture, Electroacupuncture, Electric Stimulation, Shiatsu, Laser Acupuncture and Moxibustion

Acupuncture originates from China. Acupuncture is known from over 3600 years old Hieroglyphs, and acupuncture needles made from stone have been found in stone age graves. In Chinese acupuncture is called ZHENJIU. But acupuncture is known already from ancient Egypt and Turkey. Acupuncure is at least 5000 years old. Nowadays there are hundreds of diseases where acupuncture is used. Normally a very thin metallic needle is used, and they are needled to different acupuncture points. There are 364 official acupuncture points, but there are also some 2000 so called EXTRA acupuncture points. Acupuncture is officially accepted by the WHO.

Besides normal acupuncture, there is also electroacupuncture, where small frequency, 2 – 10 Hz alternating current is fed to the metallic acupuncture needles, with low current. Nowadays there are also very many handheld electric stimulators, which can find the acupuncture points, and give electric stimulation to the acupuncture points. These devices show by sound and LED light, when the acupuncture point is located correctly. Shiatsu is acupressure, where the acupuncture points are stimulated by fingers or wooden stick. In Laser acupuncture, the stimulation is made by Laser light. In Moxibustion, the stimulation is made by heat, using small Moxa cones, which are made from the dried leaves of Mugwort, Artemisia Vulgaris.

There exists thousands of acupuncture books and research articles. All the acupuncture points can be found in acupuncture maps. There has been found over 3000 years old human like models, where all the acupuncture points are correctly shown. In China, the traditional medicine is based on thousands of medicinal herbs and acupuncture and functional diet therapy. The old Chinese acupuncture books say, that if acupuncture does not help, use Moxibustion.

The first ever acupuncure book is written about 2300 years ago. This is the most famous Chinese medicine book, "Yellow Emperor's Inner Canon", in Chinese: HUANGDI NEIJING. The book consists of 2 separate volumes, SUWEN and LINGSHU. In LINGSHU, detailed description about acupuncture and Moxibustion methods can be found.

The location of acupuncture points is rather easy, using the CUN ("Tsun") measure, which is the width of the distal inter-phalangeal joint of the thumb. This CUN is a specific measure for each individual, and using it, every acupoint in the body can be found, using the acupoint maps. The electrical resistance of acupoints are different from the resistance of skin outside the acupoints. Also when making palpation, the acupoints feel differently, like they were more painful, compared to the area around the acupoints.

Acupuncture is extremely easy and cheap method, which has only very minimal side effects, compared to any classical medicine method or medicinal compound. Everybody can easily learn Shiatsu or use handheld electrical acupoint stimulators, which are very cheap.

Acupuncture, Shiatsu, electroacupuncture, Laser acupuncture, Moxibustion and electrical acupuncture have
  – Blood pressure decreasing properties

There exists over 40 effective acupuncture points against high blood pressure. The most important of these are: Neiguan (PC6), Zusanli (ST36), Fengchi (GB20), Renying (ST9), Hegu (LI4), Quchi (LI11), Taichong (LR3), Sanyinjiao (SP6), Xingjian (LR2), Shenshu (BL23), Ganshu (BL18), Baihui (GV20), Qihai (CV6), Fenglong (ST40), Yintang (EXTRA, EX-HN-3), Taiyang (EXTRA, EX-HN-5), Guanyun (CV4), Zhongwan (CV12), Jianshi (PC5), Daling (PC7), Laogong (PC8), Taixi (KI3), Shenmen (HT7), Groove for lowering blood pressure (In the ear), Xin Qu Chi (EXTRA, New LI11), Xue Ya Dian (BP Point), Chi Yi (EXTRA, Red Doctor), Shih-Hsuan (EXTRA, EX-UE-11), Chonggu (EXTRA, EX-HN-18).

When 30 hypertensive volunteers were given acupuncture 17 times during 8 weeks, systolic blood pressure decreased by 14.7 mmHg (136.8 mmHg → 122.1 mmHg; $p < 0.01$) and diastolic blood pressure decreased by 6.9 mmHg (83.7 mmHg → 76.8 mmHg; $p < 0.01$), compared to the placebo group (Yin et.al. 2007). This was a double blind experiment. The acupoints used were: ST36, LI11, BL25, SP3, LU9, BL13, KI7, KI2, CV4, GV14, GB20, PC6, HT7.

When 27 volunteers were given electrical acupoint stimulation 2 times weekly, for 5 weeks, systolic blood pressure decreased by 7.7 mmHg (117.8 mmHg → 110.1 mmHg; $p < 0.05$) and diastolic blood pressure decreased by 3.6 mmHg (77.4 mmHg → 74.8 mmHg), compared to the control group (Zhang et.al. 2009). The acupoints used were: Hegu (LI4) and Quchi (LI11).

When 29 volunteers were given acupuncture once weekly, for 7 weeks, of 25 minutes duration each, systolic blood pressure decreased by 24.4 mmHg (153 mmHg → 128.6 mmHg; $p < 0.001$) and diastolic blood pressure decreased by 9.1 mmHg (85.9 mmHg → 76.8 mmHg; $p < 0.001$), compared to the control group (Weil et.al. 2007). The acupoints used were: SP6, SP9, PC8, PC3, PC6, PC4.

When 50 volunteers were given 30 minutes acupuncture, systolic blood pressure decreased by 18 mmHg (169 mmHg → 151 mmHg; $p < 0.01$) and diastolic blood pressure decreased by 5 mmHg (77 mmHg → 72 mmHg; $p < 0.01$), compared to the control group. The plasma Renin decreased by 35.3% ($p < 0.01$) (Chiu et.al. 1997).

When 72 hypertensive volunteers were given 30 minutes acupuncture, 22 times, during 6 weeks, systolic blood pressure decreased by 6.4 mmHg ($p < 0.001$) and diastolic blood pressure decreased by 3.7 mmHg ($p < 0.001$), compared to the control group (Flachskampf et.al. 2007). The acupoints used were: GB20, CV4, CV6, CV12, LI4, LI11, ST36, ST40, SP6, GV20, LR2, LR3, SP9, BL18, BL23.

When 45 volunteers were given Laser acupuncture 8 minutes, 12 times, during 90 days, systolic blood pressure decreased by 7.1 mmHg (129.6 mmHg → 122.5 mmHg; $p < 0.01$) and diastolic blood pressure decreased by 8.4 mmHg (85.6 mmHg → 77.2 mmHg; $p < 0.001$), compared to the control group (Zhang et.al. 2008). The acupoints used were: Hegu (LI4) and Quchi (LI11).

When 18 hypertensive volunteers were given 30 minutes of electroacupuncture one time each week, for 8 weeks, systolic blood pressure decreased by 18 mmHg ($p < 0.05$), compared to the control group (Li et.al. 2010). The acupoints used were: PC5, PC6, ST36, ST37.
The blood pressure stayed down up to 4 weeks, after the last treatment. The frequency of the used current was 2 Hz.

When 10 hypertensive volunteers were given totally 4 minutes electrical stimulation, diastolic blood pressure decreased by 7 mmHg ($p < 0.05$), compared to the control group (Williams et.al. 1991). The acupoints used were: LR3, ST36, LI11 and "Groove for lowering blood pressure". The used frequency was 10 Hz.

The blood pressure decreasing effect of acupuncture has been validated in several tens of experiments, during the last 60 years (Ayannusi et.al. 2004; Anshelevich et.al. 1985; Guo et.al. 2003; Wan et.al. 2009; Diao et.al. 2011; Yang et.al. 2010; Wu et.al. 2004 etc …). The most often used acupoints in these experiments were: PC5, PC6, LI4, LU7, LI11, LR3 etc.

It seems to be, that the best results using electroacupuncture and electrical acupoint stimulation, is achieved using low 2 Hz frequency and low 0.3 – 0.5 mA current.

Aerobic exercise

Question: What is the "Medicine", which
- Decreases blood pressure
- Increases HDL-cholesterol
- Decreases total cholesterol
- Decreases LDL-cholesterol
- Decreases triglycerides
- Decreases body weight and makes body slim
- Decreases body fat-%
- Increases heart stroke volume
- Decreases heart pulse
- Slows down aging process
- Increases lifespan
- Keeps body youthful

- Removes stress
- Increases Testosterone, Growth hormone, beta-Endorphin
- Increases muscle strength
- Has absolutely no side effects, if taken continuously, for whole lifetime

Answer: Aerobic exercise, at least 3 times weekly, at least 1 hour/exercise, all around the year, every year.

In a meta-analysis with 29 different experiments, at least 4 weeks duration each, aeroic exercise decreased systolic blood pressure by an average of 4.7 mmHg and diastolic blood pressure by an average of 3.1 mmHg (Halbert et.al. 1997).

Much higher decrements in blood pressure can be achieved with aerobic exercise. When female volunteers made aerobic exercise regularly, for 12 weeks, systolic blood pressure decreased by an average of 10 mmHg, and diastolic blood pressure decreased by an average of 5 mmHg, compared to the control group (Seals et.al. 1997).

In a meta-analysis with 49 different experiments, aerobic exercise decreased total cholesterol by an average of 2% ($p < 0.001$), LDL-cholesterol decreased by an average of 3% ($p < 0.001$), triglycerides decreased by an average of 9% ($p < 0.001$), but HDL-cholesterol increased by an average of 2% ($p < 0.001$) (Kelley et.al. 2006). The average number of exercises was 3.4 per week, for at least 22 weeks duration. The average duration of one exercise was 36 minutes.

In another meta-analysis with 25 different experiments, it was noticed, that aeroic exercise increases significantly the HDL-cholesterol (Kodama et.al. 2007). It was noticed, that for every increase of exercise time by 10 minutes, HDL-cholesterol increases by 0.036 mmol/L.

African Mango

(Irvinga Gabonensis)

African Mango originates from Central Africa. Its fruit and large seed are edible, and they are an important food item in local cultures. The seeds are very rich in protein,

African mango seeds have
- Total cholesterol decreasing properties
- LDL-cholesterol decreasing properties
- Triglycerides decreasing properties
- HDL-cholesterol increasing properties
- Body weight decreasing properties

When 28 volunteers were given 3.15 grams of African Mango seeds daily, for 4 weeks, body weight decreased by 5.6% ($p < 0.0001$), total cholesterol decreased by 39.2% (215 mg/dl → 130.7 mg/dl; $p < 0.05$), LDL-cholesterol decreased by 45.6% (121.4 mg/dl → 66.1 mg/dl; $p < 0.05$) and triglycerides decreased by 44.5% (162 mg/dl → 89 mg/dl; $p < 0.05$), but HDL-cholesterol increased by 45.9% (61.2 mg/dl → 89.9 mg/dl; $p < 0.05$), compared to the placebo group (Ngondi et.al. 2005). This was a double blind experiment.

When 61 volunteers were given African Mango seed extract 300 mg daily, for 10 weeks, body weight decreased by 12.8% (97.9 kg → 85.1 kg; $p < 0.01$), fat-% decreased by 6.3% ($p < 0.05$), total cholesterol decreased by 39.8% (151.7 mg/dl → 111.9 mg/dl; $p < 0.05$) and LDL-cholesterol decreased by 22.5% (82.2 mg/dl → 59.8 mg/dl; $p < 0.05$), compared to the placebo group (Ngondi et.al. 2009). This was a double blind experiments.

When 24 volunteers were given African Mango seed extract 500 mg and Cissus Quadrangularis extract 300 mg daily, body weight decreased by 3.0% ($p < 0.05$), total cholesterol decreased by 17.6% ($p < 0.05$) and LDL-cholesterol decreased by 28.5% ($p < 0.05$), compared with the group, which were given only Cissus Quadrangularis extract 300 mg daily (Oben et.al. 2008). This was double blind experiment.

Ajwain

(Carum Copticum)

Ajwain is very popular spice and medicinal plant in Asia, especially in Indian and Pakistan. It can also be purchased from Ethnic Markets and Shops.

Ajwain has
- Blood pressure lowering properties
- Total cholesterol lowering properties
- Triglycerides lowering properties
- HDL-cholesterol increasing properties

When rabbits were given Ajwain 1% in their daily diet, for 4 weeks, total cholesterol decreased by 42.5%, triglycerides decreased by 38.5% but HDL-cholesterol increased by 70.2%, compared to the control group (Agrewala et.al. 1986).

Ajwain decreases blood pressure both in rats and cats. The blood pressure lowerig effect increases with increasing dose (Gilani et.al. 2005; Devasankaraiah et.al. 1974).

Alcohol

Alcohol has been used possibly as long as the humans have lived on the earth. Alcohol can be prepared in principle from any berries, fruits, grains, roots etc.

Alcohol has
- Blood pressure increasing properties
- Triglycerides increasing properties
- HDL-cholesterol increasing properties

In a meta-analysis of 15 different experiments and 2234 volunteers, it was noticed, that alcohol use increases systolic blood pressure by an average of 3.31 mmHg, and diastolic blood pressure by an average of 2.04 mmHg, compared to control group (Xin et.al. 2001).

The blood pressure increasing properties of alcohol has been noticed also in another meta-analysis, with 28848 men and 13455 women (Sesso et.al. 2008).

Persons, who use daily large amounts of alcohol, the alcohol withdrawal can result in quick and strong decrease of blood pressure. When 65 alcoholics were without alcohol in hospital for 4 days, systolic blood pressure decreased by 15 mmHg (137 mmHg → 122 mmHg; $p < 0.001$) and diastolic blood pressure decreased by 6 mmHg (82 mmHg → 76 mmHg; $p < 0.001$), only in 4 days (Bannan et.al. 1984). Also plasma Aldosterone decreased by 49.9% ($p < 0.005$) and plasma Cortisol decreased by 29.2% ($p < 0.005$).

In a meta-analysis with 42 experiments, it was noticed, that daily 30 gram alcohol dose increases HDL-cholesterol by an average of 3.99 mg/dl, or about 8.3% increase. Triglycerides increased by an average of 5.69 mg/dl ($p = 0.001$), or about 5.9% increase (Rimm et.al. 1999).

Also in another meta-analysis with 63 different experiments, it was noticed, that alcohol increases HDL-cholesterol significantly (Brien et.al. 2011).

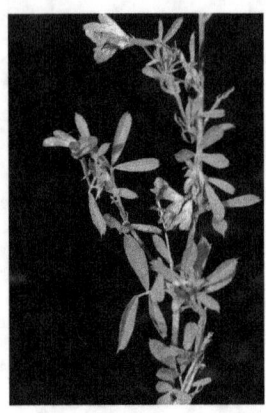

Alfalfa

(Medicago Sativa)

Alfalfa has been cultivated allready in ancient times for food and fodder. Alfalfa seed sprouts are very popular food.

Alfalfa seed sprouts have:
- Total cholesterol lowering properties.
- LDL-cholesterol lowering properties
- Triglycerides lowering properties

When 15 hyperlipidemic volunteers were given 120 grams Alfalfa seeds daily, total cholesterol, decreased by 17% and LDL-cholesterol decreased by 18%. The biggest individual decrease in total cholesterol was 26% and in LDL-cholesterol 30% (Molgaard et.al. 1987).

The same kind of results have been noticed in many animal experiments with chickens, rabbits and monkeys. In all the experiments Alfalfa seeds decrease strongly triglycerides, total cholesterol and LDL-cholesterol (Malinow et.al. 1980; Dixit et.al. 1985; Dixit et.al. 1986).

Almond

(Prunus Amygdalus)

Almond is known to everybody as a very delicious nut. Almond has a lot of mono- and polyunsaturated fatty acids, protein and L-Arginine.

Almond has
- Total cholesterol lowering properties
- LDL-cholesterol lowering properties
- HDL-cholesterol increasing properties
- Triglyceride lowering properties

When 30 volunteers with high cholesterol levels, were given Almond 25 grams daily, for 4 weeks, total cholesterol decreased by 3.0% (p < 0.05), LDL-cholesterol decreased by 5.6% (p < 0.01) and triglycerides decreased by 14.6%, but HDL-cholesterol increased by 8.6%, compared to the control group (Tamizifar et.al. 2005).

When 38 volunteers with high cholesterol levels, were given Almond 100 grams daily, for 4 weeks, total cholesterol decreased by 6.8% (247 mg/dl → 230 mg/dl; p < 0.01) and LDL-cholesterol decreased by 11.8% (160 mg/dl → 141 mg/dl; p < 0.002), compared to the control group (Spiller et.al. 2003).

When 27 volunteers were given Almond 73 grams daily, for 4 weeks, total cholesterol decreased by 5.9% (6.60 mmol/L → 6.21 mmol/L; p < 0.01), LDL-cholesterol decreased by 9.9% (4.45 mmol/L → 4.01 mmol/L; p < 0.01), but HDL-cholesterol increased by 3.4% (1.40 mmol/L → 1.45 mmol/L; p < 0.05), compared to the control group (Jenkins et.al. 2002).

When 20 diabetic volunteers were given Almond 60 grams daily, for 12 weeks, total cholesterol decreased by 6.0% (p < 0.05) and LDL-cholesterol decreased by 11.5% (p < 0.05), compared to the control group (Li et.al. 2011).

The same kind of results have been noticed in another experiment (Jalali-Khanabadi et.al. 2010).

Aloe

(Aloe Vera, Aloe Barbadensis)

Aloe is the gel, which is obtained from the inner part of leaf of different Aloe species. Aloe has very many medicinal uses, and it is used for high blood pressure, inflammation, wounds, burnt skin, allergy and asthma etc. There are many effective compounds in Aloe, like Aloeemodin, Aloin A etc.

Aloe has
- Blood pressure lowering properties
- Total cholesterol lowering properties
- LDL-cholesterol lowering properties

When rats were give Aloeemodin either 0.5 mg/kg, 1 mg/kg or 3 mg/kg, the mean average blood pressure (MAP) decreased by 28%, 52% and 79% (Saleem et.al. 2001).

When 30 diabetic volunteers were give Aloe gel 600 mg dail, for 8 weeks, both total cholesterol (p < 0.05) and LDL-cholesterol (p < 0.004) decreased significantly, compared to the control group (Huseini et.al. 2011). This was a doubble blind experiment.

When rats were give Aloe gel 300 mg/kg daily, for 3 weeks, total cholesterol (p < 0.05), LDL-cholesterol (p < 0.05), VLDL-cholesterol (p < 0.05) and triglycerides (p < 0.05) decreased significantly, compared to the control group (Rajasekaran et.al. 2006).

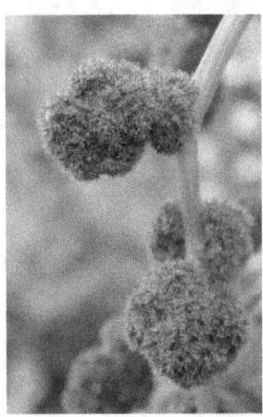

Amaranth

(Amaranthus Sp.)

Amaranth is known all over the World as an edible plant food. Both Amaranth seeds and leaves are edible and they contain large amounts of nutrients. Amaranth seeds contain about 9% of high quality oil. Amaranth seeds and seed oil contains very large amounts of Squalene, about 100 mg Squalene in 3 ml of oil. Amaranth is also a medicinal plant. There are many different Amaranth species, but they are all edible and easy to cultivate. Amaranth has been cultivated already several thousands of years.

Amaranth seeds, leaves and seed oil have
- Blood pressure lowering properties
- Total cholesterol lowering properties
- LDL-cholesterol lowering properties
- Triglycerides lowering properties
- HDL-cholesterol increasing properties

When 125 volunteers were given Amaranth oil 3 – 18 ml daily, for 3 weeks, total cholesterol (p < 0.05) and both systolic blood pressure (p < 0.05) and diastolic blood pressure (p < 0.05) decreased significantly, compared to the conrol group (Martirosyan et.al. 2007).

In Africa the leaves of the following Amaranth species are used as a food and to decrease high blood pressure: Amaranthus Hybridus and Amaranthus Cruentus (Omujal et.al. 2010).

The leaf extracts of the following Amaranth species inhibit strongly ACE: Amaranthus Dubius and Amaranthus Hybridus (Ramesar et.al. 2008).

When rats were fed pure Squalene daily for 4 weeks, blood pressure, total cholesterol and triglycerides decreased significantly (p < 0.05 in all parameters), compared to the control group (Liu et.al. 2009). Amaranth seeds and oil contain large amount of Squalene, 100 mg/3 ml oil.

In many animal experiments with rabbits and rats, it has been verified, that Amaranth seeds and leaves decrease total cholesterol, LDL-cholesterol, triglycerides and blood pressure, but increase HDL-cholesterol (Chaturvedi et.al. 1993; Fritz et.al. 2011; Girija et.al. 2011; Kim et.al. 2006; Kabiri et.al. 2011; Czerwinski et.al. 2004; Kabiri et.al. 2010; Mendonca et.al. 2009; Mendonca et.al. 2009).

The following Amaranth species have been used in these experiments: Amaranthus Esculentus, Amaranthus Caudatus, Amaranthus Viridis, Amaranthus Spinosus, Amaranthus Hypochondriacus.

Amla, Indian Gooseberry

(Emblica Officinalis)

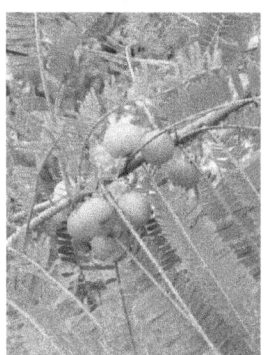

(Author: L. Shyamal)

Amla is a very famous berry from India. It has been used for thousands of years as a functional food in India. The berry contains large amounts of vitamin C, and also large amounts of Tannis and Ellagic acid. Amla has been used for several thousands of years also for medicinal purposes.

Amla has
- Blood pressure lowering properties
- Total cholesterol lowering properties
- LDL-cholesterol lowering properties
- Triglycerides lowering properties

When Amla was given to hypertensive rats either 75 mg/kg, 150 mg/kg or 300 mg/kg daily, for 5 weeks, blood pressure decreased significantly, compared to the control group (Bhatia et.al. 2011). Also heart rate decreased.

When rats were given Amla water extract, both the mean average blood pressure (MAP) and heart rate decreased significantly, compared to the control group (Ishaq et.al. 2005).

When rats were given Amla Flavonoids 10 mg/kg daily, for 3 months, total cholesterol (p < 0.01) and LDL-cholesterol (p < 0.01) decreased significantly, compared to the control group (Anila et.al. 2002).

When volunteers were given dried Amla 2 – 3 grams daily, for 3 weeks, both total cholesterol (p < 0.05) and triglycerides (p < 0.05) decreased significantly, compared to the control group (Akhtar et.al. 2011).

When volunteers were given Amla as a fresh berry daily, for 28 days, total cholesterol decreased significantly, compared to the control group (Jacob et.al. 1988).

When rabbits were given Amla juice 5 ml/kg daily, for 2 months, total cholesterol decreased by 82%, triglycerides decreased by 66% and LDL-cholesterol decreased by 90%, compared to the control group (Mathur et.al. 1996).

When rats were given Ethylacetate extract of Amla at a dose between 10 – 40 mg/kg daily, for 100 days, systolic blood pressure decreased significantly, compared to the control group (Yokozawa et.al. 2007).

When rabbits were fed either cholesterol or cholesterol and Amla daily, for 4 months, total cholesterol decreased by 57.9% (630 mg/dl $\rightarrow$ 205 mg/dl; $p < 0.01$) in the Amla group, compared to the cholesterol group (Thakur et.al. 1988).

The total choleterol and LDL-cholesterol lowering effect of Amla has been verified in many other experiments with rats (Kim et.al. 2005; Yokozawa et.al. 2007; Kim et.al. 2010).

Apigenin

Apigenin is a Flavonoid, which is a very strong antioxidant. Apigenin is found in many plants, especially in Celery and Parsley. Parsley is the best source of Apigenin.

Apigenin has
- Blood pressure lowering properties

Apigenin inhibits ACE (Loizzo et.al. 2007; Sui et.al. 2010).

When rats were given Apigenin 0.03, 0.05 or 0.11 g/kg daily, for 4 weeks, blood pressure decreased significantly in each group, compared to the control group (Sui et.al. 2009).

Apigenin is also a strong vasorelaxant (Xu et.al. 2007).

Both Celery and Parsley are known to be diuretic and lower blood pressure.

Apocynin

Apocynin is a Flavonoid, which exists in the famous medicinal plants Apocynum Venetum, Apocynum Lancifolium and Picrorhiza Kurroa. Apocynum plant species are known to decrease blood pressure. Apocynin is a specific inhibitor of NADPH Oxidase, which produce the Superoxide oxygen radical, which destroys living cells. Apocynin is a very strong antioxidant.

Apocynin has
- Blood pressure decreasing properties

When hypertensive rats were given Apocynin 33 micrograms/kg daily, for 5 weeks, blood pressure increased in the control group 40 mmHg during this time, but Apocynin inhibited this rise by 78% (Jimenez et.al. 2007).

Apocynin decreases blood pressure by stimulating NO concentration and increasing eNOS activity (Baumer et.al. 2007).

The blood pressure decreasing properties of Apocynin has been verified in many experiments (Tain et.al. 2012; Liu et.al. 2008; Hu et.al. 2006; Banappa et.al. 2009; Pechanova et.al. 2009).

Apple

(Malus Domestica)

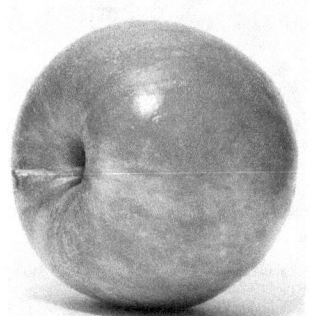

(Author: Abhijit Tembhekar)

Apple is a very popular fruit all around the World. In Russia and China it is used in diet, to decrease high blood pressure.

Apple has:
- Blood pressure lowering properties.
- Total cholesterol lowering properties.

In a meta-analysis with 4 trials in Humans, total cholesterol decreased by 5-8%, when the daily amout of Apple in diet was between 2-3 (Jensen et.al. 2009).

In another meta-analysis with 9 trials with test animals, plasma total cholesterol decreased by an average 11-43%, and liver cholesterol decreased by and average of 23-67% (Jensen et.al. 2009).

The skin of Apple inhibits ACE (Balasyriya et.al. 2011).

Red Apples and their skins are strong vasodilators (Fitzpatrick et.al. 1995).

Apple is one of the best dietary sources of the Flavonoid Quercetin. Quercetin is known to decrease both blood pressure and cholesterol.

Remember always to eat Apple with its skin, after washing.

Arjuna (Terminalia Arjuna)

Arjuna is a large tree, which grows naturally in India. The Arjuna bark powder has been used several hundreds of years as a cardiotonic, against hypertension and against asthma. Arjuna contains Tannis, Flavonoids, Phytosterols and Triperpine Saponins (Arjunic acid, Arjunolic acid, Arjungenin etc.).

Arjuna has
- Blood pressure decreasing properties
- Total cholesterol decreasing properties
- LDL-cholesterol decreasing properties
- Triglycerides decreasing properties

When hyperlipidemic rabbits were fed Arjuna bark powder 500 mg/kg daily, for 45 days, total cholesterol decreased by 50.3% ($p < 0.05$) and triglycerides decreased by 35.3% ($p < 0.05$), compared to the control group (Shaila et.al. 1998).

When 10 young, healthy volunteers were given Arjuna bark powder 500 mg daily, for 8 weeks, systolic blood pressure decreased by 5.2 mmHg (123.0 mmHg → 117.8 mmHg; $p < 0.0001$), compared to the control group (Sandhu et.al. 2010).

When 10 heart patients were given Arjuna bark powder 200 mg daily, for 3 months, triglycerides decreased by 24% ($p < 0.05$), VLDL-cholesterol decreased by 6.1% ($p < 0.05$), LDL-cholesterol decreased by 20% ($p < 0.05$) and total cholesterol decreased by 12% ($p < 0.05$), compared to the control group (Varalakshmi et.al. 2010).

When 35 heart patients were given Arjuna bark powder 500 mg daily, for 30 days, total cholesterol decreased by 9.7% ($p < 0.01$) and LDL-cholesterol decreased by 25.6% ($p < 0.01$), compared to the control group (Gupta et.al. 2001).

The hypotensive property of Arjuna has been verified in many experiments with human volunteers (Dwivedi et.al. 1994; Yegnanarayan et.al. 1997).

The hypotensive and cholesterol decreasing property of Arjuna has also been verified in many animal experiments (Reddy et.al. 2011; Chander et.al. 2004; Patil et.al. 2011; Subramamian et.al. 2011; Nammi et.al. 2003; Takahashi et.al. 1997; Asha et.al. 2012).

Artichoke

(Cynara Scolymus)

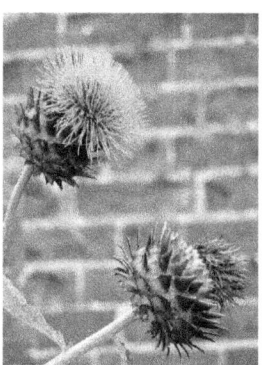

Artichoke is a familiar vegetable all over the World. It has also many medicinal applications, especially to lower high blood pressure and high cholesterol levels. Artichoke contains many pharmacologically effective comounds, especially Luteolin and Chlorogenic acid, which are known to decrease blood pressure.

Artichoke has
  - Blood pressure lowering properties
  - Total cholesterol lowering properties
  - LDL-cholesterol lowering properties
  - HDL-cholesterol increasing properties
  - Triglycerides lowering properties

When 30 diabetic volunteers were given 6 grams of dried Artichoke globes daily, for 3 months, total cholesterol (236.7 mg/dl → 225.9 mg/dl; $p < 0.01$), triglycerides (163.2 mg/dl → 146.3 mg/dl; $p < 0.01$) and LDL-cholesterol (161.6 mg/dl → 143.2 mg/dl; $p < 0.01$) decreased, but HDL-cholesterol (34.6 mg/dl → 43.4 mg/dl; $p < 0.01$) increased significantly, comparred to the control group (Nanzi et.al. 2006).

When hypertensive volunteers were given Artichoke leaf juice either 50 mg or 100 mg daily, for 12 weeks, both systolic ($p < 0.05$) and diastolic ($p < 0.05$) blood pressure decreased significantly, compared to the control group (Dehkord et.al. 2009). This was a double blind experiment.

Artichoke leaf extract is known to inhibit cholesterol synthesis (Gebhardt 1996).

When 302 volunteers were given 320 mg standardized Artichoke leaf extract (Hepar SL Forte, Germany) daily, for a long time, total cholesterol decreased by 11.5% (264.2 mg/dl → 233.9 mg/dl; $p < 0.001$) and triglycerides decreased y 12.5% (215.0 mg/dl → 188.1 mg/dl; $p < 0.01$), compared to the control group (Fintelmann 1996).

Also in other experiments, including meta-analysis with double blind experiments, it has been noticed, that Artichoke decreases both total cholesterol and LDL-cholesterol (Wider et.al. 2009; Skarpanska-Stejnborn et.al. 2008; Lupatelli et.al. 2004).

Ashitaba

(Angelica Keiskei)

Ashitaba originates from south Japan. The leaves and stalks are used as vegetables. Ashitaba has many medicinal properties. Many Ashitaba compounds with anticarcinogenic and hypotensive properties have been studied. Most of these are Chalcone compounds and Coumarins, which do not exist in other Angelica species. Ashitaba is regarded as a healthy functional, anti-aging vegetable. Its cultivation is very easy.

Ashitaba has
- Blood pressure lowering properties
- LDL-cholesterol lowering properties
- VLDL-cholesterol lowering properties
- HDL-cholesterol increasing properties

When hypertensive rats were given 0.2% Ashitaba in their daily diet, for 6 weeks, both blood pressure and liver triglycerides decreased, but serum HDL-cholesterol increased significantly, compared to the control group (Ogawa et.al. 2003).

The coumarin Laserpitin isolated from Ashitaba increases significantly the HDL-cholesterol in serum (Ogawa et.al. 2005).

When rats were given 4-Hydroxyderricin isolated from Ashitaba, at a dose of 0.7% of daily diet, for 7 weeks, systolic blood pressure and VLDL-cholesterol decreased significantly, but HDL-cholesterol increased significantly, compared to the control group (Ogawa et.al. 2005).

The ethanol extract of Ashitaba inhibits ACE, and it is hypotensive in rats, when given both acutely and chronically (Shimizu et.al. 1999).

Xanthoangenol D, isolated from the roots of Ashitaba, inhibits Endothelin-1 (ET-1), which is a known hypertensive compound (Sugi et.al. 2005).

Xanthoangenol from Ashitabe decreases both LDL-cholesterol and total cholesterol in rats (Ogawa et.al. 2007).

There are 5 different Chalcones isolated from Ashitaba, which all are vasodilators and decrease blood pressure (Matsumura et.al. 2001).

Astaxanthin

Astaxanthin is a naturally occuring carotenoid. Astaxanthin can be purchased from ordinary Supermarkets.

Astaxanthin has
- Blood pressure lowering properties
- Triglycerides lowering properties
- HDL-cholesterol increasing properties

In experiments with rats, Astaxanthin decreased significantly blood pressure (Hussein et.al. 2005; Monroy-Ruiz et.al. 2011).

When 61 volunteers were given Astaxanthin at different dosages, 6 – 18 mg daily, for 12 weeks, triglycerides decreased significantly, but HDL-cholesterol increased significantly, compared to the control group (Yoshida et.al. 2009). This was a doubble blind experiment. The minimum effective dosage was 6 mg daily.

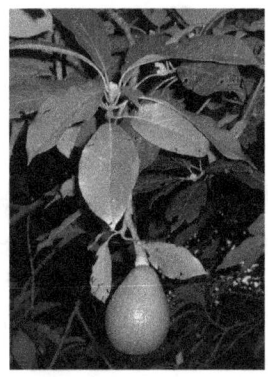

Avocado seed

(Persea Americana)

Avocado is a very popular fruit, which has a large amount of different nutritional factors. The fruit pulp contains large amounts of Monounsaturated fatty acids, vitamin E, beta-Sitosterol and GSH (Reduced Glutathione).

Normally only the pulp is eaten, and the seed is thrown away. But the seed is totally eatable, and it has a very positive influence to high blood pressure and high cholesterol values.

The Avocado Seed has
- Blood pressure lowering properties
- Total cholesterol lowering properties
- LDL-cholesterol lowering properties
- Triglycerides lowering properties
- HDL-cholesterol increasing properties

In experiments with rats, the Avocado seed extract decreases very strongly the blood pressure (Imafidon et.al. 2009).

In another experiment, rats were fed Avocado dried seed daily, for 4 weeks. Both systolic and diastolic blood pressure decreased ($p < 0.05$) significantly (Imafidon et.al. 2010).

With rabbits, the Avocado seed given daily decreased strongly total cholesterol, LDL-cholesterol and triglycerides (Nwaoguikpe et.al. 2011).

In experiments with rats, the Avocado seed extract significantly decreases total cholesterol, LDL-cholesterol and triglycerides, but increases HDL-cholesterol (Asaolu et.al. 2010).

The seed does not taste very good, but it can be broken and dried, and used as such or it can be added to foods or drinks.

Avocado fruit

(Persea Americana)

Avocado is well known fruit to everybody, and it can be purchased all around the year in supermarkets. Avocado contains large amounts of Polyunsaturated fatty acids, typically 9.8 grams/100 grams fruit. Avocado is also the richest known fruit source of beta-Sitosterol, typically 76 mg/100 grams fruit. It has been known since 1950, that beta-Sitosterol decreases cholesterol.

Avocado fruit has
- Total cholesterol decreasing properties
- LDL-cholesterol decreasing properties
- Triglycerides decreasing properties
- HDL-cholesterol increasing properties

When 30 hyperlipidemic volunteers were given Avocado daily amount, which gave 49 grams monounsaturated fatty acids for every 2000 kcal energy intake, for 7 days, total cholesterol decreased by 17% ($p < 0.01$), LDL-cholesterol decreased by 22% ($p < 0.01$) and triglycerides decreased by 22% ($p < 0.01$), but HDL-cholesterol increased by 11% ($p < 0.01$), compared to the control group (Lopez et.al. 1996).

When 16 hyperlipidemic volunteers were given daily Avocado so, that 75% of daily fat came from Avocados, for 4 weeks, total cholesterol ($p < 0.05$) and LDL-cholesterol ($p < 0.05$) decreased significantly, but HDL-cholesterol ($p < 0.05$) increased significantly, compared to the control group (Caranza et.al. 1995).

When rats were given Avocado 28% in their daily diet, for 5 weeks, triglycerides decreased by 27% ($p < 0.05$), but HDL-cholesterol increased by 17% ($p < 0.05$), compared to the control group (Perez et.al. 2007).

When 16 diabetic volunteers were given daily 1 Avocado fruit and 4 teaspoons of Olive oil, for 4 weeks, total cholesterol decreased by 7.47% (5.22 mmol/L $\rightarrow$ 4.83 mmol/L; $p < 0.05$) and triglycerides decreased by 28.7% (1.75 mmol/L $\rightarrow$ 1.25 mmol/L; $p < 0.05$), compared to the control group (Lerman-Garber et.al. 1994).

When 8 volunteers were given daily at lunch Avocado an amount, which gives 30 ml of Avocado oil, for 30 days, total cholesterol decreased by 9.0% (226.8 mg/dl → 206.3 mg/dl; $p < 0.05$), LDL-cholesterol decreased by 7.5% (146.8 mg/dl → 135.7 mg/dl; $p < 0.05$), VLDL-cholesterol decreased by 13.4% (43.3 mg/dl → 37.5 mg/dl) and triglycerides decreased by 10.2% (215 mg/dl → 193 mg/dl; $p < 0.05$), but HDL-cholesterol increased by 6.3% (31.5 mg/dl → 33.5 mg/dl; $p < 0.05$), compared to the control group (Ester et.al. 2009).

When 13 volunteers were for 4 weeks either a vegetarian diet or vegetarian diet, where 75% of daily fat came from Avocado fruits, triglycerides decreased by 8.1% ($p < 0.05$), LDL-cholesterol decreased by 5.7% ($p < 0.05$) but HDL-cholesterol increased by 17.9% ($p < 0.05$) in Avocado group, compared to the pure vegetarian group (Carranza et.al. 1997).

When 15 volunteers were given by an average 1 Avocado fruit daily, for 3 weeks, total cholesterol decreased by 8.2% (6.10 mmol/L → 5.60 mmol/L; $p < 0.05$), compared to the initial level (Colquhoun et.al. 1992).

Azukibean

(Vigna Angularis)

Azukibean has been cultivated in Asia allready over 3000 years. It is a very popular bean in Japan, second after Soybean. Azukibean contains large amounts of functionally healthy Polyphenols.

Azukibean has
- Blood pressure lowering properties
- Total cholesterol lowering properties
- Triglycerides lowering properties

When rats were given in their daily diet 0.9% Azukibean, for 8 weeks, systolic blood pressure decreased significantly by 25 mmHg (158 mmHg → 133 mmHg; $p < 0.05$), compared to the control group (Mukai et.al. 2009).

Same blood pressure lowering effect of Azukibean has been noticed also in other experiments with rats (Mukai et.al. 2009; Sato et.al. 2008).

When young women were given daily drink made from Azukibeans, 150 grams daily, triglycerides decreased by 17.9%, compared to the control group (Maruyama et.al. 2008).

When rats were fed water extract of Azukibeans daily, for 2 weeks, both total cholesterol ($p < 0.05$) and triglycerides ($p < 0.05$) decreased significantly, compared to the control group (Itoh et.al. 2009).

When rats were fed ethanol extract of Azukibeans, the serum total cholesterol decreased significantly, compared to the control group (Kojima et.al. 2006).

When rats were fed Azukibeans daily for 4 weeks, total cholesterol, LDL-cholesterol and triglycerides decreased significantly, compared to the control group (Han et.al. 2005).

Bahera

(Terminalia Bellerica)

Bahera is a very famous medicinal plant from India. It is a large growing tree, which has edible fruits. Bahera fruits contain large amount of pharmacological compounds, such as Ellagic acid, Gallic acid, beta-Sitosterol, Mannitol, Belleric acid, Arjungenin etc. Bahera fruits have been used for thousands of years in India against many different diseases, such a Asthma, hypertension, liver disease, bacterial infections etc.

Bahera has
- — Blood pressure decreasing properties
- — Total cholesterol decreasing properties
- — LDL-cholesterol decreasing properties
- — Triglycerides decreasing properties
- — HDL-cholesterol increasing properties

When rats were given intravenously water extract from Bahera fruit 70% methanol extract, at doses of 10 mg/kg, 30 mg/kg and 100 mg/kg, the mean average blood pressure (MAP) decreased by 15.6 mmHg, 25.1 mmHg and 44.7 mmHg, compared to the control group (Khan et.al. 2008).

The same hypotensive property of Bahera fruit has been verified in other experiments too (Srivastava et.al. 1992; Dwivedi et.al. 1994).

Bahera fruit extract inhibits very strongly ACE (Somanadhan et.al. 1999).

When hyperlipidemic rabbits were given Bahera fruit 1 g/kg daily, for 16 weeks, total cholesterol decreased by 61.9%, compared to the control group (630 mg/dl $\rightarrow$ 240 mg/dl; $p < 0.001$) (Thakur et.al. 1988).

The total cholesterol, LDL-cholesterol and triglycerides decreasing but HDL-cholesterol increasing property of Bahera fruit has been verified in other experiments too with rabbits and mice (Shaila et.al. 1995; Makihare et.al. 2011; Latha et.al. 2010).

Banana

(Musa Paradisiaca, Musa Sapientum, Musa Sp.)

Banana has been cultivated allready over 4000 years and there exists hundreds of different Banana species and types.

Banana has:
- Blood pressure lowering properties.

In very many African countries Banana is used generally in Folk Medicine to lower high blood pressure (Aiyeola et.al. 2006).

In Banana there exists ACE inhibitory properties (Rao et.al. 1999).

With test volunteers, who were under cold stress, daily Banana intake significantly decreased both systolic ($p < 0.005$) and diastolic ($p < 0.025$) blood pressure, compared to the control group. Also Banana inhibited ACE (Sarkar et.al. 1999).

Banana is extremely rich source of Potassium. The average amount of Potassium in one Banana is 460 mg. Potassium is known to decrease blood pressure.

Barberry

(Berberis Vulgaris)

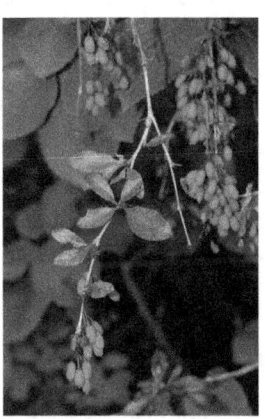

Barberry is a common plant in Europe and Asia. The berries can be eaten, and they contain high amounts of nutrients and Berberin, which is known to lower blood pressure.

Barberry has
- Blood pressure lowering properties
- Total cholesterol lowering properties
- LDL-cholesterol lowering properties
- Triglycerides lowering properties
- HDL-cholesterol increasing properties

The blood pressure lowering effect of Barberry in rats has been shown in 3 different studies (Fatehi et.al. 2005; Fatehi-Hassanabad et.al. 2005; Azmat et.al. 2009).

When volunteers were given Barberry daily, for 8 weeks, LDL-cholesterol decreased 22.5 mg/dl and also the total cholesterol/HDL-cholesterol ratio (2.56) decreased significantly, but HDL-cholesterol increased by 12.33 mg/dl (p < 0.05), compared to the control group (Mamaghani et.al. 2009).

When chicken were fed with Barberry daily, for 4 weeks, total cholesterol decreased significantly (p < 0.01), but HDL-cholesterol increased significantly (p < 0.014) (Kermamshah et.al. 2006).

With diabetic rats Barberry decreased both the serum total cholesterol and triglycerides (Meliani et.al. 2011).

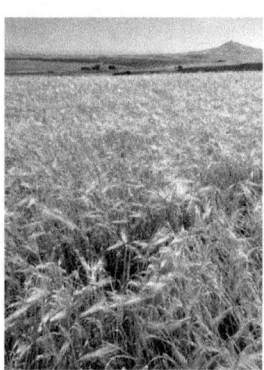

Barley

(Hordeum Vulgare)

Barley is an ancient food plant, which is grown all over the World. Barley contains large amounts of beta-Glucans, and extremely large amounts of functionally healthy Polyphenols.

Barley has
- Blood pressure lowering properties
- Total cholesterol lowering properties
- LDL-cholesterol lowering properties
- Triglycerides lowering properties
- HDL-cholesterol increasing properties

When hyperlipidemic volunteers were given 30 grams of barley bran daily, for 30 days, total cholesterol decreased 0.60 mmol/L (p < 0.0001) and LDL-cholesterol decreased by 6.5% (p < 0.036), compared to the control group (Lupton 1994).

When 18 hyperlipidemic volunteers were given daily amount of Barley, corresponding to 6 grams of soluble fiber/2000 kcal energy, for 5 weeks, total cholesterol decreased by 20%, LDL-cholesterol decreased by 16%, but HDL-cholesterol increased by 18%, compared to the control group (Behall et.al. 2004).

Also, when 27 volunteers were given daily amount of Barley, corresponding to 6 grams of beta-Glucans, for 5 weeks, total cholesterol (p < 0.0001) and LDL-cholesterol (p < 0.0001) decreased significantly, compared to the control group (Behall et.al. 2004).

When 21 hyperlipidemic volunteers were given daily amount of Barley, corresponding to 6 grams of soluble fiber/2800 kcal energy, for 5 weeks, systolic blood pressure (120 mmHg → 114 mmHg; p < 0.0004) and diastolic blood pressure (74 mmHg → 72 mmHg; p < 0.015) decreased significantly, compared to the control group (Hallfrisch et.al. 2003).

Barley grass

(Hordeum Vulgare)

Dried Barley grass flour is nowadays a very popular food supplement.

Barley grass has
- Total cholesterol lowering properties
- LDL-cholesterol lowering properties
- Triglycerides lowering properties
- HDL-cholesterol increasing properties

When 32 diabetic volunteers were given Barley grass flour 15 grams daily, for 4 weeks, total cholesterol (7.0 mmol/L → 6.4 mmol/L; $p < 0.05$), LDL-cholesterol (4.5 mmol/L → 3.9 mmol/L; $p < 0.05$) and triglycerides (2.3 mmol/L → 2.1 mmol/L; $p < 0.05$) decreased significantly, but HDL-cholesterol (1.4 mmol/L → 1.5 mmol/L; $p < 0.05$) increased, compared to the control group (Yu et.al. 2002).

When 40 hyperlipidemic volunteers were given Barley grass flour 15 grams daily, for 4 weeks, total cholesterol (8.15 mmol/L → 7.35 mmol/L; $p < 0.05$) and LDL-cholesterol (5.1 mmol/L → 4.55 mmol/L; $p < 0.05$) decreased significantly, but HDL-cholesterol (1.1 mmol/L → 1.35 mmol/L; $p < 0.05$) increased significantly, compared to the control group (Yu et.al. 2004).

When 59 diabetic volunteers were given Barley grass flour 1.2 grams daily, for 2 months, total cholesterol, LDL-cholesterol and triglycerides decreased significantly, but HDL-cholesterol increased significantly, compared to the control group (Venugopal et.al. 2010).

Basil

(Ocimum Basilicum)

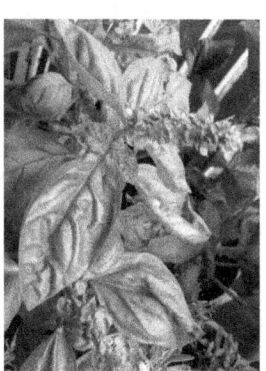

Basil is extremely popular spice and vegetable all around the World. It can be purchased both as dry and fresh, and its cultivation is very easy.

Basil has
- Blood pressure lowering properties
- Total cholesterol lowering properties
- LDL-cholesterol lowering properties
- Triglycerides lowering properties

When rats were fed Basil with different dosages between 100 – 400 mg/kg daily, for 4 weeks, systolic blood pressure decreased by 20 mmHg and diastolic blood pressure decreased by 15 mmHg, compared to the control group (Umar et.al. 2010).

The water extracts of Basil are strongly vasorelaxant (Amrani et.al. 2009).

The ethanol extract of Basil inhibits cholesterol synthesis in Human Macrophages (Bravo et.al. 2008).

In experiments with rats, Basil decreases significantly total cholesterol, LDL-cholesterol and triglycerides, but increases HDL-cholesterol (Amrani et.al. 2006).

Berberine

Berberine is an alkaloid, which occurs naturally in many plants, especially in Berberis Vulgari (Barberry) and other Berberis species. There are tens of different Berberis species in the World. Barberry fruits can be eaten raw, and Barberry fruits and roots are used in for medicinal purposes, all over the World. Berberine can be also purchased in Supermarkets. Berberine is known to decreae blood pressure in animal experiments, and it has also anti-obesity properties. It is strongly antibacterial and antiviral.

Berberine has
- Blood pressure lowering properties
- Total cholesterol lowering properties
- LDL-cholesterol lowering properties
- Triglycerides lowering properties
- Body weight lowering properties

When 16 diabetic volunteers were given Berberine 1.0 gram daily, for 3 months, systolic blood pressure decreased by 7 mmHg (124 mmHg → 117 mmHg; $p < 0.001$), diastolic blood pressure decreased by 4 mmHg (81 mmHg → 77 mmHg; $p < 0.05$), triglycerides decreased by 35.8% (2.51 mmol/L → 1.61 mmol/L; $p < 0.001$), total cholesterol decreased by 18% (5.31 mmol/L → 4.35 mmol/L; $p < 0.001$) and LDL-choleterol decreased by 21% (3.23 mmol/L → 2.55 mmol/L; $p < 0.001$), compared to the control group (Zhang et.al. 2008). Also body weight decreased by 2.3 kg (68.7 kg → 66.4 kg; $p < 0.001$).

When mice were given 0.75 mg/kg, 1.5 mg/kg or 3.0 mg/kg Berberine daily, for 36 days, triglyceride decreased by 31.2%, 25.2% and 37.8%. Total cholesterol decreased by 18.7%, 22.2% and 28.0% ($p < 0.05$ in all groups), compared to control group (Hu et.al. 2010). Also body weight decreased significantly, compared to the control group.

Bergamot

(Citrus Bergamia)

Bergamot is a Citrus fruit, which originates from Calabria, South Italy. The famous Bergamot oil is made from this fruit. Bergamot juice and pulp contain many unique Flavonoids, such as: Naringin, Rutin, Neoeriocitrin, Neohesperedin, Neodesmin, Rhoifolin, Poncirin, Melitidine and Brutieridine.

Bergamot has
- Total cholesterol lowering properties
- LDL-cholesterol lowering properties
- Triglycerides lowering properties
- HDL-cholesterol increasing properties

When 237 hyperlipidemic volunteers were given Bergamot flavonoids either 500 mg or 1000 mg daily, for 30 days, total cholesterol decreased by 21.8% ($p < 0.001$), LDL-cholesterol decreased by 24.1% ($p < 0.001$) and triglycerides decreased by 30.3% ($p < 0.001$), but HDL-cholesterol increased by 22.3% ($p < 0.001$) in the 500 mg group, compared to the control group. In the 1000 mg group, total cholesterol decreased by 29.4% ($p < 0.001$), LDL-cholesterol decreased by 36.0% ($p < 0.001$) and triglycerides decreased by 39.4% ($p < 0.001$), but HDL-cholesterol increased by 40.1% ($p < 0.001$), compared to the control group (Mollace et.al. 2011). This was a double blind experiment.

With Bergamot very large decreases in cholesterol- and triglyceride levels can be achieved within very short time period, and the effect increases, when the dose increases.

Similar cholesterol- and triglycerides lowering properties has been seen also in experiments with rats (Mollace et.al. 2011; Miceli et.al. 2007; Di Donna et.al. 2009).

Black Chokeberry

(Aronia Melanocarpa)

Black Chokeberry is a very popular berry in Eastern-Europe, especially in Russia, where it is grown in large amounts. Black Chokeberry contains extremely high amounts of functionally healthy Polyphenols. It has been given to patients with cardiovascular disease, such as high blood pressure.

Black Chokeberry has
- Blood pressure lowering properties
- Total cholesterol lowering properties
- LDL-cholesterol lowering properties
- Triglycerides lowering properties

When 25 patients with metablic syndrome were given Black Chokeberry extract 300 mg daily, for 8 weeks, the systolic blood pressure (143.4 mmHg → 131.8 mmHg; $p < 0.01$), diastolic blood pressure (87.2 mmHg → 82.1 mmHg; $p < 0.05$), total cholesterol (242.8 mg/dl → 227.96 mg/dl; $p < 0.01$), LDL-cholesterol (158.7 mg/dl → 146.2 mg/dl; $p < 0.01$) and triglycerides

(215.9 mg/dl → 187.58 mg/dl; p < 0.05) decreased significantly, compared to the control group (Broncel et.al. 2010).

When 41 diabetic patients were given Black Chokeberry juice at a dose of 2.0 desiliters daily, for 12 weeks, the total cholesterol (6.45 mmol/L → 5.05 mmol/L; p < 0.01) and triglycerides (2.92 mmol/L → 1.7 mmol/L; p < 0.01) decreased significantly (Simeonov et.al. 2002).

In many trials with rats, the Black Chokeberry has decreased the total cholesterol, LDL-cholesterol and triglycerides (Jurgonski et.al. 2008; Valcheva-Kuzmanova et.al. 2007; Valcheva-Kuzhmanova et.al. 2007).

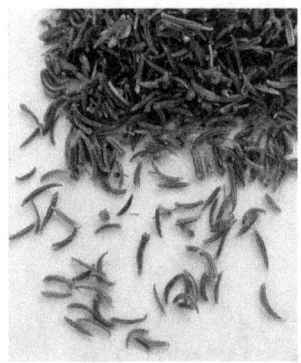

Black Cumin

(Nigella Sativa)

Black Cumin is an Ancient spice and medicinal plant, which is very popular in Asia and Arabic countries. It is very easy to cultivate. The Black Cumin seeds and seed oil has been used much in Asthma and Bronchitis.

Black Cumin has
- Blood pressure lowering properties
- Total cholesterol lowering properties
- Triglycerides lowering properties

When rats were given Black Cumin seed extract daily, for 15 days, the amount of urine increased by 16% and mean average blood pressure (MAP) decreased by 22% (Zaoui et.al. 2000).

The blood pressure lowering properties of Black Cumin has been noticed also in other rat experiments (Tahiir et.al. 1993; Khattab et.al. 2007). The cholesterol and triglycerides lowering properties of Black Cumin has been noticed in several experiments (Zaoui et.al. 2002; El-Dakhakhny et.al. 2000; Kocyigit et.al. 2009).

When volunteers with high cholesterol levels were given Black Cumin seeds 1 gram daily, for 2 months, both triglycerides (p = 0.002) and total cholesterol (p = 0.002) decreased significantly (Bhatti et.al. 2009).

Black Currant leaves

(Ribes Nigrum)

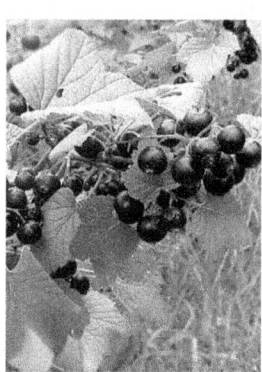

Black Currant leaves are much used in making herbal teas. Black Currant leaves are also used medicinally in Europe, especially in France. In folk medicine it is used to lower high blood pressure.

Black Currant leaves have more Flavonoids, than the Black Currant berry (Jessica et.al. 2006).

Black Currant leaves have
- Blood pressure lowering properties.

The blood pressure lowering property of Black Currant has been verified in a French Doctor Thesis (Ifansyah et.al. 1982). The blood pressure lowering effect was due to the total Flavonoids.

The main Flavonoids, in Black Currant leaves are Rutin, Hyperoside, Kaempferol-compounds and Isoquercetin (Ifansayah et.al. 1986; He et.al. 2010).

Isoquercetin is strongly diuretic and decreases blood pressure, and inhibits ACE (Gasparatto et.al. 2011; Gasparatto et.al. 2011).

Black rice

(Oryza Sativa)

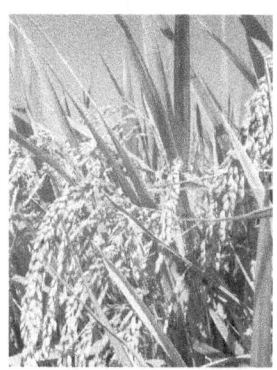

(Author: IRRI Images)

There exists different colored Rice, white Rice, brown Rice, red Rice and black Rice. Black Rice has been used in China for thousands of years as a functional food. It has much more functionally healthy Anthocyanides, than white or brown Rice.

Black Rice has
- Total cholesterol lowering properties

- LDL-cholesterol lowering properties
- Triglycerides lowering properties
- HDL-cholesterol increasing properties

When rabbits were fed black Rice daily, for 10 weeks, serum HDL-cholesterol increased significantly ($p < 0.05$), compared to the control group, which was fed with white Rice (Ling et.al. 2001).

The same results with rabbits were found in another experiment with black Rice fed daily for 10 weeks. HDL-cholesterol increased significantly ($p < 0.05$), compared to the control group (Abdel-Moemin et.al. 2011).

When mice were fed black Rice Anthocyanide fraction 300 mg/kg daily, for 20 weeks, total cholesterol ($p < 0.05$), LDL-cholesterol ($p < 0.05$) and triglycerides ($p < 0.05$) decreased significantly, compared to the control group (Xia et.al. 2006).

When mice were fed black Rice daily, for 10 weeks, HDL-cholesterol increased ($p < 0.05$) significantly, compared to the control group, which was fed with white Rice (Chiang et.al. 2006).

When rats were fed daily with black Rice, for 8 weeks, total cholesterol, LDL-cholesterol and triglycerides decreased significantly, but HDL-cholesterol increased significantly, compared to the control group, which was fed with white Rice (Kim et.al. 2006).

Black Sesame

(Sesame Indicum var. Nigra)

Sesame is an Ancient food, which is used all around the World. Together with the normal yellow Sesame, there exists the Black Sesame, which has been used in China for thousands of years as a functional food. Sesame contains Lignans, especially Sesamin and Sesaminol.

Black Sesame has
- Blood pressure lowering properties
- Total cholesterol lowering properties
- LDL-cholesterol lowering properties

When 28 volunteers were given Black Sesame 2.5 grams daily, for 4 weeks, the systolic blood pressure decreased (129.3 mmHg → 121.0 mmHg; $p < 0.05$) significantly, compared to the control group (Wichitsranol et.al. 2011).

When 12 volunteers were given 60 mg Sesamin daily, for 4 weeks, the systolic blood pressure decreased (137.6 mmHg → 134.1 mmHg; $p < 0.044$) and also the diastolic blood pressure decreased (87.7 mmHg → 85.8 mmHg; $p < 0.045$) significantly, compared to the control group (Miyawaki et.al. 2009).

When 21 volunteers with high cholesterol levels were given 40 grams of Sesame daily, for 4 weeks, the total cholesterol decreased by 6.4% and the LDL-cholesterol decreased by 9.5%, compared to the control group (Chen et.al. 2005).

The cholesterol lowering effect of Sesame has been noticed also in many animal tests (Biswas et.al. 2010; Dhar et.al. 2007).

Black Soy bean

(Glycine Max var. Nigra)

Black Soy bean has been used in China for thousands of years as a functional food. Black Soy bean has large amounts of functionally healthy Anthocyanides, much more than in the ordinary Yellow Soy beans. Black Soy bean has a stronger effect to high serum cholesterol- and triglyceride levels, thanyellow Soy bean, which also has good effect to these values.

Black Soy bean has
- Total cholesterol lowering properties
- LDL-cholesterol lowering properties
- Triglycerides lowering properties
- HDL-cholesterol increasing properties
- Body weight lowering properties

When rats were given in their daily diet 10% black Soy beans or 0.037% of black Soy bean Anthocyanides corresponding to 10% black Soy beans, triglycerides decreased ($p < 0.05$) significantly, but HDL-cholesterol increased ($p < 0.05$) significantly, compared to the control group (Kwon et.al. 2007). Also the body weight decreased ($p < 0.05$) significantly, compared to the control group.

When rats were fed either yellow Soy beans or black Soy beans in their daily diet, for 10 weeks, total cholesterol, LDL-cholesterol and triglycerides decreased significantly in the black Soy group, compared to the yellow soy group (Byun et.al. 2010).

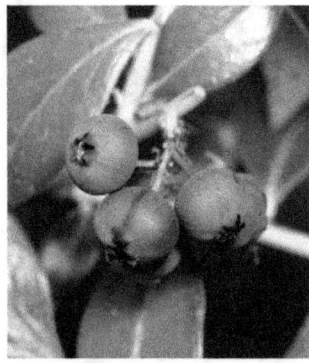

Blueberry

(Vaccinium Myrtillus)

Blueberry is an Ancient food- and medicinal plant, which has been used against stomach problems, diarrhea, inflammation and so on.

Blueberry has
- – Blood pressure lowering properties
- – Triglycerides lowering properties

Blueberry is a strong inhibitor of ACE (Persson et.al. 2009).

When 48 volunteers were fed 50 grams of Blueberry daily, for 8 weeks, systolic blood pressure decreased by 4% and diastolic blood pressure decreased by 6%, compared to the control group (Basu et.al. 2010).

When rats were given daily food, which contained 3% of dried Blueberry, for 8 weeks, systolic blood pressure decreased 30% compared to the control group (Shaughnessey et.al. 2009).

When rats were fed extract of Blueberry leaves daily, for 4 weeks, plasma triglycerides decreased by 39%, compared to the control group (Cignarella et.al. 1996).

Bodyweight reduction

Obesity increases both blood pressure and cholesterol values. Bodyweight reduction is extremely efficient method to decrease high blood pressure and high cholesterol values.

Bodyweight reduction has
- – Blood pressure decreasing properties
- – Total cholesterol decreasing properties
- – LDL-cholesterol decreasing properties
- – VLDL-cholesterol decreasing properties
- – HDL-cholesterol increasing properties
- – Triglycerides decreasing properties

In a meta-analysis with 11 different experiments, it was noticed, that for every 1.0 kg decrease in bodyweight, systolic blood pressure decreases by an average of 1.6 mmHg and diastolic blood pressure decreases by an average of 1.3 mmHg (Staessen et.al. 1989). This means, that an obese person, who reduces his or her bodyweight by 10 kg, can decrease systolic blood pressure by an average of 16 mmHg and diastolic blood pressure by an average of 13 mmHg.

In a meta-analysis with 70 different experiments, it was noticed, that bodyweight reduction decreases significantly total cholesterol, LDL-cholesterol, VLDL-cholesterol and triglycerides, but increases HDL-cholesterol (Dattilo et.al. 1992). The correlations between bodyweight reduction and cholesterol values were highly significant: TC ($r = 0.32$), LDL ($r = 0.29$), VLDL ($r = 0.38$), TG ($r = 0.32$).

The average bodyweight reduction was 16.6 kg, and the corresponding changes in cholesterol levels were:

Total cholesterol:	5.93 mmol/L $\rightarrow$ 5.14 mmol/L ($p < 0.01$)
LDL-cholesterol:	3.44 mmol/L $\rightarrow$ 3.05 mmol/L ($p < 0.01$)
VLDL-cholesterol:	1.09 mmol/L $\rightarrow$ 0.69 mmol/L ($p < 0.01$)
Triglycerides:	2.05 mmol/L $\rightarrow$ 1.39 mmol/L ($p < 0.01$)
HDL-cholesterol:	1.17 mmol/L $\rightarrow$ 1.20 mmol/L ($p < 0.01$)

Bottle Gourd

(Lagenaria Siceraria)

Bottle Gourd is an ancient, very popular vegetable and medicinal plant, which is much used especially in India and Pakistan. Its cultivation is very easy.

Bottle Gourd has
- Blood pressure lowering properties
- Diuretic properties
- Total cholesterol lowering properties
- LDL-cholesterol lowering properties
- Triglycerides lowering properties
- HDL-cholesterol increasing properties

When rats were given Bottle Gourd dried pulp 500 mg/kg daily, for 51 days, both systolic blood pressure (109.7 mmHg $\rightarrow$ 91.1 mmHg; $p < 0.05$) and diastolic blood pressure (98.6 mmHg $\rightarrow$ 79.7 mmHg; $p < 0.05$) decreased significantly, compared to the control group (Maliet et.al. 2010). Also heart rate decreased.

When rats were fed Bottle Gourd juice 5 ml daily, for 4 weeks, total cholesterol decreased by 16.3% ($p < 0.05$), LDL-cholesterol decreased by 23.6% ($p < 0.05$) and triglycerides decreased by 18.2% ($p < 0.05$), compared to the control group, which were given water (Nainwsal et.al. 2010).

Also in many other experiments Bottle Gourd decreases total cholesterol, LDL-cholesterol, VLDL-cholesterol and triglycerdes, but increases HDL-cholesterol (Ghule et.al. 2009; Ghule et.al. 2006; Kaisal et.al. 2011).

The diuretic activity of Bottle Gourd is very strong, when compared to the standard diuretic Furosemide (Ghule et.al. 2007).

Brahmi

(Centella Asiatica)

Brahmi has been used as a food and medicinal plant for thousands of years in Asia. Brahmi leaves are used as salad or vegetable. Brahmi is used medicinally to decrease high blood pressure, to improve memor and skin problems. It is very easy to cultivate, even indoors in home.

Brahmi has
- Blood pressure lowering properties
- Diuretic properties
- LDL-cholesterol lowering properties
- Triglycerides lowering properties
- HDL-cholesterol increasing properties

Brahmi inhibits very strongly ACE (Hansen et.al. 1995). Both the water extract and ethanol extract inhibit ACE.

When 60 volunteers were given Brahmi 1000 mg daily, for 6 months, diastolic blood pressure decreased (85.5 mmHg $\rightarrow$ 78.5 mmHg; $p < 0.05$), significantly, compared to the control group (Tiwari et.al. 2008).

In experiments with rats, Brahmi strongly stimulates the GABA content of Brains (Chatterjee et.al. 1992). GABA is an amino acid, which decreases strongly blood pressure.

When rats were given Brahmi either 0.3% or 5.0% of their daily diet, for 25 weeks, both LDL-cholesterol ($p < 0.05$) and triglycerides ($p < 0.05$) decreased significantly, but HDL-cholesterol ($p < 0.05$) increased significantly, compared to the control group (Hussin et.al. 2009).

Broad bean

(Vicia Faba)

Broad bean has been cultivated for thousands of years as a food plant. Broad beans contain large amounts of protein and fiber. They also contain large amounts of the amino acid L-Dopa, typically 280 mg/100 g (Vered et.al. 1997).

Broad bean has
- Blood pressure lowering properties

- Total cholesterol lowering properties
- LDL-cholesterol lowering properties
- VLDL-cholesterol lowering properties
- Triglycerides lowering properties
- HDL-cholesterol increasing properties
- Diuretic properties

Broad bean is strongly diuretic (Veed et.al. 1997).

When 40 volunteers were given in their daily diet 90 grams of Broad beans, for 4 weeks, triglycerides ($p < 0.0001$), total cholesterol ($p < 0.0001$), LDL-cholesterol ($p < 0.0001$) and VLDL-cholesterol ($p < 0.0001$) decreased significantly, but HDL-cholesterol ($p < 0.0001$) increased significantly, compared to the control group (Fruhbeck et.al. 1997).

Broad bean contains 280 mg/100 g L-Dopa. When 36 hypertensive volunteers were given L-Dopa orally at a dose of 250 mg, blood pressure decreased significantly, compared to the control group (Saito et.al. 1991).

Broad bean contains GABA, which is known to decrease blood pressure. When Broad beans are germinated, the GABA content increases up to 48 times, being up to 241 mg/100 g in the Broad bean sprouts (Li et.al. 2010).

Also in other human experiments, researchers have noticed the cholesterol lowering properties of Broad beans (Weck et.al. 1983). They noticed, that Broad beans were as good as Soy beans, to lower cholesterol.

In experiments with rats, Broad beans lower total cholesterol, LDL-cholesterol, VLDL-cholesterol and triglycerides (Nacarulla et.al. 2001; Mengheri et.al. 1985).

Broccoli sprouts

(Brassica Oleracea var. Italica)

Broccoli sprouts are very popular functional food nowadays. They are intensively researched, because they contain anticancer Isothiocyanates (Glucoraphanin, Sulforaphane). The content of Isothiocyanates reaches maximum in the 3 – 4 days old sprouts.

Broccoli sprouts have
- Blood pressure lowering properties
- Total cholesterol lowering properties
- LDL-cholesterol lowering properties
- HDL-cholesterol increasing properties

When hypertensive rats were given Sulforaphane in their daily diet, for 4 months, blood pressure decreased by 11%, compared to the control group (Gamarallage et.al. 2012).

When rats were given Broccoli sprouts 2000 mg/kg daily, 5 days a week, for 14 weeks, blood pressure decreased by 20 mmHg (p < 0.05), compared to the control group (Wu et.al. 2004).

When 40 hypertensive volunteers were given 10 grams of Broccoli sprouts daily, for 4 weeks, the systolic blood pressure decreased by 9 mmHg (153 mmHg → 144 mmHg), compared to the control group (Christiansen et.al. 2010).

When 81 diabetic volunteers were given 10 grams Broccoli sprouts daily, for 4 weeks, oxidised LDL-cholesterol decreased (p = 0.03) significantly, compared to the control group (Bahadoran et.al. 2011). This was a double blind experiment.

When 12 volunteers were given Broccoli sprouts 100 grams daily, for 7 days, both total cholesterol and LDL-cholesterol decreased significantly, but HDL-cholesterol increased significantly, compared to the control group (Murashima et.al. 2004).

Broccoli sprouts decrease cholesterol also in experiments with hamsters (Rodriguez et.al. 2011).

Buckwheat

(Fagopyrum Esculentum, Fagopyrum Tataricum)

Buckwheat is extremely popular food, especially in Russia, China, Korea and Japan. It has been grown over 3000 years. It has a very high nutritional value, and it contains large amounts of Flavonoids, especially Rutin. There are two different kind of Buckwheat in cultivation: The ordinary Buckwheat (Fagopyrum Tataricum) and the Tartary Buckwheat (Fagopyrym Tataricum). The Tartary Buckwheat contains much more Rutin than the ordinary Buckwehat. In China Buckwheat is used against high blood pressure and high cholesterol.

Buckwheat has
  – Blood pressure lowering properties
  – Total cholesterol lowering properties
  – LDL-cholesterol lowering properties
  – Triglycerides lowering properties

The ACE inhibitory property of Buckwheat has been noticed in many experiments (Higasa et.al. 2011; Li et.al. 2010).

Buckwheat has also vasorelaxing properties (Ushida et.al. 2008).

When 60 volunteers were fed Buckwheat 40 grams daily, for 8 weeks, both systolic and diastolic blood pressure decreased. Also total cholesterol, LDL-cholesterol and triglycerides decreased, but HDL-cholesterol increased (Xiping et.al. 1995).

When rats were fed the protein fraction of Buckwheat daily, for 8 weeks, total cholesterol decreased by 22.0%, compared to Casein protein group (Tomoke et.al. 2001).

Buckwheat sprouts

(Fagopyrum Esculentum, Fagopyrum Tataricum)

Buckwheat sprouts contain large amounts of Flavonoids Rutin and Quercitrin (=Quercetin-3-O-Rhamnoside). From 1 kg of Buckwheat man can get 8.9 kg of Buckwheat sprouts. The Flavonoid content of Buckwheat sprouts is much larger than in the seeds: Rutin content is 2236 mg/100 g and Quercitrin content is 2312 mg/100 g. Rutin content increases 35 times and Quercitrin content increases 65 times in sprouts, compared to seeds. The Flavonoids content reaches maximum in sprouts after 7 days (Kim et.al. 2004).

Buckwheat sprouts have
  – Blood pressure lowering properties
  – Total cholesterol lowering properties

Quercitrin inhibits strongly ACE (IC50 = 0.67 Mm) (Hansen et.al. 1996).

Quercitrin is strongly diuretic (Fukuda 1932). Also Quercitrin is known to decrease blood pressure in rats (Fukunaga et.al. 1989) and dogs (Novoa et.al. 1985).

When rats were fed Buckwheat seed extract or Buckwheat sprouts extract 600 mg/kg daily, for 5 weeks, systolic blood pressure was lower in the Buckwheat sprout group (Kim et.al. 2009).

When diabetic mice were fed either 5% or 10% of Buckwheat sprouts daily, for 3 weeks, total cholesterol decreased significantly, compared to the control group (Watanabe et.al. 2010).

Butter

Butter has been used for hundreds of years as food and also together with bread, in baking etc. Butter consists mostly of saturated fatty acids. Butter also contains large amounts of free cholesterol, typically 95 mg/100 g. The energy content of butter is very high, typically 740 calories/100 g. Butter also contains a lot of salt.

Butter has
  – Total cholesterol increasing properties
  – LDL-cholesterol increasing properties
  – Triglycerides increasing properties
  – HDL-cholesterol increasing properties
  – Body weight increasing properties

In North-Karelia, Finland, there was a huge amount of deaths due to heart attacks before 1970. The strongest single factor for this was the very high consumption of saturated fat, mostly butter, and whole fat milk, which increased the cholesterol levels very significantly. Later on this will cause blocking of the arteries. Over 90% of population in North-Karelia used Butter year 1972, but nowadays only 5% of population in North-Karelia uses butter. At the same period, deaths due to heart attacks have decreased by 80% (Puska 2009).

When 19 volunteers were given 40 grams butter daily, for 4 weeks, total cholesterol increased by 8.9% (5.6 mmol/L → 6.1 mmol/L; $p < 0.05$) and LDL-cholesterol increased by 14.7% (3.4 mmol/L → 3.9 mmol/L; $p < 0.05$), compared to the control group (Nestel et.al. 2005).

When 15 volunters were given 20 grams butter daily, for 20 days, triglycerides increased by 49.3% (112.8 mg/dl → 168.5 mg/dl; $p = 0.026$) and HDL-cholesterol increased by 16.8% (40.4 mg/dl → 47.2 mg/dl; $p = 0.050$), compared to the control group (Gorgue et.al. 2005). LDL-cholesterol increased by 15.56% and total cholesterol increased by 6.7%.

This means, that already relatively small amounts of butter increase strongly cholesterol- and triglyceride levels, already within a short time period.

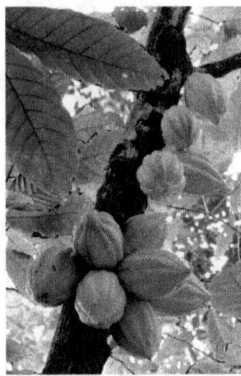
(Author: Luisovalles)

Cacao

(Theobroma Cacao)

and dark Chocolate

Cacao is an extremely popular drink all over the World. Also dark chocolate made from Cacao flour is popular everywhere. Cacao contains large amounts of functionally healthy Polyphenols.

Cacao and dark chocolate have
- Blood pressure lowering properties
- Total cholesterol lowering properties
- LDL-cholesterol lowering properties
- Triglycerides lowering properties
- Oxygenated oxLDL cholesterol lowering properties
- HDL-cholesterol increasing properties

When 16 volunteers were given dark Chocolate 75 grams, ACE activity decreased by 18%. In experiments with cells, ACE activity was strongly inhibited ($p < 0.01$) and NO concentration was increased ($p < 0.01$) significantly (Persson et.al. 2011).

In a meta-analysis with 5 doubble blind experiments, with averageg duration of 2 weeks and 173 volunteers, Cacao decreased systolic blood pressure by 4.7 mmHg ($p < 0.02$) and diastolic blood pressure by 2.8 mmHg ($p < 0.006$) (Taubert et.al. 2007).

When 44 volunteers were given 6.3 grams dark Chocolate daily, for 18 weeks, systolic blood pressure decreased by 2.9 mmHg ($p < 0.01$) and diastolic blood pressure decreased by 1.9 mmHg ($p < 0.01$) (Daubert et.al. 2007). This was a doubble blind experiment.

In a systematic meta-analysis with 24 doubble blind experiments and 1106 volunteers, Cacao decreased systolic blood pressure by an average of 1.63 mmHg (p < 0.033). LDL-cholesterol decreased by 0.077 mmol/L (p < 0.038) and HDL-cholesterol increased by 0.046 mmol/L (p < 0.038) (Shrime et.al. 2011).

When hypertensive rats were given Cacao Polyphenol extract 80 mg/kg, systolic blood pressure decreased by 39.1 mmHg, in 6 hours (Quinones et.al. 2011).

When 42 volunteers were given 40 grams of Cacao flour daily, for 4 weeks, HDL-cholesterol increased 2.67 mg/dl (p = 0.008) and oxidised oxLDL-cholesterol decreased (p = 0.001) significantly, compared to the control group (Khan et.al. 2011).

When rats were fed Cacao extract 3% of their daily diet, for 4 weeks, total cholesterol (p < 0.05), LDL-cholesterol (p < 0.05) and triglycerides (p < 0.05) decreased significantly, but HDL-cholesterol (p < 0.05) increased significantly, compared to the control groups (Ruzaidi et.al. 2005).

In a meta-analysis with 10 doubble blind experiments and 320 volunteers, and between 2 – 12 weeks duration, both Cacao and dark Chocolate decreased LDL-cholesterol by 5.90 mg/dl and total cholesterol by 6.23 mg/dl, compared to control groups (Tokede et.al. 2011).

Caffeine

Caffeine is the stimulant compound in Coffee, which can also be bought as pills.

Caffeine has
   – Blood pressure increasing properties

When 182 volunteers, of which part had normal blood pressure, part were little hypertensive and part were hypertensive, were given Caffeine 250 mg acutely, systolic blood pressure increases in different groups by 6 mmHg, 8 mmHg and 10 mmHg, and diastolic blood pressure increased in different groups by 5 mmHg, 7 mmHg and 8.5 mmHg (p < 0.0001 in all groups) (Hartley et.al. 2000).

The same results have been obtained also in other experiments (Hartley et.al. 2004).

So: Pure Caffeine increases strongly both systolic and diastolib blood pressure, and the increase is biggest in the hypertensive persons.

Caigua

(Cyclanthera Pedata)

Caigua is a vine, which is grown for its edible fruits. The fruits are used as vegetables. Caigue originates from Peru. It has been cultivated for hundreds of years for food and medicine.

Caigua fruit and fruit seeds have
- Blood pressure lowering properties
- Total cholesterol lowering properties
- LDL-cholesterol lowering properties
- HDL-cholesterol increasing properties

There are many scientific expertiments made in Peru about Caigua medicinal properties, concerning high blood pressure and high cholesterol values.

Caigua inhibits strongly ACE (Ranilla et.al. 2010).

When 42 female volunteers were given dried Caigua 6 pills (400 mg/pill) daily, for 12 weeks, total cholesterol decreased by 22% and LDL-cholesterol decreased by 33%, but HDL-cholesterol increased by 33%, compared to the control group (Gonzales et.al. 1995).

When volunteers were given 300 grams of fresh Caigua daily, for 30 days, total cholesterol decreased by 17.5%, compared to the control group (Rodriguez et.al. 1987).

When 25 hyperlipidemic male volunteers were given Caigua either 800 mg or 1600 mg daily, for 390 days, total cholesterol decreased by and average of 33.8% (93 mg/dl) and LDL-cholesterol decreased by an average of 44.5% (88 mg/dl), compared to the control group (Rosario et.al. 1997).

The cholesterol lowering properties of Caigua have been verified in other experiments too (Gonzales et.al. 1994; Gonez et.al. 1997; Gavez et.al. 2004).

Especially the seeds of Caigue are used generally in Peru to decrease high blood pressure. The seeds contain Cucurbitacin Glycosides (Tommasi et.al. 1996). Cucurbitacines are known to lower blood pressure.

Calcium

Calcium is an essential Macro mineral for humans. Good sources of Calcium are milk products, cheese, yoghurt etc.

Calcium has:
- Blood pressure lowering properties.

When 120 volunteers were given 800 mg Calcium daily, for 5 weeks, systolic blood pressure decreased by 4.7 mmHg (p = 0.027) and diastolic blood pressure decreased by 2.7 mmHg (p = 0.074), compared to control group (Pan et.al. 2000).

When 14 volunteers, who first got salt free food for 7 days, and then food with salt, were given 2160 mg Calcium daily, for 7 days, blood pressure increased less (2.85%) due to salt, than control group (8.63%), which did not get extra Calcium (Saito et.al. 1989).

In experiments with rats, added Calcium, between 1.1 – 2.5% of daily food, for 23 weeks, decreased significantly blood pressure, compared to control group (Sallinen et.al. 1996).

Capers

(Capparis Spinosa)

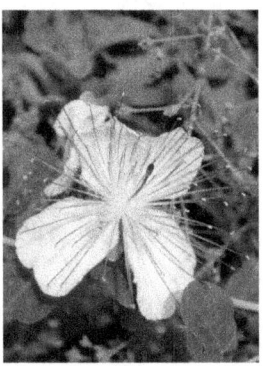

Capers are an ancient food-, spice- and medicinal plant, which is used all around the Mediterranian sea, in Europe and in Asia. The flower buds and fruits are used. Capers have extremely large amounts of Flavonoids, Rutin, Kaempferol and Quercetin. Quercetin content is higher than in any other plant, except the leaves of Blueberry. Capers are used in many countries, like Morocco and Saudi Arabia, to decrease high blood pressure (Sher et.al. 2010).

Capers have
- Blood pressure lowering properties
- Diuretic properties
- Total cholesterol lowering properties
- Triglycerides lowering properties

Capers have strong diuretic property, when compared to the standard drug Furosemide. When rats were given water extract of Capers at a dose of 500 mg/kg/hour, the urine volume increased significantly (p < 0.001), compared to the controls (Zeggwagh et.al. 2007).

When hypertensive rats were given water extract of Capers at a dose of 140 mg/kg daily, for 20 days, systolic blood pressure decreased by 13.5 mmHg (p < 0.01), compared to the control group (Zeggwagh et.al. 2007). Also urine volume increased significantly (p < 0.01).

When rats were given water extract of Capers at a dose of 20 mg/kg daily, for 2 weeks, both total cholesterol (p < 0.05) and triglycerides (p < 0.05) decreased significantly, compared to the control group (Eddouks et.al. 2005).

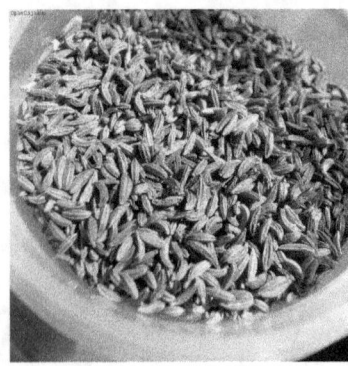

Caraway seed

(Carum Carvi)

Caraway seed is an ancient spice, which grows wildly in Europe. Its cultivation is very easy.

Caraway seed has
- Blood pressure lowering properties
- Total cholesterol lowering properties
- LDL-cholesterol lowering properties
- Triglycerides lowering properties

When rats were fed Caraway seed water extract, it had a strong diuretic activity (Lahlou et.al. 2007).

Oil from Caraway seeds decreases both blood pressure and heart rate (El-Tahir et.al. 1994).

Caraway seed water extract given to rats decreases strongly both total cholesterol ($p < 0.01$) and triglycerides ($p < 0.01$), compared to the control group (Lemhadri et.al. 2006).

When rats were given 1 g/kg Caraway seeds in their daily diet, for 3 weeks, both total cholesterol ($p < 0.036$) and LDL-cholesterol ($p < 0.01$) decreased significantly, compared to the control group (Haldari et.al. 2011).

Cardamom

(Elattaria Cardemomum)

Cardamom is a very common spice all around the World. It is also used medicinally in many Asian countries.

Cardamom has
- Blood pressure lowering properties
- Total cholesterol lowering properties
- LDL-cholesterol lowering properties
- VLDL-cholesterol lowering properties
- Triglycerides lowering properties
- Diuretic properties

When rats were given 70% methanol extract of Cardamom, in doses of 3, 10, 30 or 100 mg/kg, the mean average blodo pressure (MAP) decreased by 6.81 mmHg, 16.49 mmHg, 36.78 mmHg and 52.6 mmHg (Gilani et.al. 2008). The researchers also noticed a strong diuretic property of Cardamom.

When 20 hypertensive volunteers were given 3 grams of Cardamom daily, for 12 weeks, systolic blood pressure (154.2 mmHg → 134.8 mmHg; $p < 0.001$) and diastolic blood pressure (91.8 mmHg → 79.6 mmHg; $p < 0.05$) decreased significantly, compared to the control group. Also total cholesterol decreased by 34%, LDL-cholesterol decreased by 25%, VLDL-cholesterol decreased by 15% and triglycerides decreased by 15% (Varma et.al. 2009).

Carob flour

(Ceratonia Siliqua)

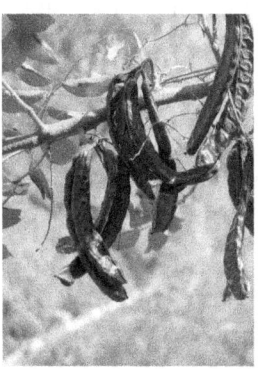

Carob flour is manufactured from the Carob tree, Ceratonia Siliqua, beans. Carob flour is very popular in food industry as an additive.

Carob flour has:
- Total cholesterol lowering properties.
- LDL-cholesterol lowering properties
- Triglyceride lowering properties

When 88 volunteers, who had high cholesterol levels, were given 8 grams of Carob flour daily, for 4 weeks, the total cholesterol decreased by 17.8% ($p < 0.05$), the LDL-cholesterol decreased by 22.5% ($p < 0.001$) and triglycerides decreased by 16.3% ($p < 0.05$) (Ruiz-Roso et.al. 2010). This was a Doubble Blind experiment.

When 58 volunteers with high cholesterol levels were given 15 grams of Carob flour daily, for 6 weeks, the LDL-cholesterol decreased by 10.5% ($p = 0.010$). Triglycerides decreased by 11.3% ($p = 0.030$) (Zunft et.al. 2003). This was a doubble blind experiment.

The same cholesterol and triglyceride lowering properties of Carob flour was seen also in an other experiment, with 17 high cholesterol and 10 normal cholesterol volunteers (Zavoral et.al. 1983). The used amount of Carob flour was between 8 – 30 grams daily.

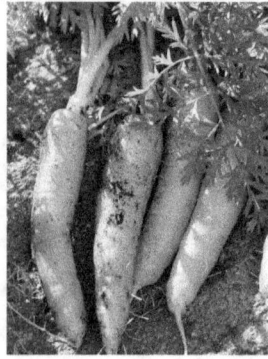

Carrot

(Daucus Carota)

Carrot is an ancient food- and medcinal plant. All parts of Carrot are edible: Root, seeds, leaves. Besides ordinary Carrot, there exists also Purple Carrot or Black Carrot, which contains up to 28 times more functionally healthy Anthocyanides, than ordinary Carrot. In Russia and China Carrot is used to decrease high blood pressure.

Carrot and especially Black or Purple Carrot has:
- – Blood pressure lowering properties.
- – Total cholesterol lowering properties.
- – Triglycerides lowering properties.

When adult volunteers were given Carrot juice 4.5 dl daily, for 3 months, systolic blood pressure decreased significantly ($p < 0.06$) (Potter et.al. 2011).

When rats were fed large amounts of fat and carbohydrates, they got metabolic syndrome, with hypertension and hyperlipidemia. When they were fed Black Carrot, both blood pressure and high cholesterol values decreased significantly (Poudyal et.al. 2010).

When rats were given food with 10% Carrot fiber in their daily diet, both total cholesterol and triglycerides decreased significantly, but HDL-cholesterol increased (Metwalli et.al. 1994).

When mice were fed in their food 0.25% Cholesterol, and were also given 20% dried Carrot daily, for 4 weeks, total cholesterol decreased by 41% and triglycerides decreased by 49%, compared to the control group. The liver total cholesterol decreased by 41% and liver triglycerides decreased by 30% (Nicolle et.al. 2004).

Carrot contains Chlorogenic acid, which is a strong antioxidant (Sun et.al. 2009). It is known, that Chlorogenic acid decreases blood pressure.

From the aerial parts of Carrot there has been found Coumaringlycosides, which strongly decrease blood pressure (Gilani et.al. 2000).

So, when cultivating Carrots, eat also the aerial parts in salad or chop it to food.

Celery

(Apium Graveolens)

Celery is an ancient vegetable, known all around the World. All parts of Celery can be eaten: The roots, the stalks, the leaves and the seeds. Celery contains big amounts of the Flavonoid Apigenin.

Celery has
- Blood pressure lowering properties
- Total cholesterol lowering properties
- LDL-cholesterol lowering properties
- Triglycerides lowering properties

When anesthetized rabbits were give intravenously aqueous extract of Celery, the blood pressure decreased by 14.3%, and when they were given the ethanolic extract of Celery, their blood pressure decreased by 45% (Btrankovic et.al. 2010).

When rats were fed Celery extract daily, for 8 weeks, the total cholesterol decreased by 23.6%, compared to the control group (Tsi et.al. 2000).

The total cholesterol, LDL-cholesterol and triglyceride lowering effect of Celery extract has been noticed in other experiments also (Tsi et.al. 1995; Tsi et.al. 1996).

One of the main active compound, which lowers both blood pressure and cholesterol, is 3-n-Butylphthalide. Celery contains also a lot of Apigenin, which is a strong Antioxidant and also lowers blood pressure.

Chayote

(Sechium Edule)

Chayote is an edible vegetable, which looks like melon or cucumber. It originates from Mexico, but it is nowadays cultivated all around the World. All parts are edible, fruit, leaves, seeds and roots. Its cultivation is very easy. Chayote is used to decrease high blood pressure.

Chayote has
- Blood pressure lowering properties
- Diuretic properties

The fruit and fruit skin decreases blood pressure in rats (Gordon et.al. 2000).

The fruit has also a strong diuretic property (Rozriguez et.al. 1984).

When volunteers were given daily 5 dl Chayote juice, for 4 weeks, the mean average blood pressure (MAP) decreased by 10.4 mmHg (100.74 mmHg → 90.35 mmHg) (Obaidy 2007).

Chicken and Turkey meat

In Asian countries, especially in Japan, China and Korea, chicken meat extract is processed into a Functional food. This extract is called Brand Essence of Chicken, or BEC.

Both chicken and turkey meat contain large quantities of L-Carnosine (beta-Alanyl-L-Histidine) and Anserine (beta-Alanyl-L-n-Methylhistidine), which both have blood pressure lowering properties. Both are strong antioxidants.

BEC has:
- Blood pressure lowering properties

Japanese researchers have noticed, that only a small, 1 microgram intravascular injection of Anserine decreases strongly blood pressure in rats (Tanida et.al. 2010).

When rats were fed 0.1% BEC in their daily diet, for 5 weeks, the systolic blood pressure in rats decreased significantly (Tanida et.al. 2010).

When rats were fed 0.1% BEC in their daily diet, for 5 weeks, the systolic blood pressure decreased to 139 mmHg, from the 181 mmHg of control rats ($p < 0.010$) (Matsumura et.al. 2001).

When rats were fed 100 mg/kg BEC daily, for 19 weeks, systolic blood pressure decreased to 238 mmHg, from the 263 mmHg of control rats ($p < 0.05$) (Matsumura et.al. 2002).

The same blood pressure lowering effect of BEC was also obtained in another experiment with rats ($p < 0.011$) (Sim 2011).

Chickpea

(Cicer Arietinum)

Chickpea is an ancient food plant, which has been cultivated for thousands of years in Asia and around Mediterranian sea. Chickpea is very rich in protein and fiber, and it can be bought from every Supermarket.

Chickpea has
- Total cholesterol lowering properties
- LDL-cholesterol lowering properties
- Triglycerides lowering properties
- HDL-cholesterol increasing properties

When 47 volunteers were given Chickpea daily, for 5 weeks, total cholesterol decreased by 3.9% ($p < 0.01$) and LDL-cholesterol decreased by 4.6% ($p < 0.01$), compared to the control group (Pittaway et.al. 2006).

When 27 volunteers were given Chickpea daily, for 5 weeks, total cholesterol decreased by 0.25 mmol/L ($p < 0.01$) and LDL-cholesterol decreased by 0.20 mmol/L ($p = 0.02$), compared to the control group (Pittaay et.al. 2007).

When hyperlipidemic rats were fed Chickpea daily, total cholesterol decreased by 54%, triglycerides decreased by 70%, LDL-cholesterol decreased by 54% and VLDL-cholesterol decreased by 70%, compared to the control group (Zulet et.al. 1995).

When rats fed with fat were fed Chickpea daily, for 8 months, triglycerides ($p < 0.05$) and LDL-cholesterol ($p < 0.05$) decreased significantly, compared to the control group (Yang et.al. 2007).

The cholesterol lowering compounds in Chickpea are Isoflavonoids Biochanin-A and Formonetin, which in experiments with rats and rabbits decrease total cholesterol, LDL-cholesterol and triglycerides, but increase HDL-cholesterol (Siddiqui et.al. 1976; Gopalan et.al. 1991).

Chinese Bellflower

(Platycodon Grandiflorum)

Chinese Bellflower roots are edible, and they have been used as food and medicine in Asia, especially in China, Korea and Japan, for hundreds of years. As a medicine, it is used in Asthma, Bronchitis, Colds, to loose mucus, against hypertension and high cholesterol levels. Its cultivation is very easy. Chinese Bellflower contains large amounts of Inulin and Saponins. The effective compounds are Saponins.

Chinese Bellflower roots have
- Total cholesterol decreasing properties
- LDL-cholesterol decreasing properties
- Triglycerides decreasing properties
- HDL-cholesterol increasing properties
- Body weight decreasing properties

When hyperlipidemic rats were given in their daily diet 5% of Chinese Bellflower roots, for 3 weeks, total cholesterol ($p < 0.05$), LDL-cholesterol ($p < 0.05$) and triglycerides ($p < 0.05$) decreased significantly, but HDL-cholesterol ($p < 0.05$) increased significantly, compared to the control group (Kim et.al. 1995).

When fat and slim rats were given Chinese Bellflower root 5% in their daily diet, for 4 weeks, triglycerides decreased by 49% ($p < 0.05$) and total cholesterol decreased by 29% ($p < 0.05$) in the fat rat group. In the slim rat group, triglycerides decreased by 40% ($p < 0.05$) and body weight decreased by 10.4% ($p < 0.05$), compared to the control group (Kim et.al. 2000).

When rats were given Chinese Bellflower root 5% in their daily diet, for 8 weeks, body weight decreased by 21.4% ($p < 0.05$), compared to the control group. Triglycerides also decreased ($p < 0.05$) significantly, compared to the control group (Han et.al. 2000).

When hyperlipidemic rats were given Chinese Bellflower root water extract at a dose of 150 mg/kg daily, for 7 weeks, total cholesterol decreased by 44% ($p < 0.05$), triglycerides decreased by 50% ($p < 0.05$) and body weight decreased by 33% ($p < 0.05$), compared to the control group (Park et.al. 2007).

When hamsters were given Chinese Bellflower root Saponins either 0.3% or 0.5% of their daily diet, total cholesterol decreased by 13% ($p < 0.05$) and 28% ($p < 0.05$), compared to the control group (Zhao et.al. 2008).

Also in experiments with mice, Chinese Bellflower root Saponins decreased triglycerides, total cholesterol and body weight significantly, compared to the control groups (Kim et.al. 2009; Han et.al. 2002). The same has been verified in experiments with rats too (Zhao et.al. 2005; Park et.al. 2005).

Chives

(Allium Schoenoprasum)

Chives are excellent, fully eatable onion species, which is used as spice and vegetable all around the Northern Hemisphere. It is very easy to cultivate. In Indonesia it is used against high blood pressure.

Chives have
- Blood pressure lowering properties
- LDL-cholesterol lowering properties
- Triglycerides lowering properties
- HDL-cholesterol increasing properties

When rats were given intravascularly water extract of Chives at a dose of 25 mg/kg, systolic blood pressure decreased by 17.2 mmHg ($p < 0.05$) and diastolic blood pressure decreased by 15.2 mmHg ($p < 0.05$), compared to the control group (Fidrianny et.al. 2003). Also the Butanol extract and Ethylacetate extract decreased blood pressure.

When rats were given ethanol extract of Chives at a dose of 100 mg/kg, the serum NO level increased by 137.8% ($p < 0.05$), compared to the control group (Amalia et.al. 2008), which might explain the blood pressure lowering property of Chives.

When rats were fed Chives at a dose of 6.25% of their daily diet, LDL-cholesterol ($p < 0.05$) and triglycerides ($p < 0.05$) decreased significantly, but HDL-cholesterol increased ($p < 0.05$) significantly, compared to the control group (Roghani et.al. 2010).

Chlorella

(Chlorella Pyrenoidosa, Chlorella Sp.)

Chlorella is a single cell, dark green freshwater algae, which is extremely popular as a functional food.

Chlorella has
- Blood pressure lowering properties
- Total cholesterol lowering properties
- LDL-cholesterol lowering properties
- Triglycerides lowering properties

When 80 hypertensive volunteers were given Chlorella daily, for 12 week, systolic blood pressure ($p < 0.01$) decreased significantly, compared to the control group. Also diastolic blood pressure decreased (Shimida et.al. 2009). This was a double blind experiment.

When rats were fed Chlorella daily, for 21 week, both blood pressure and total cholesterol decreased significantly, compared to the control group (Sansawa et.al. 2006).

When 24 volunteers were given Chlorella 10 grams daily, both blood pressure and total cholesterol decreased in most of the volunteers (Merchart et.al. 2002; Merchant et.al. 2011).

When hypertensive rats were given intravenously Chlorella alkaline extract, blood pressure decreased 69 mmHg. In the normal blood pressure group, Chlorella alkaline extract decreased blood pressure by 32 mmg, 1 hour after dose (Okamoto et.al. 1975).

When 17 volunteers were given Chlorella daily, for 12 weeks, total cholesterol decreased significantly, compared to the control group (Mizoguchi et.al. 2008).

When rats and hamsters were fed Chlorella daily for 8 weeks, triglycerides, total cholesterol and LDL-cholesterol decreased significantly, compared to the control group (Cherng et.al. 2006).

When rats were given 10% Chlorella in their daily diet, for 9 weeks, both total cholesterol ($p < 0.05$) and triglycerides ($p < 0.05$) decreased significantly, compared to the control group (Lee et.al. 2008).

When rats were fed Chlorella in their daily diet, for 2 weeks, total cholesterol decreased significantly, compared to the control group (Shibata et.al. 2007).

Also in many other experiments the total cholesterol and triglycerides lowering properties of Chlorella has been noticed (Sano et.al. 1988; Hidaka et.al. 2004; Shibata et.al. 2001).

Chlorogenic acid

Chlorogenic acid is a natural, strong antioxidant, which exists in green Coffee beans, Apple seeds and in many other plants.

Chlorogenic acid has
- Blood pressure lowering properties

When rats were given Chlorogenic acid in doses between 30 – 300 mg/kg, it decreased blood pressure both acutely and chronically (Suzuki et.al. 2006).

Chlorogenic acid inhibits ACE (Geng et.al. 2010).

When green Coffee bean water extract was given to 177 volunteers, at a dose of 185 mg daily, systolic blood pressure decreased by 5.6 mmHg ($p < 0.01$) and diastolic blood pressure decreased by 3.9 mmHg ($p < 0.01$), compared to the control group (Kozuma et.al. 2005). This was a double blind experiment.

When 28 volunteers were given 140 mg Chlorogenic acid daily, both systolic and diastolic blood pressure decreased significantly, compared to the control group (Watanabe et.al. 2006).

Roasted Coffee beans contain also Chlorogenic acid, but in roasting there is a synthesis of Hydroxyhydroquinone (=HHQ), which inhibits the blood pressure lowering effect of Chlorogenic acid.

When 203 volunteers were given 1 cup of Coffee daily, with different concentrations of HHQ, it was noticed, that normal Coffee had no effect on blood pressure, but HHQ free Coffee, which contained Chlorogenic acid, decreased significantly blood pressure, compared to the control group (Yamaguchi et.al. 2008). This was a doubble blind experiment.

Chromium Picolinate and Biotin

Chromium in the form of Chromium Picolinate is a very popular food supplement, which can be bought from every Supermarket. Chromium is an essential trace mineral in human nutrition, and it plays a very important role in sugar- and fat metabolism. Picolinic acid is a metabolite of the essential amino acid L-Tryptophan. Biotin is an essential B-vitamin in human nutrition.

Chromium Picolinate and Biotin have
- Total cholesterol decreasing properties
- LDL-cholesterol decreasing properties
- VLDL-cholesterol decreasing properties

- HDL-cholesterol increasing properties
- Triglycerides decreasing properties

When 28 volunteers were given Chromium Picolinte, corresponding to 200 micrograms Chromium daily, for 42 days, total cholesterol (7.1 mmol/L → 6.5 mmol/L; $p = 0.0003$) and LDL-cholesterol (5.7 mmol/L → 5.0 mmol/L; $p = 0.0003$) decreased significantly, compared to the control group (Press et.al. 1990). This was a double blind experiment.

When 20 healthy students were given Chromium Picolinate 1000 micrograms daily, for 13 weeks, both total cholesterol ($p < 0.001$) and LDL-cholesterol ($p < 0.001$) decreased significantly, compared to the control group (Boyd et.al. 1998). This was a double blind experiment.

When 30 diabetic volunteers were given Chromium Picolinate daily, for 2 months, triglycerides decreased by 17.4% ($p < 0.05$), compared to the control group (Lee et.al. 1994). This was a double blind experiment.

When 23 volunteers were given Chromium 218 micrograms daily, for 6 months, LDL-cholesterol decreased ($p < 0.01$) significantly, but HDL-cholesterol increased ($p < 0.05$) significantly, compared to the control group (Vinson et.al. 1984).

Much more positive results have been achieved in cholesterol- and triglycerides values, when volunteers are given Chromium Picolinate together with Biotin, which is an essential B-vitamin in human nutrition.

When volunteers were given Biotin 5 mg daily, for 4 weeks, total cholesterol decreased significantly (Dokusova et.al. 1972).

Same kind of results have been achieved, when volunteers were given only 0.9 mg Biotin daily, for a long period (Marshal et.al. 1980).

When 33 volunteers, of which 15 were diabetics, were given 15 mg Biotin daily, for 4 weeks, VLDL-cholesterol decreased by 0.11 mmol/L ($p < 0.005$) in the diabetic group, and 0.18 mmol/L ($p < 0.005$) in the normal group. Also triglycerides decreased significantly ($p = 0.005$), compared to the placebo group (Revilla-Monsalve et.al. 2006).

When 348 volunteers, of which 122 were diabetics, were given 600 micrograms Chromium Picolinate and 2 mg Biotin daily, for 3 months, total cholesterol ($p < 0.05$), LDL-cholesterol ($p < 0.05$) and VLDL-cholesterol ($p < 0.05$) decreased significantly, compared to the control group (Albarracin et.al. 2007). This was a double blind experiment.

In another experiment with 36 diabetic volunteers, who were given daily 600 micrograms Chromium Picolinate and 2 mg Biotin, for 4 weeks, total cholesterol, LDL-cholesterol and VLDL-cholesterol decreased significantly, compared to the control group (Geohas et.al. 2007).

Chrysanthemum flower

(Chrysamthemum Morifolium, Chrysanthemum Indicum)

Chrysanthemums have been cultivated in China for over 2000 years. Chrysanthemum flower, Flos Chrysanthemum, or JU HUAN, as the Chinese call it, is extremely popular functional food in China, Korea and Japan. In China it is officially registered as a functional food, and Chrysanthemum flower tea is used for high blood pressure and other diseases. Chrysanthemum flower is also officially registered in Chinese pharmacopeia. Chrysanthemum flower tea and dried Chrysanthemum flowers can be purchased from Chinese Supermarkets all around the World. Chrysanthemum flowers contain at least 55 different flavonoids, and also other compounds, such as Chlorogenic acid, which is known to decrease blood pressure (Lin et.al. 2010).

Chrysanthemum flower has
   - Blood pressure lowering properties

Chrysanthemum flower ethylacetate extract is a strong vasodilator (Jiang et.al. 2005).

When rats were given Chrysanthemum flower flavonoids at a dose of 57 mg/kg, blood pressure decreased significantly. The main components in the flavonoids fraction were Luteolin-7-O-D-Glucoside, Apigenin-7-O-Beta-Glucoside and Acacetin-7-O-Beta-Glucoside, which all separately decreased blood pressure in rats (Dai et.al. 2001).

When rats were given Chrysanthemum flower in their daily diet at a dose of $1 - 2$ g/kg, for 4 weeks, the mean average blood pressure (MAP) decreased significantly ($p < 0..05$), compared to the control group (Zhao et.al. 2008).

When rats were given Radish (Raphanus Sativus) seed and Chrysanthemum ethanol extract, which contained 1.5% flavonoids, blood pressure decreased both acutely and chronically, given daily for 28 days. Depending on dose, blood pressure decreased acutely by an average of 20 mmHg, and the duration was between $5 - 6$ hours. When given chronically, the blood pressure was $25 - 30$ mmHg lower, than in the control group, for the whole duration of the test, 28 days (Suhong et.al. 2007).

Cinnamon

(Cinnamomum Zeylanicum)

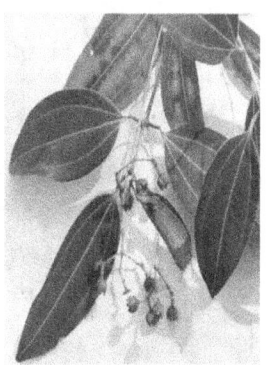

Cinnamon is a very old spice and medicinal plant which is used all around the World.

Cinnamon has
- Blood pressure lowering properties
- Total cholesterol lowering properties
- LDL-cholesterol lowering properties
- Triglycerides lowering properties

When 58 Diabetic patients were given Cinnamon at a dose of 2.0 grams daily, for 12 weeks, the systolic blood pressure decreased (132.6 mmHg → 129.2 mmHg; $p < 0.001$), and also the diastolic blood pressure decreased (85.2 mmHg → 80.2 mmHg; $p < 0.001$) significantly, compared to the control group (Akilen et.al. 2010).

Also in rats Cinnamon decreases significantly the blood pressure (Preuss et.al. 2006).

When 60 Diabetic patients were given either 1 gram, 3 grams or 6 grams of Cinnamon daily, for 40 days, the triglycerides decreased by 23% - 30%, the LDL-cholesterol decreased by 7% - 27% and the total cholesterol decreased by 12% - 26%, compared to the control group (Khan et.al. 2003).

Clove

(Syzygium Aromaticum)

and Eugenol

Clove is a very common spice, which is used all around the world as a spice in meat foods. The Clove oil main component is Eugenol. Eugenol content in Clove oil is between 70 – 90%.

Clove and Eugenol have
- Blood pressure decreasing properties

When rats were given intravenously Eugenol at doses between 1 – 10 mg/kg, the mean average blood pressure (MAP) decreased by 5 – 40%, compared to the control group (Lahou et.al. 2004).

The blood pressure lowering effect of Eugenol has been seen also in other experiments (Lahlou et.al. 2004; Interaminense et.al. 2005).

Coffee

(Coffea Arabica)

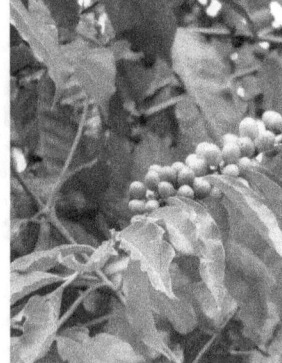

(Author: Forest & Kim Starr)

Coffee is an Ancient, stimulating drink, which is used all over the World.

Coffee has
 - Blood pressure increasing properties
 - Total cholesterol increasing properties
 - LDL-cholesterol increasing properties
 - Triglycerides lowering properties

Coffee increases mildly blood pressure (Nurminen et.al. 1999; Klag et.al. 2003). Systolic blood pressure increases about 0.2 mmHg, and diatolic blood pressure increases about 0.3 mmHg, for each cup of coffee drank (Klang et.al. 2002).

Acutely Coffee can increase blood pressure even by 10 – 15 mmHg (Bättik et.al. 1992). The rise is bigger with hypertensive persons.

The serum total cholesterol level increases steadily, the more Coffee is drank (Stensvold et.al. 1989; Strandhagen et.al. 2002).

The serum LDL-cholesterol correlates positively with the amount of Coffee drank, but serum triglycerides correlate negatively with the amount of Coffee drank (Miyake et.al. 1999).

Coriander

(Coriandrum Sativum)

Coriander seeds have a long history as a spice. Also the Coriander leaves are used in cooking.

Coriander seeds have
 - Blood pressure lowering properties
 - Total cholesterol lowering properties
 - LDL-cholesterol lowering properties
 - Triglycerides lowering properties
 - HDL-cholesterol increasing properties

When rats were fed Coriander seeds at a dose of 10% of their daily diet, for 75 days, total cholesterol decreased by 44.4% and triglycerides decreased by 50.0%, compared to the control group (Chitra et.al. 1997).

In other experiments, it has been shown, that Coriander seeds lower total cholesterol, LDL-cholesterol and triglycerides, but increase HDL-cholesterol (Dhanapakiam et.al. 2008; Lal et.al. 2004; Aissaoul et.al. 2011; Al-Jaff et.al. 2011).

In rabbits and rats, Coriander seed extracts decrease blood pressure (Jabeen et.al. 2009; Medhin et.al. 1986).

Corn Silk

(Zea Mays)

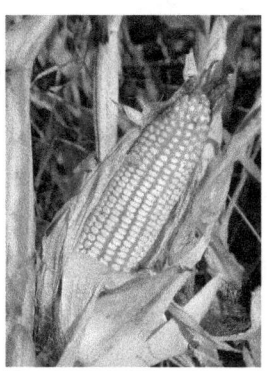

Corn Silk is known all around the World for its diuretic and hypotensive properties.

Corn Silk has
- Blood pressure lowering properties

When dogs were given intavascularly water extract of Corn Silk at doses between 1.37 – 22 mg/kg, diastolic blood pressure decreased by 14.5% - 53.8% (Martin et.al. 1991). Also the heart rate decreased.

When rats were given ethanol extract of Corn Silk at doses of 3.0 mg/kg, 30 mg/kg or 100 mg/kg, the mean average blood pressure (MAP) decreased by 10.6% ($p < 0.05$), 22.79% ($p < 0.05$) and 26.40% ($p < 0.05$), compared to the control group (Aftab 1995). This research was a Doctor Thesis.

Because Purple Maize seeds have also blood pressure lowering properties, it would be wice to cultivate Purple Maize as a Functional food for its seeds and Corn Silk.

Cumin seed

(Cyminum Cyminum)

Cumin seed is a very popular spice in Asia; in India and Iran, and also in Greece and Italy. In India it is called Jeera.

Cumin seed has
- – Total cholesterol lowering properties
- – LDL-cholesterol lowering properties
- – Triglycerides lowering properties
- – HDL-cholesterol increase properties

These properties have been documented in great many experiments (Dhandapani et.al. 2002; Akila et.al. 2010; Shirke et.al. 2009; Al-Kasi et.al. 2010).

Curry

(Murraya Koenigii)

Curry originates from Asia. It is an Ancient spice, which has been used for thousands of years also as a medicine for different ailments.

Curry has:
- – Total cholesterol lowering properties.
- – VLDL-cholesterol lowering properties
- – HDL-cholesterol increasing properties
- – Triglycerides lowering properties.

In tests with mice, they were given 80 mg/kg of Curry leaf extract daily, for 10 days. The total cholesterol decreased by 34.43% (Xie et.al. 2006).

When rats were given Curry 300 mg/kg daily, for 2 weeks, both total cholesterol and triglycerides decreased significantly (Birari et.al. 2010).

In another experiment with rats, Curry given daily for 30 days decreased both total cholesterol and triglycerides, but HDL-cholesterol increased (Kesari et.al. 2007).

When 20 volunteers were given Curry extract daily, for 2 months, the VLDL-cholesterol decreased by 15% ($p < 0.05$) (Dineshkumar et.al. 2010).

Dietary cholesterol

Cholesterol exists in all animal products, in different quantities. But there is no Cholesterol in plant products, like berries, fruits, grains, beans etc. Cholesterol in food is absorbed as such and increases the Cholesterol level of serum. In some countries it is recommended to limit the daily dietary cholesterol to not more than 200 – 400 mg.

Dietary Cholesterol has
  – Cholesterol increasing properties

In a meta-analysis with 27 different experiments, it was noticed, that the serum cholesterol and dietary cholesterol have a very strong correlation ($p < 0.0005$; $r = 0.617$) (Hopkins 1992). The research showed, that dietary Cholesterol increases serum Cholesterol approximately according to the following table:

Dietary Cholesterol (mg/daily)	Serum Cholesterol (mmol/L)
0	0.000
100	0.155
300	0.408
500	0.602
700	0.749
900	0.861
1000	0.907
1200	0.981
1500	1.061
2000	1.139
3000	1.199

The following table shows the average amount of Cholesterol of different foods, in units of milligrams per 100 grams food. (Source: USDA Nutrient database for Standard Reference, Release 15)

Food	Cholesterol (mg/100g)
Fruit	0
Berries	0
Nuts	0
Vegetables	0
Plant products generally	0
Egg, raw	425
Egg, yolk	1283
Egg, whites	0
Beef liver	482
Chicken liver	632
Sardines in oil	141
Chicken breast, Broiler	85
Turkey	75
Pork meat	121
Lamb meat	121
Beef	106
Milk	29
Haddock	74
Rainbow Trout	68
Cod, Atlantic	55
Halibut, Atlantic, Ocean	41
Tuna in water	30
Tuna in oil	17
Herring, Atlantic	13
Salami	65
Butter, salted	218
Cheese, Cheddar	105
Cheese, Camembert	71
Cheese, Feta	88
Cheese, Mozzarella	77

According to this table, hyperlipidemic persons should avoi all liver products, eggs, egg yolk and butter. Also meat should be replaced mostly by chicken, turkey and fish.

Dietary fiber

Dietary soluble fiber is essential to human beings, especially for the health of colon and gastrointestinal tract. Soluble fiber is fermented by bacteria. The following food elements are rich in dietary soluble fiber: Grains, beans, fruits and vegetables. The amount of dietary fiber should be at least 20 – 40 grams daily, but most people get far less than this amount daily, normally even under 10 grams daily.

Dietary soluble fiber has
- Blood pressure decreasing properties
- Total cholesterol decreasing properties
- LDL-cholesterol decreasing properties
- Triglycerides decreasing properties
- HDL-cholesterol increasing properties

In a meta-analysis with 67 different experiments, it was noticed, that every 10 grams increase of soluble fiber in diet daily, decreases total cholesterol by an average of 0.45 mmol/L and LDL-cholesterol by an average of 0.57 mmol/L (Brown et.al. 1999).

When 28 patients with cardiovascular diseases were given Psyllium (Plantago Ovata) husk 10.5 grams daily, for 8 weeks, triglycerides decreased by 6.7% ($p < 0.02$), total cholesterol/HDL-cholesterol ratio decreased by 10.6% ($p < 0.002$), LDL-cholesterol/HDL-cholesterol ratio decreased by 14.2% ($p < 0.003$) but HDL-cholesterol increased by 6.7% ($p < 0.006$) (Sola et.al. 2007). This was a double blind experiment.

In a meta-analysis with 24 separate experiments, it was noticed, that dietary soluble fiber significantly decreases blood pressure. Especially with hypertensive volunteers, an average of 11.5 grams of dietary soluble fiber daily decreased systolic blood pressure by an average of 4.5 mmHg and diastolic blood pressure by an average of 2.4 mmHg (Martinette et.al. 2005).

Dill

(Anethum Graveolens)

Dill is a very old culinary spice, which is also used as a medical herb. In Iran it is used to lower high cholesterol levels. Dill is extremely rich source of the Flavonoid Isorhamnetin. Isorhamnetin is a very strong antioxidant.

Dill has
- Total cholesterol lowering properties
- LDL-cholesterol lowering properties
- Triglycerides lowering properties
- HDL-cholesterol increasing properties

When rats were given either Dill oil or dried Dill daily, for 2 – 4 weeks, total cholesterol, LDL-cholesterol and triglycerides decreased, but HDL-cholesterol increased (Yazdanparast et.al. 2008; Hajhashemi et.al. 2008).

Dioscorin

There are many different Yams species (Dioscorea) in the World, such as the Purple Yams (Dioscorea Alata), Chinese Yams (Dioscorea Opposita) etc. They are ancient food plants. The big roots are used as food, normally after cooking. The biggest roots may weight several tens of kilos. The roots contain a protein called Dioscorin.

Dioscorin has
- Blood pressure lowering properties

Dioscorin inhibits very strongly ACE (IC50 = 41.1 micrograms/ml) (Nagai et.al. 2008).

The ACE inhibitory property of Dioscorin has been verified also in other experiments (Hsu et.al. 2002).

When rats were orally fed Dioscorin at a dose of 40 mg/kg, the mean average blood pressure (MAP) decreased by 21.5 mmHg, after 4 hours. When rats were fed Dioscorin 40 mg/kg daily, for 25 days, systolic blood pressure decreased by 27.7 mmHg and diastolic blood pressure decreased by 28.3 mmHg, compared to the control group (Lin et.al. 2006).

When 27 volunteers were given 140 mg Dioscorin daily, for 5 weeks, systolic blood pressure decreased by 6.52 mmHg ($p < 0.05$) and diastolic blood pressure decreased by 4.76 mmHg ($p < 0.05$), compared to the control group (Liu et.al. 2008).

Du-Zhong tea

(Eucommia Ulmoides)

Eucommia Ulmoides is a tree, which grows in Asia, China, Korea and Japan. Du-Zhong tea is made from the leaves and park. This tea has been used for hundreds of years as a functionally healthy tea. Du-Zhong tea decreases high blood pressure and high cholesterol levels.

Du-Zhong tea has
- Blood pressure lowering properties
- Total cholesterol lowering properties
- Triglycerides lowering properties
- HDL-cholesterol increasing properties

When 30 hypertensive volunteers were given Du-Zhong tea extract 1 gram, 3 times daily, for 3 weeks, systolic blood pressure decreased by 7.5 mmHg ($p < 0.008$) and diastolic blood pressure decreased by 3.9 mmHg ($p < 0.008$), compared to the control group (Grenway et.al. 2011).

Earlier in experiments with human volunteers, Du-Zhong tea has decreased systolic blood pressure by 25 mmHg and diastolic blood pressure by 14 mmHg, compared to the control group (Shchepotin et.al. 1983).

In a double blind experiment with 103 human volunteers in Japan, it was verified, that Du-Zhong tea is hypotensive. Du-Zhong tea has been since 1997 officially accepted as a functional food in Japan (Kawasaki et.al. 2000).

The blood pressure lowering effect of Du-Zhong tea has been verified also in other experiments (Lang et.al. 2005; Luo et.al. 2010).

When diabetic mice were given 1.0% Du-Zhong tea in their daily diet, for 6 weeks, total cholesterol decreased by 24.1% ($p < 0.001$) and triglycerides decreased by 38.5% ($p < 0.01$), but HDL-cholesterol increased by 41.5% ($p < 0.05$), compared to the control group (Park et.al. 2006).

The triglycerides lowering property of Du-Zhong tea has been verified also in another experiment (Kobayashi et.al. 2012).

Eggplant

(Solanum Melongena)

Eggplant is a very popular vegetable, and it is in use all around the World.

Eggplant has:
- Blood pressure lowering properties.
- Total cholesterol lowering properties.
- LDL-cholesterol lowering properties.
- Triglycerides lowering properties.
- HDL-cholesterol increasing properties.

When rabbits were fed 10% Eggplant of their total food daily, for 6 weeks, total cholesterol decreased by 65.4%, LDL-cholesterol decreased by 85% and triglycerides decreased by 47.7%, but HDL-cholesterol increased by 24.7%, compared to the control group (Odetola et.al. 2004).

When rats were fed Eggplant Flavonoids mixture, 1 mg Flavonoids/100 gram body mass, daily for 45 days, both total cholesterol and triglycerides decreased significantly ($p < 0.01$), compared to the control group (Sudheesh et.al. 1997).

When 38 volunteers were given dried Eggplant 20 grams daily, for 35 days, both total cholesterol and LDL-cholesterol decreased significantly (Gulmares et.al. 2000).

Eggplant inhibits ACE (Kwon et.al. 2008).

In tests with rats, Eggplant lowers blood pressure, depending on dose (Shum et.al. 1991).

Egyptian Luffa

(Luffa Aegyptica)

Egyptian Luffa is an annual plant, which has edible fruits. The fruits are used as vegetable in Asia and Africa. Fruits alre also used in folk medicine to cure high blood pressure and high cholesterol levels. The plant is very easy to cultivate, and seeds are readily available through seed companies. There are many different Luffa species in the World.

Aegyptian Luffa and other Luffa species have
- Total cholesterol lowering properties
- LDL-cholesterol lowering properties
- Triglycerides lowering properties
- HDL-cholesterol increasing properties

When hyperlipidemic rabbits were fed Aegyptian Luffa methanol extract at a dose of 300 mg/kg daily, for 8 weeks, total cholesterol decreased by 29% ($p < 0.01$), LDL-cholesterol decreased by 22% ($p < 0.01$), triglycerides decreased by 52% ($p < 0.01$) but HDL-cholesterol increased by 38% ($p < 0.01$), comapred to the control group (Thayyli et.al. 2011). The effect was the same as Atorvastatin, which is used to lower high cholesterol values.

Exactly same kind of cholesterol lowering effect has been achieved in other experiments also with other edible Luffa species, such as Luffa Tuberosa (Yeligar et.al. 2007) and Luffa Cylindrica (Pai et.al. 2011).

Ellagic acid

Ellagic acid is a very strong antioxidant, which occurs naturally in many berries and fruits. Strawberry, Pomegranate and Red Raspberry contain large amounts of Ellagic acid. The Ellagic acid content is especially high in Strawberry and Red Raspberry leaves.

Ellagic acid has
- Blood pressure lowering properties

When given intravenously, Ellagic acid decreases blood pressure in both mice (Bhargava et.al. 1969) and rats (Bhargava et.al. 1968).

Ellagic acid inhibits ACE (Pinto et.al. 2010).

Ellagic acid content in Red Raspberry leaves is between 2.62 – 6.87% (Gudej et.al. 2009).

Ellagic acid content in Strawberry leaves is between 8.08 – 32.30 mg/g (Maas et.al. 1991).

False Daisy

(Eclipta Alba, Syn. Eclipta Prostrata)

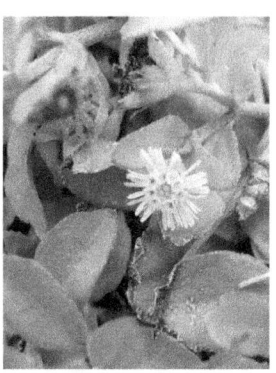

(Authors: Forest & Kim Starr)

False Dairy is a very famous medicinal plant from India and China. The plant is a small size with small Daisy like flowers. Its cultivation is very easy. False Daisy is used medicinally in Asthma, hepatic diseases, inflammation, skin problems and to increase hair growth and darken hair.

False Daisy has
- Blood pressure lowering properties
- Total cholesterol lowering properties
- LDL-cholesterol lowering properties
- VLDL-cholesterol lowering properties
- Triglycerides lowering properties
- HDL-cholesterol increasing properties
- Diuretic properties

When 60 hypertensive volunteers were given 3 grams False Daisy daily, for 60 days, the mean average blood pressure (MAP) decreased 15%, total cholesterol decreased by 17%, LDL-cholesterol decreased by 24%, VLDL-cholesterol decreased by 14% and triglycerides decreased by 14%, compared to the control group ($p < 0.05$ in all properties). Also urine output increased by 34% and the Sodium content in urine increased by 24% (Rangineni et.al. 2007).

When rats were given water extract of False Daisy at a dose of 100 mg/kg daily, for 45 days, total cholesterol decreased by 41.6% ($p < 0.05$), triglycerides decreased by 53.3% ($p < 0.05$) but HDL-cholesterol increased by 30.6% ($p < 0.05$), compared to the control group (Dhandapani 2007).

Exactly same kind of results has been verified in other experiments too (Kumari et.al. 2006; Kim et.al. 2006).

Fatty Fish

Fatty fish contain large amounts of polyunsaturated Omega-3 fatty acids, EPA and DHA, which lower blood pressure and triglycerides. With resent research also the fish protein itself decreases blood pressure and cholesterol.

Fatty fish has
- Blood pressure decreasing properties
- Total cholesterol decreasing properties
- LDL-cholesterol decreasing properties
- VLDL-cholesterol decreasing properties
- HDL-cholesterol increasing properties
- Heart rate decreasing properties

When 27 volunteers were given dried Bonito fish (Katsuwomus Pelamis) about 125 grams daily, for 4 weeks, systolic blood pressure decreased by 6.4 mmHg (128.1 mmHg → 121.6 mmHg; p = 0.037), compared to the control group (Umeki et.al. 2008).

When 36 volunteers, of which 21 were hypertensive, were given daily Vinegar and dried Bonito fish, for 12 weeks, systolic blood pressure decreased by 5.5 mmHg (p < 0.05), compared to the control group (Tanaka et.al. 2009). This was a double blind experiment.

When 142 volunteers were given 2 weekly fish portions, which gave 4.5 grams of EPA and DHA Omega-3 fatty acids, for 24 weeks, plasma triglycerides decreased (p < 0.05) significantly, compared to the control group (Moore et.al. 2006).

When 324 volunteers were given 150 grams of Salmon, 3 times weekly, for 8 weeks, systolic blood pressure decreased by 4.4 mmHg (p < 0.001) and diastolic blood pressure decreased by 4.1 mmHg (p < 0.001), compared to the control group (Ramel et.al. 2010).

When 63 obese, hypertensive volunteers were given daily 54 – 200 grams of fatty fish (Salmon, Tuna, Anchovy), which gave about 3.65 grams of Omega-3 fatty acids, for 16 weeks, systolic blood pressure decreased by 6.0 mmHg and diastolic blood pressure decreased by 3.0 mmHg, compared to the control group. Also heart rate decreased by 3.1 beats/minute (p = 0.036) (Bao et.al. 1998).

When 48 healthy volunteers were given 125 grams Salmon daily, for 4 weeks, systolic blood pressure decreased by 4% (p = 0.001), diastolic blood pressure decreased by 4% (p = 0.007), triglycerides decreased by 15% (p = 0.040), LDL-cholesterol decreased by 7% (p = 0.051), VLDL-cholesterol decreased by 14% (p = 0.042), but HDL-cholesterol increased by 5% (p = 0.031), compared to the control group (Lara et.al. 2007).

The blood pressure, cholesterol and triglycerides lowering properties of fatty fish have been verified in a number of other experiments with animals (Yahia et.al. 2005; Gutierrez et.al. 1994; Shukla et.al. 2006; Wergedahl et.al. 2004; Mohamed et.al. 2011; Ait-Yahia et.al. 2003; Hosomi et.al. 2011; Fukunaga et.al. 2011; Kouno et.al. 2005).

The following fatty fish should be eaten several times every week by hypertensive or hyperlipidemic persons: Salmon, Trout, Bonito, Mackerel, Anchovy, Tuna, Rainbow Trout etc.

Fennel

(Foeniculum Vulgare)

Fennel is a very popular spice, which is in use all over the World. In Folk medicine it is used against high blood pressure.

Fennel seeds and leaves have
- Blood pressure lowering properties
- Diuretic properties

When rats were given water extract of Fennel leaves intravasculary at a dose of 6 mg/kg, the mean average blood pressure (MAP) decreased significantly by 18% (109 mmHg → 89 mmHg; $p = 0.025$), compared to the control group (Abdul-Ghani et.al. 1988).

When hypertensive rats were given water extract of Fennel seeds at a dose of 190 mg/kg, for 5 days, systolic blood pressure decreased about 10 mmHg ($p < 0.05$), compared to the control group (El-Bardai et.al. 2001). At the same time there was a significant 80% increase in urine, compared to the control group.

Fenugreek

(Trigonella Foenum-Graecum)

Fenugreek is an ancient food plant, which is much used in Asia, especially in India, Iran etc. Normally the Fenugreek seeds or sprouts are used as a food. Fenugreek is also a very old medicinal plant, which is used for example in Diabetes care.

Fenugreek seeds have
- Blood pressure lowering properties
- Total cholesterol lowering properties
- LDL-cholesterol lowering properties
- VLDL-cholesterol lowering properties
- Triglycerides lowering properties
- HDL-cholesterol increasing properties

When 80 Diabetic, hyperlipidemic volunteers were given 100 grams of Fenugreek seed flour daily in water, for 2 months, total cholesterol decreased by 6.8% (232 mg/dl → 219 mg/dl; $p < 0.05$), LDL-cholesterol decreased by 8.15% (160 mg/dl → 147 mg/dl; $p < 0.05$), VLDL-cholesterol decreased by 15.75% (38 mg/dl → 32 mg/dl) and triglycerides decreased by 13.4% (185 mg/dl → 160 mg/dl), but HDL-cholesterol increased by 23.53% (34 mg/dl → 42 mg/dl), compared to the control group (Mtra et.al. 2006).

Same kind of results have been obtained also in other experiments with diabetic volunteers. When volunteers were given 10 grams of Fenugreek seeds daily, for 10 days, total cholesterol, LDL-cholesterol, VLDL-cholesterol and triglycerides decreased significantly, compared to the control group (Sharma et.al. 1990).

When 18 diabetic volunteers were given 10 grams of Fenugreek seeds daily, for 8 weeks, triglycerides decreased by 30% ($p < 0.05$) and VLDL-cholesterol decreased by 30.6% ($p < 0.05$), compared to the control group (Kassaian et.al. 2009).

In great many animal experiments the cholesterol- and triglycerides lowering properties of Fenugreek seeds have been clearly documented (Belguth-Hadriche et.al. 2010; Roberts 2011; Muraki et.al. 2011; Singh et.al. 2010; Petit et.al. 1995; Xue et.al. 2007; Vijayakumar et.al. 2010).

Fenugreek seeds have diuretic properties (Rohini et.al. 2009).

When Fenugreek saponin extract was given to hypertensive rats, either 100 mg/kg or 200 mg/kg, blood pressure decreased significantly (Theerthahalli et.al. 2011).

Fenugreek seed oil decreases systolic blood pressure in diabetic and hyperlipidemic rats (Talpur et.al. 2005).

When hypertensive rats were given methanolic extract of Fenugreek seeds 30 mg/kg daily, for 4 weeks, blood pressure decreased significantly (Balaraman et.al. 2006).

Fermented Yoghurt, Milk and sour Milk

When milk products are fermented with different lactic acid bacteria, results are fermented youghurt, milk or sour milk products, which have many functionally healthy properties, such as decreasing high blood pressure and high cholesterol levels and enhancing immunity.

Fermented milk products have
- Blood pressure decreasing properties
- Total cholesterol decreasing properties
- LDL-cholesterol decreasing properties
- VLDL-cholesterol decreasing properties
- Triglycerides decreasing properties
- HDL-cholesterol increasing properties

When 39 hypertensive volunteers were given 150 ml Lactobacillus Helveticus fermented milk daily, for 21 weeks, systolic blood pressure decreased by 6.7 mmHg and diastolic blood pressure decreased by 3.6 mmHg, compared to the control group (Seppo et.al. 2003).

When 70 healthy volunteers were given 450 ml Lactobacillus Acidophilus and Streptococcus Thermophilus fermented yoghurt daily, for 8 weeks, systolic blood pressure decreased by 4.4 mmHg and diastolic blood pressure decreased by 3.4 mmHg, compared to the control group (Algerholm-Larsen et.al. 2000). This was a double blind experiment.

When 80 volunteers, of which 40 were hypertensive, were given 6 capsules or 12 grams of Lactobacillus Helveticus fermented milk in dried form daily, for 4 weeks, systolic blood pressure decreased by 5 mmHg and diastolic blood pressure decreased by 11.2 mmHg, compared to the control group (Aihara et.al. 2005). This was a double blind experiment.

When 46 hypertensive volunteers were given 160 grams Lactobacillus Helveticus fermented milk daily, for 4 weeks, systolic blood pressure decreased by 5.2 mmHg, compared to the control group (Mizushima et.al. 2004). This was a double blind experiment.

When 60 volunteers were given 150 ml Lactobacillus Helveticus fermented sour milk daily, for 5 – 10 weeks, systolic blood pressure decreased by 16 mmHg and diastolic blood pressure decreased by 11 mmHg, compared to the control group (Tuomilehto et.al. 2004).

When 28 hypertensive volunteers were given 800 mg Lactobacillus Casei extract daily, for 2 months, systolic blood pressure decreased by 9 mmHg (169 mmHg $\rightarrow$ 160 mmHg; $p < 0.01$) and diastolic blood pressure decreased by 6 mmHg (100 mmHg $\rightarrow$ 94 mmHg; $p < 0.05$), compared to the control group. Also heart rate decreased by 7 heats/minute (88/min $\rightarrow$ 81/min; $p < 0.05$), and total cholesterol decreased significantly (218 mg/dl $\rightarrow$ 206 mg/dl; $p < 0.05$), compared to the control group (Nakajima et.al. 1995). This was a double blind experiment.

When 60 diabetic volunteers were given 30 grams Lactobacillus Acidophilus and Bifidobacterium Lactis fermented milk daily, for 6 weeks, total cholesterol decreased by 4.54% ($p = 0.008$) and LDL-cholesterol decreased by 7.45% ($p = 0.004$), compared to the control group (Ejtahed et.al. 2012). This was a double blind experiment.

When 30 hypertensive volunteers were given 95 ml Lactobacillus Helveticus and Saccharomyces Cerevisiae fermented sour milk daily, for 8 weeks, systolic blood pressure decreased by 14.1 mmHg ($p < 0.01$) and diastolic blood pressure decreased by 6.9 mmHg ($p < 0.01$), compared to the control group (Hata et.al. 2005). This was a double blind experiment.

When 20 young, healthy volunteers were given 200 ml Lactobacillus Casei and Streptococcus Thermophilus fermented milk daily, for 8 weeks, HDL-cholesterol increased ($p < 0.05$) significantly, but triglycerides decreased ($p < 0.05$) significantly, compared to the control group. Also systolic blood pressure decreased ($p < 0.05$) significantly, compared to the control group (Kawase et.al. 2000).

When 29 volunteers were given 300 ml Lactobacillus Acidophilus and Bifidophilus Longum fermented milk daily, for 21 weeks, HDL-cholesterol increased significantly ($p < 0.05$) by 0.30 mmol/L, but LDL/HDL-cholesterol ratio decreased (3.24 $\rightarrow$ 2.48; $p < 0.05$) significantly, compared to the control group (Kieling et.al. 2002).

Also in other human double blind experiments with fermented milk products, it has been verified, that total cholesterol and LDL-cholesterol decreases, compared to the control groups (Bertolami et.al. 1999; Anderson et.al. 1999).

Ferulic acid

Ferulic acid is a strong antioxidant, which is common in many plants, like Rice bran and Angelica Sinensis roots. Angelica Sinensis is a famous Chinese medicinal plant, which is used in cardiovascular disease.

Ferulic acid has
- Blood pressure lowering properties
- Total cholesterol lowering properties
- Triglycerides lowering properties

Ferulic acid inhibits strongly ACE (Geng et.al. 2010).

When rats were given orally and acutely Ferulic acid at a dose of 9.5 mg/kg, blood pressure decreased significantly, and was lowest after 2 hours. Plasma ACE activity decreased, and also triglycerides and total cholesterol decreased (Ardiansyah et.al. 2008).

When rats were given Ferulic acid at different doses between 1 – 100 mg/kg, systolic blood pressure decreased with increasing dose. The effect lasted 6 hours. When rats were given Ferulic acid either 10 mg/kg or 50 mg/kg daily, for 6 weeks, blood pressure decreased significantly, compared to the control group (Suzuki et.al. 2002).

When 80 diabetic volunteers were given intravenously Ferulic acid 300 mg daily, for 4 weeks, the mean average blood pressure (MAP) ($p < 0.05$), triglycerides ($p < 0.05$) and total cholesterol ($p < 0.05$) decreased significantly, compared to the control group (Chen et.al. 2006).

Fish oil, EPA, DHA

Fish contains a lot of polyunsaturated fatty acids. The most important of these are EPA (EicosaPentaenoic Acid) and DHA (DocoaHexaenoic Acid). Very good sources of fish oil are Salmon, Trout, Atlantic Herring, Sardines, Anchovy, Rainbow Trout and Mackerel. Fish oil can be purchased from every supermarket also. Fish oils EPA and DHA are called Omega-3 fatty acids, just like alpha-Linolenic acid in Flaxseed oil or Perilla oil, which in human body is converted firstly to EPA and then to DHA.

Fish oils have
- Blood pressure decreasing properties
- Total cholesterol decreasing properties
- LDL-cholesterol decreasing properties
- Triglycerides decreasing properties
- HDL-cholesterol increasing properties

When 62 elderly volunteers were given 7 grams of Omega-3 fish oil daily, for 12 weeks, total cholesterol decreased by 17.2% (p < 0.05), LDL-cholesterol decreased by 16.2% (p < 0.05) and triglycerides decreased by 39.6% (p < 0.05), but HDL-cholesterol increased by 10.3% (p < 0.05), compared to the control group. At the same time systolic blood pressure decreased by 25.9% (175.5 mmHg → 130.0 mmHg; p < 0.05), and diastolic blood pressure decreased by 13.1% (95.0 mmHg → 82.5 mmHg; p < 0.05), compared to the control group (Yam et.al. 2002). This was a double blind experiment.

When 38 volunteers were given very small amount of DHA, only 0.7 grams daily, for 3 months, diastolic blood pressure decreased by 3.3 mmHg (71.3 mmHg → 69.1 mmHg; p < 0.01), systolic blood pressure decreased by 2.1 mmHg (116.7 mmHg → 114.6 mmHg; p < 0.05) and heart rate decreased by 2 beats/minute, compared to the control group (Theobald et.al. 2007). This was a double blind experiment.

When 20 hyperlipidemic volunteers were given 20 ml fish oil daily, for 8 weeks, systolic blood pressure decreased by 12 mmHg (139 mmHg → 127 mmHg; p < 0.001) and diastolic blood pressure decreased by 9 mmHg (90 mmHg → 81 mmHg; p < 0.002), and serum triglycerides decreased by 42.4% (417 mg/dl → 240 mg/dl; p < 0.01), compared to the control group (Olivieri et.al. 1988).

In a meta-analysis with 31 different placebo controlled experiments and 1356 volunteers, it was noticed, that both systolic- and diastolic blood pressure decrease, the more the daily fih oil dose is (Morris et.al. 1992).

When 20 volunteers with very high serum triglyceride values, were given fish oil daily, for 4 weeks, total cholesterol decreased by 36% and triglycerides decreased by an average of 71%, compared to the control group. Also VLDL-cholesterol decreased significantly (Phillipson et.al. 1985).

In some cases fih oil may increase LDL-cholesterol. But when volunteers at the same time take Garlic, LDL-cholesterol decreases. When 50 volunteers were given daily either placebo, 900 mg Garlic, or 12 grams fish oil or 900 mg Garlic and 12 grams fish oil, LDL-cholesterol decreased 14.2% in the Garlic group, 9.5% in the Garlic and fish oil group, but increased 8.5% in the fish oil group. But triglycerides decreased 37.3% in the fish oil group, and 34.3% in the Garlic and fish oil group (Adler et.al. 1997).

Fish oil have a very significant positive effect in high blood pressure and high triglyceride levels.

Flaxseed

(Linum Usitatissimum)

Flaxseed is well known to everybody, an is cultivated all around the Northern Hemisphere. It is a popular supplement. Flaxseed contains large amounts, up to 60%, alpha-Linolenic acid, and Lignans, especially Secoisolariciresinol Diglucoside (SDG).

Flaxseed has
- Blood pressure decreasing properties
- Total cholesterol decreasing properties
- LDL-cholesterol decreasing properties
- Triglycerides decreasing properties
- HDL-cholesterol increasing properties

When 55 volunteers were given 30 grams Flaxseed daily, for 3 months, total cholesterol decreased by 7% and LDL-cholesterol decreased by 10%, compared to the control group (Palade et.al. 2008).

When 100 volunteers were given 543 mg Flaxseed Lignan SDG daily, for 6 months, both diastolic blood pressure ($p = 0.046$) and triglycerides ($p = 0.017$) decreased significantly, compared to the control group (Cornish et.al. 2009). This was a double blind experiment.

When 30 volunteers were given 100 mg Flaxseed Lignan SDG daily, for 12 weeks, LDL-cholesterol ($p < 0.05$) decreased significantly, compared to the conrtol group (Fukumitsu et.al. 2010). This was a double blind experiment.

In a meta-analysis of 28 different experiments, it was noticed, that Flaxseed decreases significantly both total cholesterol and LDL-cholesterol (Pan et.al. 2009).

When hyperlipidemic rabbits were given 15 mg/kg Flaxseed Lignan SDG daily, for 8 weeks, total cholesterol decreased by 33% and LDL-cholesterol decreased by 35%, but HDL-cholesterol increased by 140%, compared to the control group (Prasad 1999).

When hyperlipidemic rabbits were given Flaxseed 7.5 g/kg daily, for 8 weeks, total cholesterol decreased by 31% and LDL-cholesterol decreased by 32%, compared to the control group (Prasad et.al. 1998).

When hyperlipidemic rabbits were given 40 mg/kg Flaxseed Lignan SDG daily, for 2 months, total choleterol decreased by 20%, LDL-cholesterol decreased by 14%, but HDL-cholesterol increased by 30%, compared to the control group (Prasad 2005).

When hamsters were given in their daily diet 15% Flaxseed, for 3 months, total cholesterol decreased by 12%, compared to the control group (Lucas et.al. 2011).

When rats were given in their daily diet 25% Flaxseed, for 6 months, HDL-cholesterol increased by 47% ($p < 0.05$), but LDL-cholesterol decreased by 22% and triglycerides decreased by 23% (Daleprane et.al. 2010).

When 55 hyperlipidemic volunteers were given 600 mg Flaxseed Lignan SDG daily, for 8 weeks, both total cholesterol and LDL-cholesterol decreased by an average of 23%, compared to the control group (Zhang et.al. 2008). This was a double blind experiment.

When SDG was given intravenously to rats at doses of 10 mg/kg, 15 mg/kg or 20 mg/kg, the mean average blood pressure (MAP) decreased by 40%, 41% and 47% (Prasad 2004). SDG causes the blood pressure to be decreased for several hours.

Flaxseed oil

(Linum Usitatissimum)

Flaxseed oil contains extremely large amounts of alfa-Linolenic acid, typically between 50 – 65% of oil.

Alfa-Linolenic acid belongs to Omega-3 fatty acids. From alfa-linolenic acid, the human body makes the well known "Fish oils" EPA (EicosaPentanoic Acid) and DHA (DocosaHexanoic Acid).

Alfa-Linolenic acid has
 – Blood pressure lowering properties

When 59 hyperlipidemic volunteers were given alfa-Linolenic acid 8 grams daily, for 12 weeks, both systolic blood pressure (120 mmHg → 110 mmHg; $p < 0.016$) and diastolic blood pressure (80 mmHg → 72 mmHg; $p < 0.011$), decreased significantly, compared to the control group (Paschos et.al. 2007).

When hypertensive volunteers were given 2.6 grams alfa-Linolenic acid daily, for 12 weeks, both systolic blood pressure and diastolic blood pressure decreased significantly, compared to the control group (Takeuchi et.al. 2007).

When hypertensive rats were given 10% Flaxseed oil, in their daily diet, systolic blood pressure decreased by 59 mmHg, compared to the control group (Dierberger et.al. 1991). Also blood viscosity decreased significantly.

Alfa-Linolenic acid decreases both systolic- and diastolic blood pressure and inhibits ACE in rats (Ogawa et.al. 2009).

Folic acid

Folic acid is an essential vitamin, belonging to the vitamin B group. It exists in many plants, and especially in Brewer's yeast. Folic acid is known to decrease Homocysteine, which is a strong risk factor in cardiovascular disease. The higher the Homocysteine level is, the higher is blood pressure (Sutton-Tyrrel et.al. 1997; Florina et.al. 1998; Stehouwer et.al. 1998).

Folic acid has
- – Blood pressure decreasing properties
- – Total cholesterol decreasing properties
- – LDL-cholesterol decreasing properties
- – Triglycerides decreasing properties
- – HDL-cholesterol increasing properties

When 20 children with high levels of Homocysteine, were given 5 mg Folic acid, Homocysteine ($p < 0.001$), systolic blood pressure ($p < 0.01$) and diastolic blood pressure ($p = 0.045$) decreased significantly, compared to the control group (Papandreou et.al. 2010).

When 24 smoking volunteers were given Folic acid 5 mg daily, for 4 weeks, both Homocysteine (10.8 micromol/dl $\rightarrow$ 8.2 micromol/dl; $p < 0.001$) and diastolic blood pressure (88 mmHg $\rightarrow$ 83 mmHg; $p < 0.01$) decreased significantly, compared to the control group (Mangoni et.al. 2002).

When rats were given 10 – 20 times (=10 – 20xRDA) more Folic acid, than their daily need was, systolic blood pressure at the 190 days old rats decreased by 11.3% (230 mmHg $\rightarrow$ 204 mmHg), compared to the control group. But 5xRDA or less doses had no effect (Perez et.al. 2005).

When 10 young, healthy volunteers were given acutely Folic acid either 5 mg or 10 mg, total cholesterol decreased 4.40 mmol/L $\rightarrow$ 3.54 mmol/L $\rightarrow$ 3.12 mmol/L, LDL-cholesterol decreased 2.16 mmol/L $\rightarrow$ 1.37 mmol/L $\rightarrow$ 1.10 mmol/L, triglycerides decreased 1.79 mmol/L $\rightarrow$ 1.77 mmol/L $\rightarrow$ 0.41 mmol/L, but HDL-cholesterol increased 0.96 mmol/L $\rightarrow$ 1.74 mmol/L $\rightarrow$ 1.71 mmol/L ($p < 0.05$ in all parameters) (Owoyele et.al. 2005).

When 15 volunteers were given 7.5 mg Folic acid daily, for 4 weeks, LDL-cholesterol decreased by 9.0% ($p < 0.03$), but HDL-cholesterol increased by 6.0% ($p < 0.05$), compared to the control group (Paradisi et.al. 2004).

When Japanese Quails were given in their daily diet Folic acid 1 mg/kg, both total cholesterol and triglycerides decreased significantly, but HDL-cholesterol increased significantly, compared to the control group ($p < 0.05$ in all parameters) (Gurse et.al. 2004).

Folic acid can be bought as pills, but they contain far too low levels of Folic acid, typically 0.3 – 0.6 mg/pill. This small dose has no effect on high blood pressure or cholesterol value. The dose must be at least 5 – 10 mg/day, to be effective.

Foxtail Millet

(Setaria Italica)

Foxtail Millet is a very old food plant. It has been cultivated in Asia, especially in China and Korea, for thousands of years. It grows well in dry and nutrient free lands, and the cultivation is very easy. The average yield is 800 – 900 kg per hectare. Foxtail Millet contains lot of nutrients and large amounts of Phenolic acids, such as Ferulic acid. The total amount of Phenolic acids can be up to 390 mg/100 g (Dykes et.al. 2007). Foxtail Millet has exceptionally high HDL-cholesterol increasing property.

Foxtail Millet has
- Total cholesterol lowering properties
- LDL-cholesterol lowering properties
- VLDL-cholesterol lowering properties
- Triglycerides lowering properties
- HDL-cholesterol increasing properties

When mice were fed in their daily diet about 40% of Foxtail Millet, for 3 weeks, HDL-cholesterol increased by an average of 100% ($p < 0.05$), compared to the control group, which was fed casein (Choi et.al. 2005).

When rats were given Foxtail Millet water extract at a dose of 300 mg/kg daily, for 30 days, total cholesterol, LDL-cholesterol, VLDL-cholesterol and triglycerides decreased significantly, but HDL-cholesterol increased significantly, compared to the control group (Sireesha et.al. 2011).

When 30 diabetic volunteers were given Foxtail Millet 100 grams daily, for 4 weeks, total cholesterol decreased by 6% ($p < 0.05$), LDL-cholesterol decreased by 20% ($p < 0.05$), but HDL-cholesterol increased by 23%, compared to the control group (Thathola et.al. 2011). This was a double blind experiment. Triglycerides decreased by 9.0% and VLDL-cholesterol decreased by 9.1%.

GABA

(Gamma-Amino-Butyric Acid)

GABA is a natural amino acid, which exists in all plants and animals. Human brains contain large amount of GABA. GABA gives better sleep, and stimulates Growth Hormone. GABA is made in a reaction from L-Glutamic acid, catalysed by CAD (Glutamate decarboxylase) entzyme, and vitamin B6, Pyridoxin. CAD content decreases during aging, but it can be activated by an extra vitamin B6 (Messripour et.al. 2011). The blood pressure lowering property of GABA has been known for a long time.

GABA has
 - Blood pressure lowering properties

When 50 hypertensive volunteers, with systolic blood pressure between 120 – 180 mmHg, were given 80 mg GABA daily, for 8 weeks, systolic blood pressure decreased by 10 mmHg ($p < 0.05$) and diastolic blood pressure decreased by 5 mmHg ($p < 0.05$), compared to the control group (Matsubara et.al. 2002). This was a double blind experiment.

When hypertensive rats were given acutely, orally, 0.5 mg/kg GABA, systolic blood pressure decreased very strongly, after 4 hours it was 20.8 mmHg ($p < 0.01$) lower and after 8 hours it was 22.8 mmHg ($p < 0.01$) lower, compared to the control level (Hayakawa et.al. 2002). The duration of decreased blood pressure was 24 hours.

Galangal root

(Alpinia Galangal)

Galangal root is, just like Ginger, very popular both in Chinese and Thai food culture.

Galangal root has
 - Total cholesterol lowering properties
 - LDL-cholesterol lowering properties
 - Triglycerides lowering properties

When ethanol extract of Galangal root was given to diaetic rats 200 mg/kg daily, for 3 weeks, triglycerides decreased by 20.2% ($p < 0.001$) and LDL-cholesterol decreased 52.2% ($p < 0.001$), compared to the control group (Srividua et.al. 2010).

When rats were given ethanol extract of Galangal root 20 mg/kg daily, both triglycerides and LDL-cholesterol decreased significantly, compared to the control group (Achuthan et.al. 1997).

Garden cress

(Lepidium Sativum)

Garden cress is an ancient vegetable and medicinal plant, which is known all over the World. It is very easy to cultivate even indoors, and it grows quickly. Garden cress is used in salads and cooking, and its seeds are used in Asia in Asthma, in bronchitis, in diabetes and in high blood pressure.

Garden cress seeds have
- Blood pressure lowering properties
- Diuretic properties
- Total cholesterol lowering properties
- LDL-cholesterol lowering properties
- VLDL-cholesterol lowering properties
- HDL-cholesterol increasing properties

When hypertensive rats were given Garden cress seed water extract 20 mg/kg daily, for 3 weeks, systolic blood pressure decreased by 25 mmHg (200 mmHg → 175 mmHg; $p < 0.01$), compared to the control group (Maghrani et.al. 2005). Also a strong diuretic property was noticed, urine output increased significantly ($p < 0.01$), compared to the control group.

Diuretic property was also noticed in another experiment (Patel et.al. 2009).

When hyperlipidemic rats were given Garden cress seeds 5% of their daily diet, for 8 weeks, total cholesterol decreased by 43.3% ($p < 0.05$), triglycerides decreased by 38.0% ($p < 0.05$), LDL-cholesterol decreased by 39.5% ($p < 0.05$) and VLDL-cholesterol decreased by 38.0% ($p < 0.05$), but HDL-cholesterol increased by 54.8% ($p < 0.05$), compared to the control group (Hamedan et.al. 2010).

Garlic

(Allium Sativum)

Garlic is an ancient food, spice and medicinal plant, which has been known over 6000 years. It originates from Central-Asia. Garlic is used and cultivated all over the World, and its cultivation is very easy. Garlic has huge amounts of medicinal properties. It is antibacterial, antiviral, antifungal, anti-inflammatory and it is used all over the World to decrease high blood pressure and high cholesterol levels. Garlic contains many Sulphur containing organic compounds, like Allicin, S-Allyl-L-Cysteine, Alliin, Ajoene, Diallylsulfide, Dithin etc., which have many pharmacological actions. Garlic can be eaten raw, dried, as Garlic oil pills or aged Garlic, which do not smell at all, like Kwai, Kyolic etc. Aged Garlic is easily made by everybody, just by slicing the fresh Garlics, and putting them into strong alcohol for at least 3 months or longer time.

Garlic has
- Blood pressure decreasing properties

- Total cholesterol decreasing properties
- VLDL-cholesterol decreasing properties
- Triglycerides decreasing properties
- HDL-cholesterol increasing properties

When 41 hyperlipidemic volunteers, with their cholesterol levels between 5.7 – 7.5 mmol/L, were given 7.2 grams Garlic daily, for 6 months, total cholesterol decreased by 6.1% (p < 0.0001), LDL-cholesterol decreased by 4.6% (p = 0.0004) and systolic blood pressure decreased by 5.5% (p = 0.0001), compared to the placebo group (Steiner et.al. 1996). Also diastolic blood pressure decreased (p = 0.026) significantly, compared to the placebo group. This was a double blind experiment.

In a meta-analysis with 11 different experiments, Garlic decreased systolic blood pressure in normotensive volunteers by 4.6 mmHg (p = 0.001), but in hypertensive volunteers Garlic decreased systolic blood pressure by an average of 8.4 mmHg (p < 0.001), and diastolic blood pressure by an average of 7.3 mmHg (p < 0.001), compared to the placebo group (Ried et.al. 2008).

In another meta-analysis with 8 different experiments and 415 volunteers, Garlic decreased systolic blood pressure by an average of 5 – 7%, compared to the placebo group. The decrease in diastolic blood pressure was of the same size (Silagy et.al. 1994).

In a meta-analysis with 13 different experiments, Garlic decreased total cholesterol by an average of 0.41 mmol/L (p < 0.01), compared to the placebo group (Stevinson et.al. 2000).

In an experiment with 4 years duration, volunteers were given 900 mg standardized Garlic daily, LDL-cholesterol decreased by 4%, HDL-cholesterol increased by 8% and blood pressure decreased by 7%. These changes mean, that the probability to get a heart attack decrease by an average of 50% (Siegel et.al. 1999).

Garlic decreases blood pressure also acutely. When volunteers with diastolic blood pressure over 115 mmHg, were given 2400 mg Garlic, containing 1.3% Allicin, systolic blood pressure decreased by 7 mmHg and diastolic blood pressure decreased by 16 mmHg, already 5 hours after the dose, and the blood stayed a long time depressed, over 14 hours in case of diastolic blood pressure (p < 0.05) (McMahon et.al. 1993).

When 84 volunteers were given sustained release (Allicor time released) Garlic 600 mg daily, for 8 weeks, systolic blood pressure decreased by 7 mmHg and diastolic blood pressure decreased by 3.8 mmHg, compared to the control group (Sobenmin et.al. 2009).

When 50 volunteers were given Garlic 800 mg daily, containing 2 mg Allicin, for 6 weeks, total cholesterol decreased by 12.1% (26.82 mg/dl; p < 0.0001) and LDL-cholesterol decreased by 17.3% (22.18 mg/dl; p < 0.0001), but HDL-cholesterol increased by 15.7% (10.02 mg/dl; p < 0.0001), compared to the control group (Kojuri et.al. 2007). So the changes can be very large, even in a relatively short time period.

When 50 volunteers were given 960 mg Garlic extract containing 2.4 mg S-Allyl-L-Cysteine daily, for 12 weeks, systolic blood pressure decreased by 10.3 mmHg (p = 0.03), compared to the control group (Ried et.al. 2010).

When 23 hyperlipidemic volunters, of which 13 were also hypertensive, were given raw Garlic 10 grams daily, for 4 months, systolic blood pressure decreased by 22.1 mmHg (148.3 mmHg → 126.2 mmHg; $p < 0.05$) and diastolic blood pressure decreased by 13.4 mmHg (98.5 mmHg → 85.1 mmHg; $p < 0.05$) in the hypertensive group. In the whole group, total cholesterol decreased by 25.6% ($p < 0.01$), LDL-cholesterol decreased by 32.5% ($p < 0.05$), VLDL-cholesterol decreased by 20.2% ($p < 0.05$) and triglycerides decreased by 28.4% ($p < 0.005$), but HDL-cholesterol increased by 28.0% ($p < 0.01$), compared to the control group (Durak et.al. 2004).

So, when using at least 10 grams raw Garlic daily, very large decreases in blood pressure, cholesterol and triglycerides, and large increases in HDL-cholesterol can be achieved in a few months.

When volunteers were given 800 mg Garlic extract daily, for 4 weeks, diastolic blood pressure decreased by 9.5% (74 mmHg → 67 mmHg), compared to the control group (Kiesewetter et.al. 1991).

When 60 volunteers were given Garlic 4 grams daily, for 3 months, total cholesterol decreased by 12.8% (252.9 mg/dl → 220.5 mg/dl; $p < 0.01$), and triglycerides decreased by 15.2% (130.0 mg/dl → 110.2 mg/dl; $p < 0.01$), but HDL-cholesterol increased by 22.2% (40.5 mg/dl → 49.5 mg/dl; $p < 0.05$), compared to the control group (Bordia et.al. 1998).

Garlic Chives

(Allium Tuberosum)

Garlic Chives is a very popular vegetable in Asia, especially in China, Korea and Japan. All parts can be eaten, and besides the seeds are a very popular Sex stimulant (Aphrodisiac). It is very easy to cultivate.

Garlic Chives have
 – Total cholesterol lowering properties
 – LDL-cholesterol lowering properties
 – VLDL-cholesterol lowering properties
 – Triglycerides lowering properties

When Hamsters with high cholesterol levels were given 2 g/kg Garlic Chives daily, for 4 weeks, total cholesterol decreased by 50.5% ($p < 0.05$), LDL-cholesterol decreased by 65.3% ($p < 0.05$), VLDL-cholesterol decreased by 37.4% and triglycerides decreased y 37.3% ($p < 0.05$), compared to the control group (Choudhary et.al. 2008).

These changes were bigger than in the same experiment, where Hamsters were given ordinary Garlic 2 g/kg, for 4 weeks. With ordinary Garlic, total cholesterol decreased by 36.3% ($p < 0.05$), LDL-cholesterol decreased by 46.1% ($p < 0.05$), VLDL-cholesterol decreased by 28.5% ($p < 0.05$) and triglycerides decreased by 28.5% (Choudhary 2008).

Genistein

Genistein is an Isoflavonoid, which exists in many plants, but especially large amounts of Genistein is found in Soy beans, Red Clover, Pueraria Lobata and Psoralea Corylifolia. Soy, Red Clover and Pueraria Lobata are known to decrease blood pressure.

Genistein has
- Blood pressure lowering properties

Genistein inhibits ACE (Montenegro et.al. 2009; Xu et.al. 2006).

When hypertensive rats were given Genistein 10 mg/kg daily, for 5 weeks, systolic blood pressure decreased 10% ($p < 0.01$), compared to the control group (Vera et.al. 2007).

When hypertensive rats were given either 0.2 g, 0.5 g or 2.0 g Genistein in 1 kg of their food, systolic blood pressure decreased in these groups by 7.37%, 9.67% and 13.36%, and diastolic blood pressure decreased by 3.22%, 8.38% and 9.67% ($p < 0.05$ in all groups), compared to the control group (Si et.al. 2008)..

The blood pressure lowering effect of Genistein has been noticed in other experiments too (Taehyeon et.al. 2007).

When human volunteers were given acutely Isoflavonoids 80 mg in their meal, the plasma NO concentration increased ($p < 0.01$) significantly, causing vasodilatation.

Ginkgo
(Ginkgo Biloba)

Ginkgo, or Maidenhair tree is a famous medicinal plant, which originates from China. The tree can grow up to 30 meters, and live more than 1500 years. The leaves are full of very strong antioxidants.

Ginkgo has
- Blood pressure decreasing properties
- Total cholesterol decreasing properties

When 10 healthy young volunteers were given acutely Gincosan pills, which consist of standardized Ginkgo extract 60 mg and Ginseng extract 100 mg, 2 pills at the same time, systolic blood pressure decreased by 14.0 mmHg (137.0 mmHg → 123.0 mmHg; $p = 0.002$) and diastolic blood pressure decreased by 8.0 mmHg (84.5 mmHg → 72.6 mmHg; $p = 0.006$) and heart rate decreased by 4.8 beats/minute (77.4/min → 72.6/min), 1 hour after dose (Kiesewetter et.al. 1992).

When 70 healthy young volunteers were given 120 mg of standardized Ginkgo EGb 761 extract, 30 minutes before a 6 minutes isometric handgrip test, systolic blood pressure was about 12.5 mmHg (p < 0.05) and diastolic blood pressure about 6.5 mmHg (p < 0.05) lower in the EGb 761 group, than in the control group, after the stress test (Jezova et.al. 2002).

When 54 volunteers were given standardized Ginkgo extract 160 mg daily, for 3 months, diastolic blood pressure decreased by 5 mmmHg (73 mmHg → 68 mmHg;p = 0.04), compared to the control group (Winther et.al. 1998).

When 20 mildly hypertensive volunteers were given Ginkgo water extract 120 mg daily, for 3 months, systolic blood pressure decreased by 6% (125 mmHg → 118 mmHg; p < 0.05) and diastolic blood pressure decreased by 21% (88 mmHg → 68 mmHg;p < 0.05), compared to the control group (Kubolo 2000).

In hypertensive animals, Ginkgo extract decreases significantly both systolic and diastolic blood pressure, and it inhibits ACE, Angiotensin II and Endothelin-1, but stimulates cGMP (Yannan et.al. 2000; Mansour et.al. 2011; Umegaki et.al. 2000; Kubota et.al. 2006; Kubota et.al. 2006).

In human volunteers, Ginkgo decreases significantly serum viscosity and increases microcirculation (Galduroz et.al. 2007; Witte et.al. 1992; Koltringer et.al. 1993; Jung et.al. 1990).

Both in rats and hamsters, Ginkgo decreases significantly total cholesterol (Dubey et.al. 2005; Wojcicki et.al. 1994; Zhang et.al. 2009).

Ginseng

(Panax Ginseng)

Ginseng is possibly the most famous medicinal plant in the whole World. Ginseng root is edible, and it has been used thousands of years in Asia, especially in China and Korea, in many different diseases, such as asthma, cancer, impotence and for speeding healing from infectious diseases. Ginseng grows wildly in Russia, China and Korea, and nowadays the biggest Ginseng cultivators are Korea and China. The effective compounds are numerous Ginsenoids and Saponins.

Ginseng has
- Blood pressure decreasing properties
- Total cholesterol decreasing properties
- LDL-cholesterol decreasing properties
- Triglycerides decreasing properties
- HDL-cholesterol increasing properties
- Blood vessel elasticity increasing properties

When 8 volunteers were given Ginseng 6 grams daily, for 8 weeks, total cholesterol decreased by 12.0% (163.4 mg/dl → 155.6 mg/dl; p < 0.05), LDL-cholesterol decreased by 44.5% (85.4 mg/dl → 47.4 mg/dl; p < 0.05) and triglycerides decreased by 23.7% (!55.6 mg/dl → 118.6 mg/dl; p < 0.05), but HDL-cholesterol increased by 44.2% (50.1 mg/dl → 72.3 mg/dl; p < 0.05), compared to the control group (Kim et.al. 2003).

When 20 volunteers with stable angina pectoris were given 2.7 grams Ginseng daily, for 10 weeks, systolic blood pressure decreased by 12 mmHg (141 mmHg → 129 mmHg; $p < 0.05$) and diastolic blood pressure decreased by 3 mmHg (84 mmHg → 81 mmHg; $p < 0.05$), compared to the control group. Total cholesterol decreased by 9.6%, LDL-cholesterol decreased by 15.1% but HDL-cholesterol increased by 4.3%. LDL/HDL-cholesterol ratio decreased by 18.6%. The blood vessel elasticity increased significantly ($p < 0.05$), compared to the control group (Chung et.al. 2010).

When 17 volunteers were given acutely 3 grams Ginseng, the elasticity of blood vessels increased significantly ($p = 0.046$), compared to the control group (Jovanovski et.al. 2010). This was a double blind experiment.

When 13 volunteers were given acutely 0.84 mg Rg3 Ginsenoid, systolic blood pressure decreased by 4.3 mmHg ($p = 0.06$) and diastolic blood pressure decreased by 8.9 mmHg ($p = 0.02$) after 2 hours, compared to the control group (Stavro et.al. 2002).

When 26 hypertensive volunteers were given 4.5 grams Ginseng daily, for 8 weeks, systolic blood pressure decreased significantly ($p = 0.03$), compared to the control group (Han et.al. 1998). Diastolic blood pressure decreased also, but not significantly ($p = 0.17$).

When 30 volunteers were given Ginseng extract 200 mg daily, for 28 days, diastolic blood pressure decreased by 6.6% (75 mmHg → 70 mmHg; $p = 0.02$), compared to the control group (Caron et.al. 2002). This was a double blind experiment.

When 7 hypertensive volunteers were given 4.5 grams Ginseng daily, for 24 months, the mean average blood pressure (MAP) decreased by 10.77% (127.1 mmHg → 113.2 mmHg; $p < 0.001$), compared to the control group (Sung et.al. 2000).

Ginseng inhibits strongly ACE (Persson et.al. 2006).

When 10 young, healthy volunteers were given acutely Gincosan extract, which contains standardized extracts of Ginkgo Biloba 60 mg and Panax Ginseng 100 mg, 2 capsules at the same time, systolic blood pressure decreased by 14.0 mmHg (137.0 mmHg → 123.0 mmHg; $p = 0.002$), diastolic blood pressure decreased by 8.0 mmHg (84.5 mmHg → 72.6 mmHg; $p = 0.06$) and heart rate decreased by 4.8 beats/minute (77.4/min → 72.6/min), after 1 hour, compared to the control group (Kiesewetter et.al. 1992).

The total cholesterol, LDL-cholesterol and triglycerides lowering, but HDL-cholesterol increasing properties of Ginseng have been verified in a number of animal experiments (Jeon et.al. 2000; Hu et.al. 2011; Song et.al. 2012; Inoue et.al. 1999; El-Khayat et.al. 2011; Park et.al. 2011).

The blood pressure lowering properties of Ginseng have been verified in a number of animal experiments (Kim et.al. 1994; Toda et.al. 2001; Jeon et.al. 2000; Jeon et.al. 2000; Akasaka et.al. 1990).

GLA

(Gamma-Linolenic Acid)

GLA belongs to the omega-6 group (w-6), and it is an essential polyunsaturated fatty acid in human body. The human body synthesises GLA from Linolenic acid, which comes from food. GLA comes also from natural sources, especially Blackcurrant (Ribes Nigrum) seeds, Evening Primrose (Oenethera Biennis) seeds and Borage (Borage Officinalis) seeds are good sources of GLA. From GLA the cells make DHGLA (Di-Homo-Gamma-Linolenic Acid), from which comes Prostaglandin PGE1, which has blood pressure lowering properties.

GLA has
- Blood pressure lowering properties
- Total cholesterol lowering properties
- LDL-cholesterol lowering properties
- Triglycerides lowering properties
- HDL-cholesterol increasing properties

When 12 volunteers with high cholesterol levels were give Evening Primrose seed oil 3.0 grams daily, corresponding to 220 mg GLA and 2.2 grams Linolenic acid daily, for 4 months, total cholesterol decreased by 32% (286 mg/dl $\rightarrow$ 194 mg/dl; $p < 0.01$), LDL-cholesterol decreased by 49% (246 mg/dl $\rightarrow$ 125 mg/dl; $p < 0.01$) and triglycerides decreased by 48% (290 mg/dl $\rightarrow$ 150 mg/dl; $p < 0.001$), but HDL-cholesterol increased 22% (33 mg/dl $\rightarrow$ 42 mg/dl; $p < 0.01$), compared to the control group (Guivernan et.al. 1994).

When rats were fed in their food either 11% Sesame oil or 11% GLA-rich Borage oil daily, for 5 weeks, systolic blood pressure decreased by 12 mmHg in the GLA group, compared to the Sesame oil group (Engler et.al. 1998). Also the plasma Aldosterone level decreased in the GLA-group.

The blood pressure lowering property of GLA has been noticed also in other experiments (Engler et.al. 1992), where during a 7 week experiement with GLA-rich Evening Primrose oil, Borage oil and Black currant oil, blood pressure decreased by an average of 12 mmHg (191 mmHg $\rightarrow$ 168 mmHg), compared to the Sesame oil control group.

When 120 volunteers were given GLA 840 mg and EPA 135 mg daily, for 24 months, systolic blood pressure decreased by 7.3% (161.8 mmHg $\rightarrow$ 150 mmHg; $p < 0.05$), compared to the control group (Leng et.al. 1998).

Glucuronic acid

Glucuronic acid exists in small amounts in every animal and plant cells. Glucuronic acid is studied for its anticancer properties. Gucuronic acid can be purchased as pills in Calcium-D-Glucarate form.

Glucuronic acid has
- Total cholesterol lowering properties
- LDL-cholesterol lowering properties

When rats were fed 30 mmol Calcium-D-Glucarate daily, for 8 weeks, total cholesterol decreased by 14% ($p < 0.05$) and LDL-cholesterol decreased by 30% ($p < 0.05$), compared to the control group (Walaszek et.al. 1996).

The following foods have large amounts of Glucuronic acid:
- Spinach   112 mg/100 g
- Mung bean sprouts 146 mg/100 g
- Cauliflower   146 mg/100 g
- Tomato   209 mg/100 g
- Broccoli sprouts   270 mg/100 g
- Azuki bean sprouts 240 mg/100 g
- Alfalfa sprouts   167 mg/100 g
- Orange   129 mg/100 g
- Apricote   139 mg/100 g
- Cherries   143 mg/100 g
- Apple   340 mg/100 g
- Grapefruit   360 mg/100 g

Grape seed extract

(Vitis Vinifera)

In Wine making there is a lot of Grape seeds as a byproduct. Grape seed extracts, GSE, have many healthy properties, and GSE is under intensive research.

Grape seed extract GSE has
- Blood pressure lowering properties
- Heart rate decreasing properties
- Total cholesterol decreasing properties
- LDL-cholesterol decreasing properties

When 27 volunteers, with metabolic syndrome, were given either 150 mg or 300 mg GSE daily, for 4 weeks, systolic blood pressure decreased by 11 mmHg (134 mmHg $\rightarrow$ 123 mmHg; $p = 0.003$) and 11 mmHg (127 mmHg $\rightarrow$ 116 mmHg; $p = 0.007$), and diastolic blood pressure decreased by

6 mmHg (83 mmHg → 77 mmHg; p = 0.01) and 7 mmHg (78 mmHg → 71 mmHg; p = 0.0079), compared to the control group (Sivaprakasapillai et.al. 2009).

When 30 mildly hypertensive volunteers were given 300 mg GSE daily, for 8 weeks, systolic blood pressure decreased by 12 mmHg (134 mmHg → 126 mmHg; p = 0.003) and diastolic blood pressure decreased by 5 mmHg (79 mmHg → 74 mmHg; p < 0.05) (Robinson et.al. 2007). This was a double blind experiment.

In a meta-analysis with 9 different experiments and 360 volunteers, GSE significantly decreased systolic blood pressure (1.54 mmHg; p = 0.02) and heart pulse (2.85 beats/minute; p = 0.02) (Feringa et.al. 2011).

When 30 diabetic volunteers were given GSE 600 mg daily, for 2 months, total cholesterol decreased by 4.4% (4.5 mmol/L → 4.3 mmol/L; p = 0.05), compared to the control group (Laight et.al. 2009). This was a double blind experiment.

When 40 hyperlipidemic volunteers (Choesterol level between 210 – 300 mg/dl) were given either 100 mg GSE, or Chromium Piocolinate 200 micrograms or GSE 100 mg plus Chromium Picolinate 200 micrograms daily, for 2 months, total cholesterol decreased by 3.5%, 10.0% and 16.5% (p < 0.01) and LDL-cholesterol decreased y 3.0%, 14.0% and 20.0% (p < 0.01), compared to the control group (Preuss et.al. 2000). This was a double blind experiment. This means, that GSE and Chromium Picolinate have a synergistic effect on cholesterol levels.

When rats were given GSE 4 mg/kg daily, for 6 months, the mean average blood pressure (MAP) decreased by 15.9% (197.2 mmHg → 165.8 mmHg; p = 0.002), compared to the control group (Allers et.al. 2008).

In experiments with rats, GSE decreased significantly both total cholesterol and triglycerides (Adisakwattana et.al. 2010).

Green Tea

(Camellia Sinensis)

Green Tea originates from China, where it has been used over 4000 years. Green Tea contains very large amounts of Catechins, which are very strong antioxidants. Green Tea contains also large amounts of Flavonoids, such as Quercetin, Kaempferol etc. Also Green Tea contains large amounts of L-Theanine.

Green Tea has
  – Blood pressure decreasing properties
  – Total cholesterol decreasing properties
  – LDL-cholesterol decreasing properties
  – HDL-cholesterol increasing properties

In a meta-analysis with 14 different experiments and 1136 volunteers, it was noticed, that Green Tea decreases significantly both total cholesterol (p < 0.001) and LDL-cholesterol (p < 0.001), compared to the control group (Zheng et.al. 2011).

When researching the correlation between Green Tea drinking and blood pressure of 1507 volunteers, it was noticed, that persons, who drank 1.2 – 6.0 dl Tea daily, had 46% less probability to become hypertensive. Persons, who drank over 6.0 dl Tea daily, had 65% less probability to become hypertensive (Yang et.al. 2004).

When 78 volunteers were given Green Tea extract 1200 mg daily, for 12 weeks, LDL-cholesterol decreased by 10.7% ($p < 0.01$), triglycerides decreased by 6.0% ($p < 0.05$), but HDL-cholesterol increased by 3.7% ($p < 0.05$), compared to the control group (Hsu et.al. 2008). This was a double blind experiment.

When 240 volunteers were given Green Tea daily, containing 583 mg Catechins, for 12 weeks, systolic blood pressure decreased by 9.0 mmHg (139.8 mmHg $\rightarrow$ 130.8 mmHg; $p < 0.05$) and diastolic blood pressure decreased by 6.7 mmHg (90.3 mmHg $\rightarrow$ 83.7 mmHg; $p < 0.05$) in the hypertensive group (SBP > 130 mmHg; DBP > 85 mmHg), compared to the control group (Nagao et.al. 2007). This was a double blind experiment.

When 111 volunteers were given standardized Green Tea extract 400 mg and L-Theanine 200 mg daily, for 3 weeks, systolic blood pressure decreased by 5 mmHg ($p < 0.05$) and diastolic blood pressure decreased by 4 mmHg ($p < 0.05$), compared to the control group (Nanz et.al. 2009). This was a double blind experiment. Also total cholesterol and LDL-cholesterol decreased.

When researching the correlation between total cholesterol and daily Green Tea intake of 13916 volunteers, it was noticed, that Green Tea decreases ($p < 0.001$ for men, $p < 0.01$ for women) significantly total cholesterol (Tokunaga et.al. 2002).

Green Tea inhibits ACE (Persson et.al. 2008; Persson et.al. 2010; Liu et.al. 2003) and also Angiotensin II (Liang et.al. 2010).

In experiments with rats, Green Tea decreased significantly both blood pressure and cholesterol (Sagesaka-Mitane et.al. 1996; Liang et.al. 2010; Yang et.al. 1997; Liang et.al. 2011; Yokogoshi et.al. 1995).

Guava

(Psidium Guava)

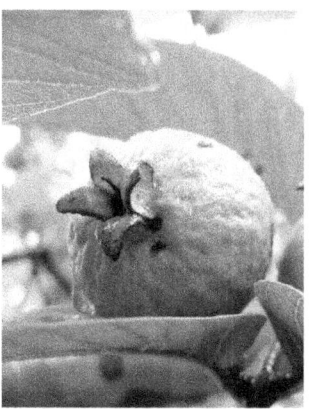

Guava is a delicious tropical fruit, which can be purchased nowadays from every Supermarket.

Guava has:
- Blood pressure lowering properties.
- Total cholesterol lowering properties.
- LDL-cholesterol lowering properties.
- Triglycerides lowering properties.
- HDL-cholesterol increasing properties.

When 120 volunteers were given daily 1 Guava fruit before meal, for 12 weeks, systolic blood pressure decreased by 9 mmHg and diastolic blood pressure decreased by 8%, compared to the control group. Total cholesterol decreased by 9.9%, triglycerides decreased by 7.7%, but HDL-cholesterol increased by 8.0%, compared to the control group (Ram et.al. 1992).

When 145 hypertensive volunteers were given 0.5 – 1.0 kg Guava daily, for 4 weeks, systolic blood pressure decreased by 7.5 mmHg, diastolic blood pressure decreased by 8.5 mmHg, total cholesterol decreased by 7.9%, and triglycerides decreased by 7.0%, but HDL-cholesterol increased by 4.6%, compared to the control group (Singh et.al. 1993).

When rats were given daily Guava fruit, for 6 weeks, systolic blood pressure decreased significantly. Total cholesterol decreased by 34.4%, triglycerides decreased by 43.59% and LDL-cholesterol decreased by 69.70%, but HDL-cholesterol increased, compared to the control group (Norazmir et.al. 2010).

Guinea pepper

(Xylopia Aethiopica)

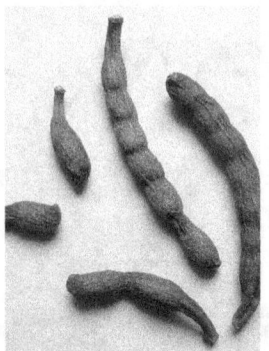

Guinea pepper originates from Africa, where it is commonly used as a spice, in many foods and also it is used medicinally.

Guinea pepper has
- – Total cholesterol lowering properties
- – LDL-cholesterol lowering properties
- – Triglycerides lowering properties
- – HDL-cholesterol increasing properties

When hyperlipidemic rats were given Guinea pepper extract 250 mg/kg daily, for 8 weeks, total cholesterol decreased by 33.7% ($p < 0.05$) and LDL-cholesterol decreased by 49.0% ($p < 0.05$), compared to the control group (Nwozo et.al. 2011).

When rats were given Guinea pepper water extract 200 mg/kg daily, for 2 weeks, total cholesterol decreased by 29.8% ($p < 0.05$), LDL-cholesterol decreased by 31.8% ($p < 0.05$) and triglycerides decreased by 23.1% ($p < 0.05$), but HDL-cholesterol increased by 6.7% ($p < 0.05$), compared to the control group (Johnkennedy et.al. 2011).

Haritaki

(Terminalia Chebula)

Haritaki is a large size tree, which originates from Asia. Its edible fruits have been used as a medicinal plant in India for thousands of years in liver- and skin diseases. The fruits contain large amounts of different compounds, such as Ellagic acid, Gallic acid, Chebulinic acid, Corilagin, Chebugalic acid etc.

Haritaki fruits have
  - Total cholesterol decreasing properties
  - LDL-cholesterol decreasing properties
  - Triglycerides lowering properties
  - HDL-cholesterol increasing properties

When hyperlipidemic rabbits were given Haritaki fruit 1 g/kg daily, for 16 weeks, total cholesterol decreased by 73.6% (630 mg/dl $\rightarrow$ 166 mg/dl; $p < 0.001$), compared to the control group (Thakur et.al. 1988).

When hyperlipidemic rabbits were given Haritaki fruit powder 500 mg/kg daily, for 45 days, total cholesterol decreased by 34.3% ($p < 0.059$) and triglycerides decreased by 26.3% ($p < 0.05$), compared to the control group (Shaila et.al. 1988).

When hyperlipidemic rats were given Haritaki fruit extract 300 mg/kg daily, for 45 days, total cholesterol decreased by 39.9% ($p < 0.05$), triglycerides decreased by 38.6% ($p < 0.05$) and LDL-cholesterol decreased by 48.0% ($p < 0.05$), but HDL-cholesterol increased by 119.2% ($p < 0.05$), compared to the control group (Israni et.al. 2010).

The Haritaki fruit total cholesterol and triglycerides decreasing but HDL-cholesterol increasing properties have been verified also in other experiments (Maruthappan et.al. 2010; Murali et.al. 2007; Ahirwar et.al. 2003).

Hawthorn

(Crataegus Oxyacantha, Crataegus Sp.)

Hawthorn is an ancient medicinal plant, which has been used in cardiovascular diseases all around the World, over 1500 years. There are many Hawthorn species, but they all contain same kind of flavonoids. There are at least 17 different Cardioactive flavonoids in Hawthorn. Hawthorn is used in Europe to decrease high blood pressure, but in China it is also used to lower high cholesterol levels, besides high blood pressure. The berry of Hawthorn is edible, but almost tastless. There are very large amount of research experiments of the blood pressure decreasing and cardioprotective properties of Hawthorn.

Hawthorn berries, flowers and leaves have
  - Blood pressure decreasing properties
  - Total cholesterol decreasing properties

- LDL-cholesterol decreasing properties
- Triglycerides decreasing properties
- HDL-cholesterol increasing properties

The blood pressure lowering properties of Hawthorn has been scientifically verified already over 70 years ago (Graham 1939; Graham 1940).

When rats were given intravenously Hawthorn water extract 31 mg/kg, systolic blood pressure decreased by 37% (p < 0.005) and diastolic blood pressure decreased by 49% (p < 0.005), compared to the control group (Abdul-Ghan et.al. 1987).

Hawthorn extract inhibits ACE strongly (Uchida et.al. 1987).

When hyperlipidemic rabbits were given Hawthorn berry 10% water extract, 10 mg/kg daily, for 6 weeks, total cholesterol decreased by 22.9%, LDL-cholesterol decreased by 21.4% and triglycerides decreased by 20.0%, compared to the control group (Khall et.al. 2008).

When hyperlipidemic rats were given Hawthorn berry 2% of their daily diet, for 4 weeks, total cholesterol decreased by 34.0% (p < 0.01), LDL-cholesterol decreased by 36.4% (p < 0.01) but HDL-cholesterol increased by 100.0% (p < 0.01), compared to the control group (Kwok et.al. 2010).

The same cholesterol decreasing property of Hawthorn has been verified also in experiments with hamsters, where it was noticed, that Ursolic acid and Oleanolic acid decreased cholesterol (Lin et.al. 2009).

Also with mice, Hawthorn significantly decreased cholesterol, when compared with Simvastatin (Xu et.al. 2009).

In double blind experiments with human volunteers, Hawthorn decreased significantly blood pressure, compared to the controls (Walker et.al. 2002; Walker et.al. 2002).

The blood pressure lowering property of Hawthorn has been verified in other human experiments too (Leuchtgens et.al. 1993; Schusslet et.al. 1995; Weikl et.al. 1996).

Hibiscus Tea

(Hibiscus Sabdariffa)

Hibiscus tea is very popular tea all around the World. It has been used for a long time to decrease high blood pressure in many countries.

Hibiscus tea has
- Blood pressure lowering properties
- Total cholesterol lowering properties
- LDL-cholesterol lowering properties
- Triglycerides lowering properties
- HDL-cholesterol increasing properties

When 60 diabetic and hypertensive volunteers were given Hibiscus tea 2 times daily, for 4 weeks, systolic blood pressure decreased by 17.1% (134.4 mmHg → 112.7 mmHg), compared to the group (Mozaffari-Khosvari et.al. 2009).

Many other researchers have noticed the blood pressure lowering properties of Hibiscus Tea (Ajay et.al. 2007; Adegunloye et.al. 1996; Haji-Faraji et.al. 1999).

When 42 volunters were given Hibiscus Tea extract daily, for 4 weeks, 71.4% of volunteers experienced an average decrease of 12% in total cholesterol value (Lin et.al. 2007).

The same total cholesterol lowering effect of Hibiscus Tea has been noticed also in rats (Chen et.al. 2004) and rabbits (Chen et.al. 2003).

In other experiments with rats, Hibiscus Tea decreased total cholesterol, LDL-cholesterol and triglycerides but increased HDL-cholesterol, compared to the control group (Ochani et.al. 2009).

Himematsukate

(A. Sylvaticus, A. Subrufescens, A. Brasiliensis)

Himematsutake is an edible mushroom, close relative to the White Mutton mushroom, Agaricus Bisporus. Himematsutake originates from Brazil, North-America and Europe, and is nowadays much cultivated in Japan, China and Korea. It has many medicinal properties, especially as an immunostimulant in cancer patients.

Himematsutake has
- Blood pressure decreasing properties
- Total cholesterol decreasing properties
- Triglycerides decreasing properties
- Body weight decreasing properties

When 28 volunteers were given hot water extract of Himematsutake, 30 mg/kg daily, for 6 months, systolic blood pressure decreased by 8.6 mmHg (127.88 mmHg → 119.23 mmHg; $p = 0.0001$) and diastolic blood pressure decreased by 7.1 mmHg (82.50 mmHg → 75.38 mmHg; $p = 0.0001$), after 3 months, compared to the control group. Total cholesterol decreased by 7.8% ($p = 0.01$) and triglycerides decreased by 7.4% ($p = 0.18$) after 6 months,compared to the control group (Fortes et.al. 2011). This was a double blind experiment.

Also in other double blind experiments with humans, the systolic- and diastolic blood pressure decreasing effect of Himematsutake has been verified (Watanabe et.al. 2003; Satoshi et.al. 2006). These experiments had totally 148 volunteers.

The total cholesterol lowering effect of Himematsutake in human volunteers has been verified also in other experiments (Liu et.al. 2007). In these experiments, Himematsutake also decreased body weight ($p < 0.01$) and fat-% ($p < 0.01$), compared to the control group.

The hypotensive and hypolipidemic effect of Himematsutake has been verified also in experiments with rats (Watanabe et.al. 2002; Fumio et.al. 1999).

Himematsutake contains 770 mg/kg dw Lovastatin, 200 mg/kg dw GABA and 79 mg/kg dw Ergothioneine (Chen et.al. 2012). Lovastatin is known to decrease cholesterol, GABA is known to decrease blood pressure and Ergothioneine is a strong antioxidant.

HMB

(beta-Hydroxy-beta-MethylButyrate)

HMB is a very popular nutritional supplement among sportsmen, because it increases fat free muscle mass and increases strength. HMB is a natural Leucine metabolite in human body.

HMB has:
- Blood pressure lowering properties.
- Total cholesterol lowering properties.
- LDL-cholesterol lowering properties

When 12 hyperlipidemic volunteers were given 3 grams HMB daily, for 4 weeks, LDL-cholesterol decreased by 28.4% (172 mg/dl → 123 mg/dl) (Coelho et.al. 2001).

In a meta-analysis of 9 controlled trials on HMB, where the average daily use of HMB was 3 grams, for 3 – 8 weeks, LDL-cholesterol decreased by 7.3% ($p < 0.01$), total cholesterol decreased by 5.8% ($p < 0.03$) and systolic blood pressure decreased by 4.4 mmHg ($p < 0.05$) (Nissen et.al. 2000).

Homocysteine

Homocysteine is synthetised in cells from the amino acid Methionine. High levels of Homocysteine is regarded as a strong risk factor in cardiovascular diseases. There is a correlation between Homocysteine and plasma cholesterol levels.

When Homocysteine levels were measured in 52 volunteers, age between 30 – 60, it was noticed a very strong correlation between Homocysteine and total cholesterol ($r = 0.47$; $p < 0.001$) and Homocysteine and triglycerides ($r = 0.40$; $p < 0.001$) and Homocysteine and Body Mass Index BMI ($r = 0.42$; $p < 0.001$) (Olszewksi et.al. 1989).

When 12 volunteers, which had survived heart attac, were given daily 150 mg B6 vitamin, 5 mg Folic acid, 0.3 mg B12 vitamin, 2 grams Choline citrate, 9 mg Riboflavin and 1 gram Rutin, for 3 weeks, Homocysteine decreased by 31.9% ($p < 0.01$), total cholesterol decreased by 21.3% (6.80 mmol/L → 5.35 mmol/L; $p < 0.01$), LDL-cholesterol by 37.0% (3.56 mmol/L → 2.24 mmol/L; $p < 0.01$) and triglycerides by 32.0% (2.53 mmol/L → 1.72 mmol/L; $p < 0.001$), compared to the control group (Olszewski et.al. 1989).

When 40 hyperlipidemic volunteers were given daily 5 mg Folic acid, for 8 weeks, Homocysteine decreased by 36.5%, compared to the control group (Shidfar et.al. 2009). This was a double blind experiment.

The following nutrients are known to decrease Homocysteine:
- Folic acid
- B6 vitamin
- B12 vitamin
- Riboflavin
- Choline
- Betaine
- Rutin
- Taurine
- L-Serine
- L-Cysteine

Honey

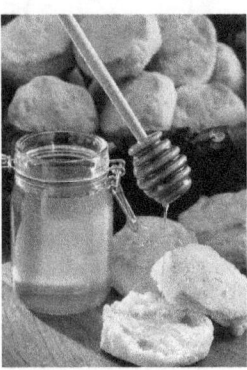

Honey has been collected by humans for thousands of years, all over the World. It has also been used for thousands of years as a medicine. Besides different sugars, Honey contains large amounts of functionally healthy Flavonoids and Polyphenols. Especially the Flavonoid Galangin is abundant in Honey. Galangin is a vasorelaxant (Morello et.al. 2006). The content of Polyphenols is higher in dark colored Honey varieties than in other Honey varieties (Kaskoniene et.al. 2009).

Honey has
  - Total cholesteol decreasing properties
  - LDL-cholesterol decreasing properties
  - Triglycerides decreasing properties
  - HDL-cholesterol increasing properties

When 48 diabetic volunteers were given Honey daily, for 8 weeks, total cholesterol ($p < 0.001$), LDL-cholesterol ($p < 0.001$) and triglycerides ($p < 0.001$) decreased significantly, but HDL-cholesterol ($p < 0.01$) increased significantly, compared to the control group (Bahrami et.al. 2009).

When volunteers were given 75 grams Honey daily, for 15 days, total cholesterol decreased by 7%, LDL-cholesterol decreased by 1%, triglycerides decreased by 2%, Homocysteine decreased by 6%, but HDL-cholesterol increased by 2%, compared to the control group (Al-Waili 2004).

When 55 obese volunteers were given Honey 70 grams daily, for 4 weeks, total cholesterol decreased by 3.15%, LDL-cholesterol decreased by 5.05%, triglycerides decreased by 15%, but HDL-cholesterol increased by an average of 3.3% ($p < 0.05$ in all parameters), compared to the control group (Yaghoobi et.al. 2008).

When 155 hyperlipidemic volunteers were given Honey and Pollen daily, total cholesterol decreased by 18.3% and LDL-cholesterol decreased by 23.9%, compared to the control group (Kasianenko et.al. 2011).

When hyperlipidemic rats were given honey 20 mg/kg daily, for 2 months, triglycerides decreased by 51.9% ($p < 0.01$), total cholesterol decreased by 44.0% ($p < 0.01$) and LDL-cholesterol decreased 62.2% ($p < 0.01$), but HDL-cholesterol increased by 62.6% ($p < 0.05$), compared to the control group (Adnan et.al. 2011).

When diabetic rats were given Honey 10 mg/kg daily, for 6 weeks, total cholesterol decreased by 19.5% ($p < 0.05$), LDL-cholesterol decreased by 43.7% ($p < 0.05$) and triglycerides decreased by 24.2% ($p < 0.05$), but HDL-cholesterol increased by 11.1% ($p < 0.05$), compared to the control group (Sheriff et.al. 2011).

When hypertensive rats were given 1.0 g/kg Honey daily, for 3 weeks, systolic blood pressure decreased by 10% (p < 0.01), compared to the control group (Erejuwa et.al. 2011).

The cholesterol decreasing properties of Honey has been verified also in many other animal experiments (Munstedt et.al. 2009; Busserolles et.al. 2002; Nemoseek et.al. 2011).

Hypocaloric protein diet

In hypocaloric protein diet people eat a lot of protein containing food, like meat, fish, chicken etc., and only very small amounts of carbohydrates and fat, so as to minimize the daily amount of calories.

Hypocaloric protein diet has
- Blood pressure lowering properties
- Total cholesterol lowering properties
- LDL-cholesterol lowering properties
- Triglycerides lowering properties
- Body weight lowering properties

When 83 diabetic volunteers were 16 weeks on protein diet or protein diet plus 3 aerobic exercise weekly, systolic blood pressure decreased by an average of 15 mmHg (139.5 mmHg → 124.5 mmHg; p < 0.001), and diastolic blood pressure decreased by 8 mmHg (81 mmHg → 73 mmHg; p < 0.001). Triglycerides decreased by an average of 23.6% (p < 0.001), total cholesterol decreased by an average of 9.2% (p < 0.001) and body weight decreased by an average of 11.4 kg, compared to control values (Wycherley et.al. 2010).

When 32 volunteers were 8 weeks on a protein diet, where they ate 4 times weekly different beans, 160 – 320 grams at a time, body weight decreased by an average of 7.8%, which was significantly (p = 0.024) more, than in the control group with the same calorific value in their diet. Also total cholesterol (p < 0.05), LDL-cholesterol (p < 0.05) and blood pressure (p < 0.05) decreased significantly, compared to the control group (Hemsdorff et.al. 2011).

When 100 volunteers were 12 weeks on protein diet, they lost body weight by an average of 7.3 kg. Triglycerides decreased by an average of 21.9% (p < 0.001), total cholesterol decreased by an average of 8.3% (p < 0.001) and LDL-cholesterol decreased by an average of 6.8% (p < 0.001). The control group was given carbohydrates (Noakes et.al. 2005).

When 215 volunteers were 12 weeks on protein diet, they lost body weight by an average of 6.8 kg. Triglycerides decreased by an average of 0.47 mmol/L, which was significantly (p < 0.001) more, than the 0.27 mmol/L in the control group (Clifton et.al. 2009).

When volunteers were 12 weeks on a protein diet, or protein diet plus 3 physical exercise weekly, body weight decreased in the protein group by 4.6 kg and in the exercised protein group by 7.0 kg. The control group lost 2.1 kg of body weight. Total cholesterol decreased significantly in both groups, and LDL-cholesterol decreased significantly in the protein group. Triglycerides decreased significantly in the protein plus exercise group (Meckling et.al. 2007).

When in hypocaloric protein diet, volunteers can easily lose at least 6 kg body weigt in 3 months.

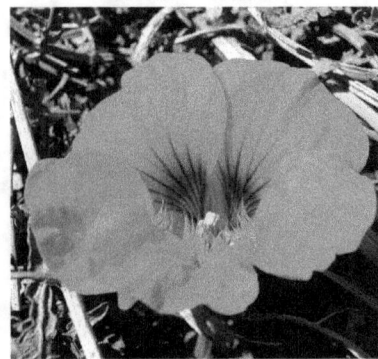

Indian Cress

(Tropaeolum Majus)

Indian Cress is a well-known, very large growing Cress species, which has large, decorative flowers. Indian Cress is eatable, and especially its flowers are used in salads. Its cultivation is very easy.

Indian Cress has
 – Blood pressure lowering properties
 – Diuretic properties

Indian Cress is used in many countries, especially in South-America and Brazil, as a diuretic, to increase the volume of urine.

This has been verified also in 2 research experiments, where Indian Cress increased significantly the urine volume and Sodium content of urine in rats (Gasparatto et.al. 2010; Gasparatto et.al. 2009).

The ethanol extract decreases significantly the mean average blood pressure (MPA) of rats (Gasparatto et.al. 2011). The effective compound is Isoquercetin, which lowers blood pressure and inhibits ACE in rats (Gasparatto et.al. 2011).

Jaffa Sweetie

(Citrus Paradisi x Citrus Grandis)

Jaffa Sweetie is a green Citrus fruit, which looks almost as Grapefruit. Its taste is sweet, and not sour like Grapefuit.

Jaffa Sweetie has
 – Blood pressure lowering properties
 – Total cholesterol lowering properties
 – LDL-cholesterol lowering properties
 – Triglycerides lowering properties

When 72 volunteers with high cholesterol values were given Jaffa Sweetie juice either 1 dl or 2 dl daily, for 30 days, total cholesterol decreased y 9.5% (8.02 mmol/L → 7.34 mmol/L), LDL-cholesterol decreased by 11.8% (6.37 mmol/L → 5.63 mmol/L, p < 0.01) and triglycerides decreased by 11.5% (2.27 mmol/L → 2.01 mmol/L) in the 1 dl group. In the 2 dl group, total cholesterol decreased by 16.1% (8.02 mmol/L → 6.73 mmol/L; p < 0.0125), LDL-cholesterol decreased y 21.0% (6.37 mmol/L → 5.03 mmol/L; p < 0.0005) and triglycerides decreased by 24.7% (2.27 mmol/L → 1.71 mmol/L; p < 0.0005) (Gorinstein et.al. 2004). The higher the juice intake, the more cholesterol- and triglyceride values decreased.

Same kind of results have been obtained also in experiments with rats (Gorinstein et.al. 2003).

When 12 volunteers were given Jaffa Sweetie juice daily for 5 weeks, both diastolic blood pressure (p = 0.04) and systolic blood pressure decreased, compared to the control group (Resherf et.al. 2005). This was a doubble blind experiment.

Japanese Honeysuckle

(Lonicera Japonica)

dried flower bud

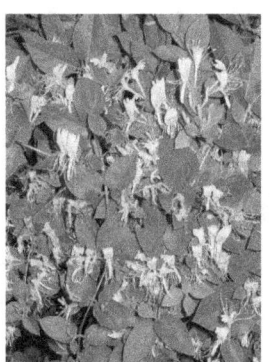

*(Author: **William Rafti of the William Rafti Institute**)*

The dried flower bud of Japanese Honeysuckle is a very famous medicinal plant in Asia, especially in China, Korea and Japan. It is strongly antibacterial and antiviral and it is used against bacterial- and viral infections, allergic inflammations and high blood pressure. The dried flower bud contains large amounts of Flavonoids Luteolin and Rutin, and also Biflavonoids and Chlorogenic acid. The Chinese call it JIN YIN HUA.

Japanese Honeysuckle has
   – Blood pressure lowering properties

The dried flower bud decreases blood pressure in both normotensive and hypertensive mice (Hsu et.al. 1994). The effective compound is Chlorogenic acid.

The methanolic extrct of the flower bud strongly inhibits ACE, and the effective compound was found to be Chlorogenic acid (Xian-Gang et.al. 2009).

Chlorogenic acid is known to lower blood pressure (Zhao et.al. 2011).

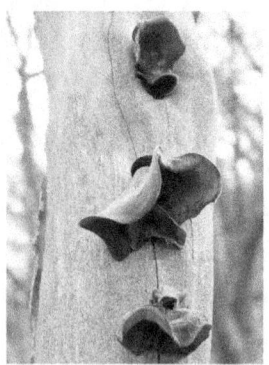

Jew's Ear

(Auricularia Auricula)

Jew's Ear is an Ancient food- and medicinal mushroom, which is widely cultivated in Asia, especially in China, Korea and Japan. It can be purchased also from Ethnic Shops.

Jew's Ear has
- Total cholesterol lowering properties
- LDL-cholesterol lowering properties
- Triglycerides lowering properties
- HDL-cholesterol increasing properties

The serum cholesterol and triglycerides lowering properties of Jew's Ear are well documented in rats, mice and rabbits.

When rats were given Jew's Ear 5% in their daily diet, for 4 weeks, total cholesterol decreased by 17% and LDL-cholesterol decreased by 24%, compared to the control group (Cheung et.al. 1996).

In other experiments, researchers have noticed, that Jew's Ear decreases total cholesterol, LDL-cholesterol and triglycerides, but increases HDL-cholesterol (Chen et.al. 2011; Ya-Ming et.al. 1989; Qwin et.al. 2010; Chen et.al. 2008).

Kale

(Brassica Oleracea var. Acephala)

Kale has been cultivated as a food for a very long time. There is both dark green Kale and red Kale. Kale has a very high amount of nutrients, especially beta-Carotene, vitamin K, vitamin C, Lutein and Zeaxanthin.

Kale has
- LDL-cholesterol lowering properties
- HDL-cholesterol increasing properties

When 32 hyperlipidemic volunteers were given 1.5 dl Kale juice daily, for 3 months, LDL-cholesterol decreased by 10% ($p < 0.0007$) and HDL-cholesterol increased by 27% ($p < 0.0001$) and HDL/LDL-ratio increased by 52% ($p < 0.0001$), compared to the control group (Kim et.al. 2008).

Kelp

(Laminaria Japonica)

Kelp is a brown algae, which consists of several different algae species, especially Laminaria Japonica and other Laminaria species. Kelp is extremely popular food in Korea, China and Japan. It has been eaten as a functional food for thousand of years.

Kelp has
- Total cholesterol lowering properties
- LDL-cholesterol lowering properties
- Triglycerides lowering properties
- HDL-cholesterol increasing properties

When rats were given 200 mg/kg Kelp flour daily, for 4 weeks, total cholesterol decreased by 10.8% ($p < 0.05$), LDL-cholesterol decreased by 7.9% ($p < 0.05$) and triglycerides decreased by 8.5% ($p < 0.05$), but HDL-cholesterol increased by 10.7% ($p < 0.05$), compared to the control group (Lee et.al. 2011).

The triglycerides, total cholesterol and LDL-cholesterol lowering but HDL-cholesterol increasing property of Kelp has been noticed in many experiments with mice, rats, rabbits and birds (Huang et.al. 2008; Huang et.al. 2010; Yuan et.al. 2010; Xu et.al. 2010; Liu et.al. 2006; Gao et.al. 2005; Tang et.al. 1989).

Ketogenic Diet

Ketogenic diet contains a lot of protein from fish, meat and chicken, and only very small amount of carbohydrates and fat, but a lot of fresh vegetables, and fruits. Olive oil or Sesame oil is used as cooking and salad oil. Red wine can be used as drink. Daily calorific value is unlimited.

Ketogenic diet is extremely effective to reduce body weight, and also very effective to reduce high blood pressure and high cholesterol values.

Ketogenic diet has
- Blood pressure lowering properties
- Total cholesterol lowering properties
- LDL-cholesterol lowering properties
- Triglycerides lowering properties
- HDL-cholesterol increasing properties
- Body weight lowering properties

When 31 obese volunteers were on Ketogenic diet for 12 weeks, body weight decreased by 14.14 kg (108.52 kg → 94.48 kg), systolic blood pressure (84.5 mmHg → 75.2 mmHg), total cholesterol (208.2 mg/dl → 186.6 mg/dl), triglycerides (218.7 mg/dl → 113.9 mg/dl) and LDL-cholesterol (114.5 mg/dl → 106 mg/dl) decreased significantly, but HDL-cholesterol (50.1 mg/dl → 54.5

mg/dl) increased significantly. The biggest drop was for triglycerides, 47.9% (Perez-Guisado et.al. 2008).

When volunteers were on Ketogenic diet for 6 weeks, body weight (86.15 kg → 79.43 kg), total cholesterol (204 mg/dl → 181 mg/dl), LDL-cholesterol (150 mg/dl → 136 mg/dl) and triglycerides (119 mg/dl → 93 mg/dl) decreased significantly, but HDL-cholesterol (46 mg/dl → 52 mg/dl) increased significantly (Paoli et.al. 2011).

When obese children, age between 12 – 15, were on Ketogenic diet for 12 weeks, body weight decreased by 15.4 kg and total cholesterol decreased 25.3% (162 mg/dl → 121 mg/dl) (Will et.al. 1998).

Typically the body weight decreases in Ketogenic diet, where daily calorific value is not limited, by an average of 1.2 kg per week.

Kidney bean

(Phaseolus Vulgaris)

The red Kidney beans are very protein- and fiber rich and healthy beans, which can be purchased in Supermarkets either as dry beans or canned, ready to use beans.

Kidney beans have
- Total cholesterol lowering properties
- LDL-cholesterol lowering properties

When volunteers were given 200 grams Kidney beans daily, for only 2 weeks, total cholesterol decreased by 6% (p < 0.05) and LDL-cholesterol decreased by 9% (p < 0.05), compared to the control group (Trinidad et.al. 2010).

The cholesterol lowering effect of Kidney bean has been verified also in experiments with rats (McPerson 1991; Rosa et.al. 1998).

Kiwifruit

(Actinidia Chinensis, Actinidia Deliciosa, Actinidia Polygama)

Kiwifruit is a very delicious fruit, which can be purchased from every supermarket. There are many different Kiwifruit species, and they originate from China, Korea and Siberia. Nowadays Kiwifruit is cultivated all around the World.

Kiwifruit has
  – Blood pressure lowering properties
  – Total cholesterol lowering properties
  – LDL-cholesterol lowering properties
  – Triglycerides decreasing properties
  – HDL-cholesterol increasing properties

When 102 volunteers were given 3 Kiwifruits daily, for 8 weeks, systolic blood pressure decreased by 10 mmHg ($p=0.019$) and diastolic blood pressure decreased by 9 mmHg ($p=0.016$), compared to the control group (Karlsen et.al. 2012). Also ACE activity was decreased by 11% ($p=0.034$).

When 43 hyperlipidemic volunteers were given daily 2 Kiwifruits, for 8 weeks, HDL-cholesterol increased ($p < 0.05$) significantly, but total cholesterol/HDL-cholesterol ratio ($p < 0.05$) and LDL-cholesterol/HDL-cholesterol ratio decreased ($p < 0.05$) significantly, compared to the control group (Chang et.al. 2009).

When volunteers were given 2 – 3 Kiwifruits daily, for 28 days, triglycerides decreased by 15% ($p < 0.05$), compared to the control group (Duttaroy et.al. 2004).

When 24 volunteers were given 2 Kiwiruits daily, for 4 weeks, triglycerides decreased by 11.6% ($p=0.05$), compared to the control group (Brevik et.al. 2011).

The 70% ethanol extract of Kiwifruit, at a dose of 10 mg/dl, inhibits ACE by 21 – 26% and HMG-CoA by 13 – 14%, and at a dose of 50 mg/ml, inhibits ACE by 46 – 49% and HMG-CoA by 19 – 30% (Jung et.al. 2005).

The water-ethanol extract of Kiwifruit (Actinidia Polygama) inhibits very strongly ACE (Nagai et.al. 2011).

L-Arginine

L-Arginine is an amino acid, which exists both in human body and in food. Peanuts, Almonds, Walnuts, Beans and Sunflower seeds are very rich in L-Arginine.

L-Arginine has
- Blood pressure lowering properties

It has been known for a long time, that acute high dose of L-Arginine causes strong hypotension in normotensive healthy volunteers (Keiichi et.al. 1992). In this trial the volunteers were given 30 grams of L-Arginine within 30 minutes. The drop in mean arterial pressure (MAP) was 10.5 mmHg (from 79.3 mmHg to 68.8 mmHg).

In a meta-analysis, which consisted of 11 separate doubble blind trials, it was noticed, that L-Arginine lowered both the systolic blood pressure (5.39 mmHg; $p < 0.01$) and the diastolic blood pressure (2.66 mmHg; $p < 0.01$) (Dong et.al. 2011). The number of volunteers was 387, and the used daily doses of L-Arginine were between 4 – 24 grams.

L-Carnitine

L-Carnitine is a B-vitamin like compound, which exists naturally in every living cell. It has a very important role in the oxidation of fatty acids. The human cells make L-Carnitine from the amino acid Lysine. Both in animal and human experiments, L-Carnitine increases aerobic endurance.

L-Carnitine has
- Blood pressure decreasing properties
- Total cholesterol decreasing properties
- LDL-cholesterol decreasing properties
- VLDL-cholesterol decreasing properties
- oxLDL-cholesterol decreasing properties
- Triglycerides decreasing properties
- HDL-cholesterol increasing properties

When 40 diabetic volunteers were given 2.0 grams L-Carnitine daily, for 3 months, LDL-cholesterol decreased by 9.0% (3.98 mmol/L → 3.53 mmol/L; $p < 0.05$) triglycerides decreased by 30.5% (3.31 mmol/L → 2.30 mmol/L; $p < 0.001$) and oxidised oxLDL-cholesterol decreased by 25.9% ($p < 0.001$), compared to the control group (Mazlaguarnera et.al. 2009).

When 36 dialysis patients were given L-Carnitine 1.0 grams daily, for 12 weeks, both total cholesterol ($p < 0.001$) and triglycerides ($p < 0.001$) decreased significantly, compared to the control group (Shakeri et.al. 2007).

When 74 hepatitis patients were given L-Carnitine 2.0 grams daily, for 24 weeks, total cholesterol decreased by 21.5% (6.09 mmol/L → 4.78 mmol/L; $p < 0.001$), LDL-cholesterol decreased by

30.3% (4.52 mmol/L → 3.15 mmol/L; p < 0.001) and triglycerides decreased by 23.8% (3.07 mmol/L → 2.34 mmol/L; p < 0.001), but HDL-cholesterol increased by 20.8% (0.96 mmol/L → 1.16 mmol/L; p < 0.001), compared to the control group (Malaguarnera et.al. 2010). This was a double blind experiment.

Also in hepatitis C patients, L-Carnitine decreases significantly both total cholesterol (p < 0.05) and triglycerides (p < 0.05), compared to the control group (Romano et.al. 2008).

When 12 dialysis patients, with high triglyceride values but low HDL-cholesterol values, were given L-Carnitine 20 mg/kg daily, for 120 days, triglycerides decreased by 50.4% (361 mg/dl → 181 mg/dl; p < 0.01) but HDL-cholesterol increased by 100.0% (31 mg/dl → 62 mg/dl; p < 0.01), compared to the control values (Vacha et.al. 1983).

When 18 dialysis patients were given L-Carnitine intravenously at a dose of 15 mg/kg, 3 times per week, for 6 months, total cholesterol decreased by 19.0% (4.57 mmol/L → 3.70 mmol/L; p = 0.03) and triglycerides decreased by 41.8% (3.06 mmol/L → 1.78 mmol/L; p = 0.004), compared to the placebo group (Mitwalli et.al. 2005).

When 40 dialysis patients were given 500 mg L-Carnitine daily, for 2 months, triglycerides decreased by 13.0% (p < 0.01) and VLDL-cholesterol decreased by 12.9% (p = 0.01), but HDL-cholesterol increased by 17.7% (p < 0.05), compared to the control group (Argani et.al. 2005).

The triglycerides, total cholesterol, LDL-cholesterol and VLDL-cholesterol decreasing but HDL-cholesterol increasing properties of L-Carnitine has been verified in a number of human experiments (Digiesi et.al. 1994; Fernandez et.al. 1992; Derosa et.al. 2011) and animal experiments (Elgazzar et.al. 2011).

In experiements with hypertensive animals, L-Carnitine decreases significantly both systolic and diastolic blood pressure (Mate et.al. 2010; Patel et.al. 2008; Rauchova et.al. 1998; Miguel-Carrasco et.al. 2010).

L-Carnitine inhibits ACE and increases eNOS activity (Miguel-Carrasco et.al. 2010).

L-Carnosine

L-Carnosine is a dipeptide, made from two amino acids, beta-Alanine and L-Histidine. L-Carnosine occurs in large amounts in muscles, heart and neural tissue. L-Carnosine is a very strong antioxidnat. It is under intensive research, due to its anti-aging properties.

Nowadays tens of antihypertensive dipeptides, tripeptides and multipeptides are known, from different food hydrolysates, which inhibit strongly ACE and lower blood pressure.

L-Carnosine can be purchased from Supermarkets.

L-Carnosine has:
   – Blood pressure lowering properties.

Japanese researchers have discovered, that L-Carnosine inhibits ACE. The effect was stronger, together with Copper or Zinc (Nakagawa et.al. 2006).

When rats were fed in their daily food either 0.0001% or 0.001% L-Carnosine, for 5 weeks, systolic blood pressure decreased significantly ($p < 0.005$), compared to the control group (Niijima et.al. 2002).

Japanese researchers have discovered, that even small intravascular doses of L-Carnosine in rats strongly decrease the mean average blood pressure (MAP) (Tanaida et.al. 2005).

L-Citrulline

L-Citrulline is a naturally occuring amino acid, which exists in food and is also synthetized in living cells from L-Arginine or Ornithine. Watermelon contains very large amounts of L-Citrulline, both in fruit pulp and fruit peel, typically between 130 – 190 mg/100 g (Rimando et.al. 2005).

L-Citrulline has
   – Blood pressure decreasing properties
   – Blood vessel elasticity increasing properties

When 17 young volunteers were given 6 grams L-Citrulline daily, for 4 weeks, systolic blood pressure decreased by 6 mmHg ($p < 0.05$), compared to the placebo group (Figueroa et.al. 2010).

When 14 hypertensive volunteers were given 6 grams L-Citrulline extracted from Watermelon daily, for 6 weeks, systolic blood pressure decreased by 11.5 mmHg ($p < 0.05$) and diastolic blood pressure decreased by 7.8 mmHg ($p < 0.05$), compared to the placebo group (Figueroa et.al. 2012).

When 9 hypertensive volunteers were given extract of Watermelon containing 2.7 grams L-Citrulline and 1.2 grams L-Arginine daily, for 6 weeks, systolic blood pressure decreased by 7 mmHg (134 mmHg → 127 mmHg; $p < 0.05$), compared to the placebo group (Figueroa et.al. 2011).

When 15 patients with heart disease were given Citrullinemalate 3 grams daily, for 2 months, systolic blood pressure decreased by 10.8% and diastolic blood pressure decreased by 8.3%, compared to the placebo group (Orozco-Gutierrez et.al. 2010). This was a double blind experiment,

When 15 healthy volunteers were given L-Citrulline 5.6 grams daily, for 7 days, blood vessel elasticity increased significantly ($p < 0.01$), compared to the control group. Plasma L-Citrulline concentration ($p < 0.05$), L-arginine concentration ($p < 0.01$) and NO concentration ($p < 0.05$) increased significantly, compared to the control group (Ochiai et.al. 2012).

In experiments with rats, L-Citrulline significantly decreases blood pressure in hypertensive rats (Koeners et.al. 2007; El-Bassossy et.al. 2012).

Arginase-entzyme converts L-Arginine to Ornithine, thus decreasing NO production via eNOS entzyme. But L-Citrulline inhibits Arginase, thus increasing NO from L-Arginine vie the eNOS entzyme (El-Bassossy et.al. 2012). NO is a strong vasodilator and decreases blood pressure.

L-Serine

L-Serine is a natural amino acid, which exists both in human cells and in food.

L-Serine has
- Blood pressure lowering properties

When L-Serine was given intravenously to rats at a dose of 1 mmol/kg, it decreased the mean average blood pressure (MAP) both in normotensive rats, with 22% decrease (108 mmHg → 84 mmHg; $p < 0.01$) and in hypertensive rats, with 34% decrease (166 mmHg → 109 mmHg; $p < 0.01$), compared to the control group (Mishra et.al. 2010).

The blood pressure lowering effect of L-Serine has been noticed in other experiments too (Mishra et.al. 2007; Mishra et.al. 2008). The blood pressure decreases more, when the L-Serine dose increases. Heart rate does not change.

Japanese researchers studied 12 normotesive volunteers and 12 hypertensive volunteers. The researchers measured 26 different amino acid contents in plasma. Only 4 amino acids, Taurine, Threonine, L-Serine and Methionine were significantly different between these 2 groups. The concentrations of these amino acids were significantly lower in hypertensive volunteers, compared to normotensive volunteers. The most significant difference was in L-Serine content (10.8 mmol/dl versus 13.4 mmol/dl; $p < 0.001$) (Ogawa et.al. 1983).

L-Serine decreases significantly the Homocysteine content in human plasma (Verhoef et.al. 2004). Homocysteine is a strong risk factor in cardiovascular diseases.

L-Tryptophan

L-Tryptophan is an essential amino acid in human diet.

L-Tryptophan has:
- Blood pressure lowering properties.

When 14 volunteers with hypertension were given 50 mg/kg L-Tryptophan, blood pressure decreased significantly 60 – 120 minutes after the dose (Feltkamp et.al. 1984).

When hypertensive rats were given L-Tryptophan, blood pressure decreased significantly after 2 hours (Sved et.al. 1982).

When hypertensive rats were given L-Tryptophan, either acutely or chronically for 3 weeks, blood pressure decreased significantly (Ardiansyah et.al. 2011).

The brains makes Melatonin from L-Tryptophan, which is known to lower blood pressure.

Lemon

(Citrus Limon)

Lemon is well known to everybody as a sour Citrus fruit. The acidity is due to Citric acid. The concentration of Citric acid in Lemon is typically 5 – 6%. The PH value is typically between 2 – 3. Besides Lemon pulp, also Lemon peel and Lemon juice are used in cooking and salads. Lemon contains large amounts of Flavonoids, especially Eriocitrin (9.5 mg/100 g), Hesperidin (15.8 mg/100 g), Naringin (0.2 mg/100 g) and Narirutin (0.8 mg/100 g) (Peterson et.al. 2006). Lemon contains large amounts of Pectin, which decreases cholesterol.

Lemon has
- – Blood pressure decreasing properties
- – Total cholesterol decreasing properties
- – LDL-cholesterol decreasing properties
- – Triglycerides decreasing properties
- – HDL-cholesterol increasing properties

When rats were fed 5% strong Lemon juice daily, for 16 weeks, blood pressure decreased significantly, compared to the control group. Also the Flavonoid fraction extracted from Lemon juice decreased significantly ($p < 0.05$) blood pressure, compared to the control group (Miyake et.al. 1998).

Both Eriocitrin and Hesperidin inhibits ACE (Miyake et.al. 1998).

In Turkey, up to 40% of hypertensive persons use Lemon juice to control their high blood pressure (Adibelli et.al. 2009).

The Flavonoid Hesperidin in Lemon decreases significantly the blood pressure of hypertensive rats (Yamamoto et.al. 2008).

Citric acid in Lemon, by itself decreases blood pressure. When rats were given Citric acid 15 mg/kg, the mean average blood pressure (MAP) decreased by 71% (Saleem et.al. 2004).

The Flavonoids in Lemon peel decrease blood pressure (Kunamoto et.al. 1985).

When volunteers were given Hesperidin 292 mg daily, for 4 weeks,diastolic blood pressure decreased by 5.3 mmHg ($p = 0.023$), compared to the control group (Morand et.al. 2011).

When volunteers were given Citrus fruit Peetin 15 grams daily, for 6 weeks, total cholesterol decreased by 8.6% in mildly hyperlipidemic volunteers, and by 16.7%, in hyperlipidemic volunteers (Ginter et.al. 1979).

When hyperlipidemic volunteers were given Hesperidin 500 mg daily, for 6 or 24 weeks, triglycerides decreased significantly in over 50% of the volunteers (Miwa et.al. 2005; Miwa et.al. 2004).

When hamsters were given 3% of Lemon peel or 3% Lemon Pectin in their daily diet, for 8 weeks, total cholesterol decreased by 16.7% in the Lemon peel group, and 22.6% in the Lemon Pectin group, compared to the control group (Tepstra et.al. 2002).

When hyperlipidemic rabbits were given Lemon juice 1 ml/kg daily, for 30 days, total cholesterol decreased by 56.3% ($p < 0.005$), LDL-cholesterol decreased by 55.1% ($p < 0.005$) but HDL-cholesterol increased by 57.7% ($p < 0.05$), compared to the control group (Khan et.al. 2010).

When hyperlipidemic rats were fed 0.35% Eriocitrin in their daily diet, for 3 weeks, LDL-cholesterol ($p < 0.05$), VLDL-cholesterol ($p < 0.05$) and triglycerides ($p < 0.05$) decreased significantly, compared to the control group (Miyake et.al. 2006).

Lemon Balm

(Melissa Officinalis)

Lemon Balm is very popular and famous tea plant, which has been used in Europe for hundreds of years. As a medicinal plant, it has been used against high blood pressure, sleep problems, as an antiviral and as an antibacterial. Lemon Balm contains a lot of Flavonoids (Luteolin, Luteolin Glucosides, Isoquercetin etc.) and also Rosmarinic acid and Ursolic acid. The Lemon Balm tea has excellent taste. Also Lemon Balm can be used as a salad component.

Lemon Balm has
   – Blood pressure lowering properties
   – Total cholesterol lowering properties

Lemon Balm water extract inhibits strongly ACE (Kwon et.al. 2006), which might explain its blood pressure lowering properties.

When rats with high cholesterol levels were given Lemon Balm at a dose of 2 g/kg daily, for 4 weeks, total cholesterol decreased by 48.3% ($p < 0.0001$) and serum total lipids decreased by 52.9% ($p < 0.0001$), compared to the control group (Bolkent et.al. 2005).

Lemon Grass

(Cymbopogon Citratus)

Lemon Grass is very popular spice and tea all around the World. In South-America it is a popular tea. In Cuba and in many other countries, it is used against high blood pressure.

Lemon Grass has
- Blood pressure lowering properties
- Total cholesterol lowering properties
- LDL-cholesterol lowering properties
- Triglycerides lowering properties
- HDL-cholesterol increasing properties

When rats were given Lemon Grass water extract 135 – 500 mg/kg daily, for 42 days, total cholesterol ($p < 0.05$), LDL-cholesterol ($p < 0.05$) and triglycerides ($p < 0.05$) decreased significantly, but HDL-cholesterol ($p < 0.05$) increased significantly, compared to the control group (Adeneye et.al. 2007).

The cholesterol lowering effect of Lemon Grass has been noticed also in experiments with mice (Costa et.al. 2011).

When rats were given Lemon Grass extract, with a 1 mg dose, the mean average blood pressure (MAP) decreased from 122 mmHg to 106 mmHg, and the blood pressure drop was equal to the blood pressure drop of ethanol extract of Garlic (Singi et.al. 2005).

When rats were given Lemon Grass extract, the mean average blood pressure (MAP) decreased significantly (Carbajal et.al. 1989). This blood pressure lowering property of Lemon Grass has been noticed also in other experiments (Bastos et.al. 2010).

Lime leaves

(Citrus Limetta)

Lime fruit is the familiar small, dark green Citrus fruit, which is grown all over the World, from Mediterranian Sea to Mexico. Lime tree leaves are used in Mexico to decrease high blood pressure.

Lime leaves have
- Blood pressure lowering properties

When mice were given Angiotensin II, to make them hypertensive, and then were given Lime leaves water extract at a dose of 125 mg/kg, systolic blood pressure decreased by 20 mmHg ($p < 0.0001$) and diastolic blood pressure decreased by 20 mmHg ($p < 0.0002$), compared to the control group. The effect was the same, as with 3.0 mg/kg Telmisartanin (Perez et.al. 2010).

Lipoic acid

Lipoic acid is a natural, essential, vitamin like compound in human body. Lipoic acid is needed in the cell energy production. Lipoic acid is a very strong antioxidant.

Lipoic acid has
- Blood pressure lowering properties
- Total cholesterol lowering properties
- LDL-cholesterol lowering properties
- Triglycerides lowering properties
- HDL-cholesterol increasing properties

In experiments with rats, Lipoic acid decreases systolic blood pressure, compared to the control group (Vasdev et.al. 2000).

In experiments with rats, Lipoic acid decreases total cholesterol, LDL-cholesterol and triglycerides, but increases HDL-cholesterol (Thirunavukkarasu et.al. 2004; Jayanthi et.al. 1992; Segermann et.al. 1991).

Luobuma tea

(Apocynum Venetum)

Luobuma tea is a very popular drink in North China. The tea is made from the leaves of Apocynum Venetum. It is cultivated in large scale in China, Korea and Japan. Luobuma tea contains large amount of Flavonoids, especially Quercetin and Apocynin. In Japan it is called Rafuma.

Luobuma tea has
- Blood pressure lowering properties
- Total cholesterol lowering properties
- LDL-cholesterol lowering properties
- HDL-cholesterol increasing properties

When 116 hypertensive volunteers were given Luobuma tea in pill form daily, for 5 weeks, systolic blood pressure decreased by 19.2 mmHg ($p < 0.01$) and diastolic blood pressure decreased by 12.9 mmHg ($p < 0.01$), compared to the control group (Gao et.al. 2010).

When 102 hypertensive volunteers were given Luobuma tea daily, for 45 days, both systolic blood pressure ($p < 0.05$) and diastolic blood pressure ($p < 0.05$) decreased significantly, compared to the control group (Dai et.al. 2010).

When rats were given Luobuma tea daily, for 40 days, total cholesterol decreased by 18.6% ($p < 0.01$), LDL-cholesterol decreased by 19.6% ($p < 0.01$) but HDL-cholesterol increased by 23.2% ($p < 0.05$), compared to the control group (Kim et.al. 1998).

The blood pressure lowering and HDL-cholesterol increasing property of Luobuma tea has been verified also in other experiments (Kim et.al. 2000; Ma et.al. 1989).

Luteolin

Luteolin is a Flavonoid, which exists in plants, especially Dandelion (Taraxacum Officinalis) and Artichoke (Cynara Scolymus) leaves. Luteolin is a strong antioxidant, and it has many pharmacological properties.

Luteolin has
- Blood pressure lowering properties

When rats were given orally 50 mg/kg Luteolin, blood pressure decreased up to 24 hours very strongly (20 mmHg; $p < 0.01$), compared to the control group (Ichimura et.al. 2006).

When pigs were given Luteolin 1.0 mg/kg, 1.5 mg/kg or 5 mg/kg, both systolic and diastolic blood pressure decreased significantly, compared to the control group (Abdalla et.al. 1994).

When cats and dogs were given Luteolin, blood pressure decreased significantly (Liyan 1986).

Luteolin inhibits strongly ACE (Loizzo et.al. 2007).

Luteolin is a good vasorelaxant (Xu et.al. 2007).

Luteolin inhibits Endothelin-1 (ET-1), which is a vasoconstrictor, and increases blood pressure (Kozakai et.al. 2005).

Luteolin stimulates eNOS enzyme, and increases plasma NO concentration, and acts like a vasodilator and decreases blood pressure (Huige et.al. 2004).

Lycopene

Lycopene is a Carotenoid, which exists especially in Tomatoes, Watermelon and Guava. Lycopene is a very strong antioxidant.

Lycopene has
- Blood pressure lowering properties
- Total cholesterol lowering properties
- LDL-cholesterol lowering properties

When 6 volunteers were given Lycopene 60 mg daily, for 3 months, LDL-cholesterol decreased by 14% (165 mg/dl → 140 mg/dl) (Fuhrman et.al. 1997).

When 100 pregnant, hypertensive women were given Lycopene 2 mg daily, for 4 weeks, systolic blood pressure (149.7 mmHg → 130 mmHg) and diastolic blood pressure (99.9 mmHg → 80.2 mmHg) decreased significantly (Aggarwal et.al. 2009).

In a meta-analysis, which consisted of 12 human experiments, of at least 2 weeks duration, it was noticed, that Lycopene decreases strongly systolic blood pressure (5.6 mmHg; p = 0.04), LDL-cholesterol 10% (10.35 mg/dl; p = 0.0003) and total cholesterol (7.55 mg/dl; p = 0.02), compared to control group, when the daily dose was at least 25 mg (Ried et.al. 2011).

Maca

(Lepidium Meyenii)

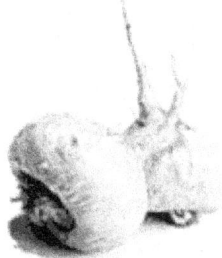

Maca is an Ancient food plant, which has been cultivated for thousands of years in South-American Andes mountains. Nowadays it can be purchased from ordinary Supermarkets.

Mace inhibits strongly ACE (Ranilla et.al. 2010).

It has been noticed, that people at Andes mountains of Peru and Ecuador, who use regularly Maca, have lower blood pressure, than those, who do not use Maca (Gonzales 2010).

When rats were given daily Maca in their food, total cholesterol, LDL-cholesterol and triglycerides decreased strongly, but HDL-cholesterol increased, compared to the control group (Vecera et.al. 2007).

When 20 women volunteers were given Maca 2 grams daily, for 4 months, total cholesterol, triglycerides and blood pressure decreased, compared to the control group (Meissner et.al. 2006). This was a doubble blind experiment.

Magnesium

Magnesium is an essential macro mineral for human beings.

Magnesium has:
  – Blood pressure lowering properties.

When 28 volunteers were given Magnesium Chloride 383 mg daily, for 6 weeks, the systolic blood pressure decreased by 7.4 mmHg (p < 0.05), compared to the control group (Purvis et.al. 1994).

When 21 volunteers were given Magnesium Oxide 1 gram daily, for 4 weeks, the mean average blood pressure (MAP) decreased significantly (Motoyama et.al. 1989).

When Magnesium is given to volunteers between 500 – 1000 mg daily, the systolic blood pressure may decrease by an average of 5.6 mmHg and the diastolic blood pressure may decrease by an average of 2.8 mmHg (Houston 2011).

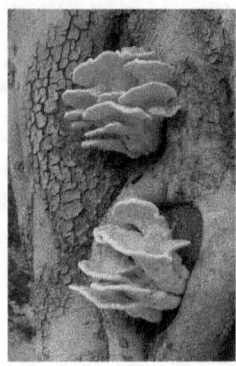

Maitake

(Grifola Frondosa)

Maitake is a very famous, eatable mushroom, which is extremely popular in Asian countries. Maitake is famous for its blood pressure decreasing properties.

Maitake has
- Blood pressure lowering properties
- Total cholesterol lowering properties
- VLDL-cholesterol lowering properties
- Triglycerides lowering properties
- HDL-cholesterol increasing properties

When hypertensive rats were given Maitake 5% of their daily diet, for 9 weeks, total cholesterol decreased by 20.8% (p < 0.01), VLDL-cholesterol decreased by 43.8% (p < 0.01) and triglycerides decreased by 6.2%, but HDL-cholesterol increased by 9.5% (p < 0.01), compared to the control group. Systolic blood pressure decreased about 7.3% (125 mmHg; p < 0.01) (Kabir et.al. 1987).

When rats were fed fiber of Maitake at a dose of 50 g/kg daily, for 4 weeks, total cholesterol decreased significantly (p < 0.05), compared to the control group (Fukushima et.al. 2001).

When rats were fed different fractions of Maitake, for 120 days, systolic blood pressure decreased 15 mmHg (p < 0.01), compared to the control group. Diastolic blood pressure decreased 13 mmHg (p < 0.05), compared to the control group (Preuss et.al. 2010).

When rats were given either Maitake or its water- or ethanol extracts, systolic blood pressure decreased by an average of 18 mmHg (p < 0.001) in different groups, compared to the control group (Talpur et.al. 2002).

Blood pressure lowering property of Maitake has been noticed also in other experiments (Talpur et.al. 2002; Kabir et.al. 1989; Kubo et.al. 1997; Adachi et.al. 1988).

Cholesterol lowering property of Maitake has been verified in other experiments also (Kubo et.al. 1996; Kubo et.al. 1997).

Mate tea

(Ilex Paraguariensis)

Mate tree is a small tree, which originates from South-America. The tea made from its leaves is called Yerba Mate in Spanish. The tea is commonly drank in Chile, Argentina, Uruguay, Paraguay and Brazil as a stimulating and healthy drink. Mate tea contains large amounts of Coffeine, Theobromine, Chlorogenic acid, Saponins and Polyphenols.

Mate tea has
- Total cholesterol decreasing properties
- LDL-cholesterol decreasing properties
- Triglycerides decreasing properties
- HDL-cholesterol increasing properties
- Body weight decreasing properties

When 72 volunteers were given 3.3 dl Mate tea, 3 times daily, for 40 days, LDL-cholesterol decreased by an average of 8.7% ($p < 0.05$) but HDL-cholesterol increased by 4.4% ($p < 0.01$), compared to the control group (de Morais et.al. 2009).

When diabetic volunteers were given Mate tea 3.3 dl, 3 times daily, for 60 days, LDL-cholesterol decreased by an average of 12.2 mg/dl ($p < 0.05$) and triglycerides decreased by 53.0 mg/dl ($p < 0.05$), compared to the control group (Klein et.al. 2011).

When diabetic mice were given Mate tea water extract 100 mg/kg daily, for 7 days, triglycerides decreased by 29.2% ($p < 0.01$) and total cholesterol decreased by 10.1% ($p < 0.01$), compared to the control group. Body weight increased by 7.2%, being significantly ($p < 0.05$) lower, than the 16.3% increase in the control group (Hussein et.al. 2011).

When mice were given Mate tea water extract 100 mg/kg daily, for 3 weeks, total cholesterol decreased by 23.1% ($p < 0.001$) and triglycerides decreased by 38.7% ($p < 0.001$), compared to the control group. Body weight increased by 3.5%, being significantly ($p < 0.05$) lower than the 5.8% increase in the control group (Hussein et.al. 2011).

When hyperlipidemic mice were given Mate tea 1.0 g/kg daily, for 8 weeks, total cholesterol decreased by 23.3% ($p < 0.01$), LDL-cholesterol decreased by 26.8% ($p < 0.01$) and triglycerides decreased by 33.4% ($p < 0.05$), compared to the control group (Arcari et.al. 2009). Body weight was 7.4% ($p < 0.05$) lower, than in the control group, after this 8 weeks test period.

The triglycerides ($p < 0.01$), total cholesterol ($p < 0.01$) and body weight ($p < 0.01$) decreasing properties of Mate tea has been verified also in experiments with rats (Przygodda et.al. 2010).

Melatonin

Melatonin is also called Sleep Hormone, The concentration of Melatonin in serum increases during sleep and darkness. Human body makes melatonin from the amino acid Tryptophan. Melatonin stimulates very strongly all the human body antioxidant systems (SOD, Catalase, GSH, GSPx, GR).

Melatonin has
- Blood pressure lowering properties
- LDL-cholesterol lowering properties
- HDL-cholesterol increasing properties

In a meta-analysis, which included 7 controlled experiments concerning the effect of Melatonin against high blood pressure, it was noticed, that Melatonin decreased systolic blood pressure by 6.1 mmHg ($p < 0.009$) and diastolic blood pressure by 3.5 mmHg ($p < 0.009$), compared to control groups. This was seen in experiments, which used Controlled Release Melatonin pills. (Grossman et.al. 2011). The number of volunteers in these experiments was 221.

When 30 volunteers with metabolic syndrome were given 5 mg Melatonin daily, for 2 hours before sleep, systolic blood presure (132.8 mmHg $\rightarrow$ 120.5 mmHg; $p < 0.01$) and diastolic blood pressure (81.7 mmHg $\rightarrow$ 75.7 mmHg; $p < 0.01$) and LDL-cholesterol (149.7 mg/dl $\rightarrow$ 139.9 mg/dl; $p < 0.05$) decreased, compared to the control group (Kozirog et.al. 2011).

In experiments with rats, Melatonin decreases significantly both LDL-cholesterol and triglycerides, but increases HDL-cholesterol (Agil et.al. 2011). Also in experiments with rats, Melatonin decreases blood pressure (Tain et.al. 2011).

Milk Thistle

(Silybum Marianum)

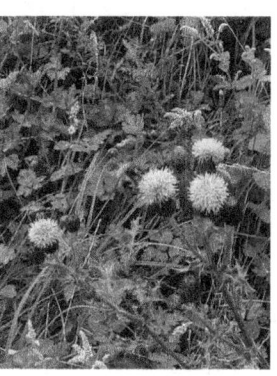

Milk Thistle is a very old medicinal- and food plant. The young leaves and seed sprouts are edible. The seed sprouts contain large amounts of Polyphenols (Vaknin et.al. 2008). From the Milk Thistle seeds a Flavonoid mixture is obtained, which is called Silymarin. The most important Flavonoids in Silymarin are: Silybin, Silydianin, Silybin A and Silybin B. Also the seeds contain Quercetin and Taxifolin, which is anticarcinogenic. Silymarin is used very much in liver diseases.

Milk Thistle seeds and Silymarin have
  – Total cholesterol decreasing properties
  – LDL-cholesterol decreasing properties
  – VLDL-cholesterol decreasing properties
  – Triglycerides decreasing properties

When 51 diabetic volunteers were given Silymarin 400 mg daily, for 4 months, total cholesterol decreased by 12.0% (225 mg/dl → 198 mg/dl; p = 0.0001), LDL-cholesterol decreased by 12.1% (140 mg/dl → 123 mg/dl; p = 0.005) and triglycerides decreased by 25.7% (294 mg/dl → 211 mg/dl; p = 0.004), compared to the control group (Huseini et.al. 1998). This was a double blind experiment.

When hyperlipidemic rats were given Silymarin either 25 mg/kg or 100 mg/kg daily, for 7 days, total cholesterol decreased by 18.8% and 36.3%, LDL-cholesterol decreased by 31.7% and 45.7%, and VLDL-cholesterol decreased by 27.8% and 25.1%, compared to the control group (Metwally et.al. 2009).

Same kind of results have been obtained also in other experiments (Sobolova et.al. 2006; Yao-Cheng et.al. 1991). In rats Silymarin decreased also blood pressure (Yao-Cheng et.al. 1991; Jadhav et.al. 2011).

Mistletoe

(Viscum Album)

Mistletoe is an ancient medicinal plant, which is commonly used in Europe, Asia and Africa against cancer and high blood pressure.

Mistletoe has
   - Blood pressure lowering properties
   - Total cholesterol lowering properties
   - LDL-cholesterol lowering properties
   - Triglycerides lowering properties
   - HDL-cholesterol increasing properties

When hypertensive rats were given Mistletoe water extract 150 mg/kg daily, for 5 weeks, the mean average blood pressure (MAP) decreased by 34.48% ($p < 0.05$), total cholesterol decreased by 20.7% ($p < 0.05$) and LDL-cholesterol decreased by 24.3% ($p < 0.05$), compared to the control group (Nkanu et.al. 2007).

When hypertensive rats were given Mistletoe daily, for 33 days, systolic blood pressure, diastolic blood pressure, total cholesterol, LDL-cholesterol and triglycerides decreased significantly, compared to the control group (Kim 2006).

When rats were given Mistletoe water extract at a dose of 200 mg/kg daily, for 10 weeks, HDL-cholesterol increased by 58.5% (0.95 mmol/L $\rightarrow$ 1.50 mmol/L; $p < 0.001$), compared to the control group (Ben et.al. 2006).

When hypertensive rats were given intravenously Mistletoe water extract either 5 mg/kg or 160 mg/kg, the mean average blood pressure (MAP) decreased by 4.8% in the 5 mg/kg group, and by 43.9% in the 160 mg/kg group (Eno et.al. 2004).

When hypertensive rats were given Mistletoe water extract 150 mg/kg daily, for 6 weeks, the mean average blood pressure (MAP) decreased significantly by 18.8% ($p < 0.001$), compared to the control group (Ofem et.al. 2007).

When hyperlipidemic rats were given Mistletoe ethanol extract 100 mg/kg daily, for 30 days, total cholesterol decreased by 59.1% ($p < 0.01$), LDL-cholesterol decreased y 24.3% ($p < 0.01$) and triglycerides decreased by 76.3% ($p < 0.01$), but HDL-cholesterol increased by 46.7% ($p < 0.001$), compared to the control group (Avei et.al. 2006).

Motherwort

(Leonurus Cardiaca)

Motherwort is an Ancient medicinal plant, which was used already in 15th century to treat cardiovascular disease, as the name "Cardiaca" tells. Motherwort is included in the Russian Pharmacopeia, and it is recommended for treating high blood pressure. Extracts of Motherwort are sold in Pharmacies in Russia, Estonia and Poland. Motherwort is easily cultivated.

Motherwort has
 – Blood pressure lowering properties

The blood pressure lowering properties of Motherwort have been shown in several experiment with humans and animals (Shikov et.al. 2011; Milkowska-Leyck et.al. 2002). One of the effective compounds is Lavandulifolioside.

Mulberry

(Morus Alba, Morus Nigra)

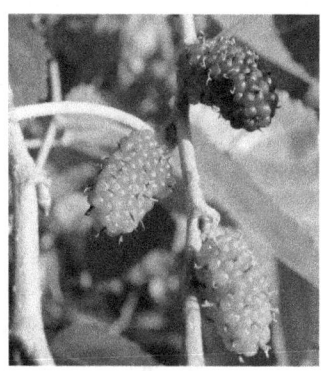

Mulberry is a famous fruit tree, whose leaves the Silkworms use as their food. The cocoon of silkworm larvae gives the famous raw silk. Mulberries are delicious berries, and they, as well the Mulberry leaves, have many medicinal uses. Both berries and leaves are used in China, Korea and Japan to decrease high blood pressure.

Mulberries have
 – Blood pressure lowering properties
 – Total cholesterol lowering properties
 – LDL-cholesterol lowering properties
 – Triglycerides lowering properties
 – HDL-cholesterol increasing properties

When 12 diabetic volunteers and 26 non-diabetic volunteers were given 100 grams fresh Mulberries daily, for 4 weeks, total cholesterol decreased in the diabetic group by 9.86% (p = 0.02) and in the non-diabetic group by 10.80% (p < 0.001). Systolic blood pressure decreased in the diabetic group by 12.18% (160 mmHg → 140.5 mmHg; p = 0.01) and in the non-diabetic group by 8.77% (123.4 mmHg → 112.6 mmHg; p < 0.001). Diastolic blood pressure decreased in the diabetic group by 5% (100 mmHg → 95 mmHg; p = 0.214) and in the non-diabetic group by 4.6% (84.2 mmHg → 80.3 mmHg; p = 0.001), compared to the control group (Abdalla et.al. 2006).

When rats were fed a diet with cholesterol and fat without Mulberries, or the same food added with 10% dried Mulberries, in their daily diet, total cholesterol decreased by 16.23% ($p < 0.05$), triglycerides decreased by 35.7% ($p < 0.05$), LDL-cholesterol decreased by 23.5% ($p < 0.05$), but HDL-cholesterol increased by 24.8% ($p < 0.05$) in the Mulberry group, compared to the control group (Yang et.al. 2010).

When rabbits were fed a diet with cholesterol and fat without Mulberries, or diet added with 5% or 10% Mulberry water extract, triglycerides decreased by 46% ($p < 0.05$) in the 5% Mulberry group, and 56% ($p < 0.01$) in the 10% Mulberry group, compared to the group without Mulberries. Also LDL-cholesterol decreased significantly in the 5% Mulberry group ($p < 0.05$) and in the 10% Mulberry group ($p < 0.01$), compared to the group without Mulberry (Chen et.al. 2005).

When rats were fed Mulberries, triglycerides decreased significantly, compared to control rats (Kim et.al. 2001).

Mung bean sprouts

(Vigna Radiata)

Mung bean sprouts are popular healthy food. They are very easy to grow home. Mung beans contain large amount of protein and dietary fiber.

Mung bean sprouts have:
- Blood pressure lowering properties
- Total cholesterol lowering properties
- Triglycerides lowering properties

Mung bean sprouts have hypotensive properties, when given both acutely and chronically to rats. When given daily for 4 weeks, systolic blood pressure decreased significantly ($p < 0.05$). At the same time the ACE activity was decreased significantly ($p < 0.05$) (Hsu et.al. 2011).

When mice were fed Mung bean sprouts 2g/kg daily, for 5 weeks, both total cholesterol and triglycerides decreased significantly (Yao et.al. 2008).

N-Acetyl-L-Cysteine

(NAC)

N-Acetyl-L-Cysteine is an amino acid. NAC is the Acetylated form of naturally in human body and food existing amino acid Cysteine.

NAC has been in use over 40 years, to help the lungs get rid of excess mucus (Mucolytic property). By this way, it is very valuable in Asthma, Chronic and Acute bronchitis etc. NAC is an extremely powerfull antioxidant.

NAC has
- Blood pressure lowering properties
- Total cholesterol lowering properties
- LDL-cholesterol lowering properties
- HDL-cholesterol increasing properties
- Triglycerides lowering properties

In experiments with rats, NAC lowers blood pressure (Fields et.al. 2009; Lahera et.al. 1993; Vasdev et.al. 1995; Cabassi et.al. 2001; Tian et.al. 2006; Pechanova et.al. 2006).

With diabetic volunteers, NAC together with L-Arginine decreases systolic blood pressure, total cholesterol, LDL-cholesterol and triglycerides, but increases HDL-cholesterol (Martina et.al. 2008).

In experiments with rats, NAC decreases triglycerides and LDL-cholesterol (Diniz et.al. 2006; Korou et.al. 2010).

In human volunteers, NAC increases significantly HDL-cholesterol by 16.2%, when the daily dose is 3600 mg NAC (Franceschini et.al. 1993).

Cysteine is essential in the biosynthesis of Reduced Glutathione, GSH, which is a tripeptide in human body. GSH is extremely powerfull antioxidant, and it inhibits strongly ACE (Wagner 1998).

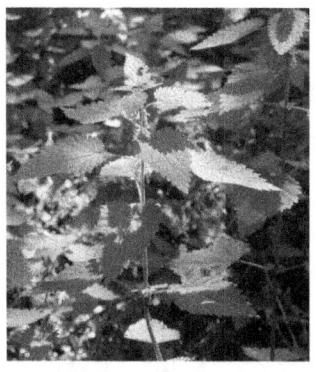

Nettle

(Urtica Dioica)

Nettle is an ancient food, fiber and medicinal plant, which is used all over the World. It has a very high content of nutrients. Young Nettles are excellent vegetables. Nettle is used in many countries in folk medicine, to decrease high blood pressure and high cholesterol and as a diuretic.

Nettle has
- Blood pressure lowering properties
- LDL-cholesterol lowering properties
- Triglycerides lowering properties
- HDL-cholesterol increasing properties
- Diuretic properties

When rats were given intravenously Nettle water extract either 4 mg/kg or 24 mg/kg dose, blood pressure decreased by 15% and 38%, urine volume increased by 11% and 84%, and Sodium in urine increased by 28% and 143%, respectively ($p < 0.001$ in all values) (Tahri et.al. 2000).

Also Nettle roots decrease blood pressure (Testai et.al. 2002).

In experiments with mice, Nettle extracts decreased LDL-cholesterol but increased HDL-cholesterol (Avci et.al. 2006).

When rats were given Nettle water extract at a dose of 150 mg/kg daily, for 30 days, both total cholesterol and LDL-cholesterol decreased significantly (Daher et.al. 2006).

Exactly same kind of cholesterol lowering results were seen in other experiments with rats, during 4 weeks test period (Nassiri-Asl et.al. 2009; Das et.al. 2011).

When 50 diabetic volunteers were given Nettle extract 100 mg/kg daily, for 8 weeks, triglycerides (143.68 mg/dl → 129.42 mg/dl; $p = 0.004$) decreased 9.92%, but HDL-cholesterol (45.29 mg/dl → 53.92 mg/dl; $p = 0.040$) increased significantly by 19.05%, compared to the control group. Systolic blood pressure (116.9 mmHg → 100 mmHg; $p = 0.06$) decreased significantly by 14.45%, compared to the control group (Namazi et.al. 2011).

Nutmeg

(Myristica Fragrans)

Nutmeg is a very old spice, which originates from Indonesian, the Moluccas Islands.

Nutmeg has
- Total cholesterol lowering properties
- LDL-cholesterol lowering properties
- Triglycerides lowering properties

The cholesterol and triglyceride lowering properties of Nutmeg has been verified in several animal experiments (Kareem et.al. 2009; Ram et.al. 1996; Sharma et.al. 1995).

Oat

(Avena Sativa)

Oat has been cultivated for a very long time, all over te Northern Hemisphere, as a human and animal food. Oat bran contains large amounts of functionally important beta-Glucans.

Whole oats and Oat bran has
- Blood pressure lowering properties
- Total cholesterol lowering properties
- LDL-cholesterol lowering properties

When volunteers were fed for 6 weeks whole oat, with a standardized amount of 5.52 grams of beta-Glucans daily, systolic blood pressure decreased 7.5 mmHg and diastolic blood pressure decreased 5.5 mmHg, compared to the control group. Total cholesterol decreased 9% and LDL-cholesterol decreased 14%, compared to the control group (Keenan et.al. 2002). This was a doubble blind experiment.

Okra

(Abelmoschus Esculentus)

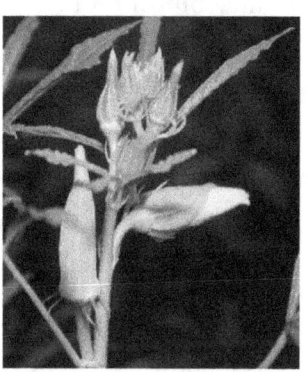

Okra is well known vegetable all over the World. The green seed pods are very healthy, and full of nutrients.

Okra seed pods have
- Total cholesterol lowering properties
- Triglycerides lowering properties
- VLDL-cholesterol lowering properties
- HDL-cholesterol increasing properties

When rats with high cholesterol levels were given methanolic extract of Okra seed pods, corresponding to 30 g/kg Okra seed pods, total cholesterol decreased by 40.50% ($p < 0.05$) and triglycerides decreased by 41.88% ($p < 0.05$), compared to the control group (Trinh et.al. 2009).

When diabetic rats were given Okra seed pods 200 mg/kg daily, for 2 weeks, total cholesterol decreased by 17.0% ($p < 0.01$), VLDL-cholesterol decreased by 45.7% ($p < 0.01$) and triglycerides decreased by 45.7% ($p < 0.01$), but HDL-cholesterol increased by 36.4% ($p < 0.01$), compared to the control group (Sabitha et.al. 2011).

Olives

(Olea Europea)

Olives are well known to everybody as the fruit of Olive tree. Olives are used in cooking all around the World. There are both green and black Olives, which are totally ripe. There are large amounts of many healthy compounds in Olives, such as Luteolin, Apigenin and especially Oleuropein and Hydroxytyrosol. These compounds are known to decrease both blood pressure and cholesterol.

Olives have
- Blood pressure decreasing properties
- Total cholesterol decreasing properties
- LDL-cholesterol decreasing properties
- HDL-cholesterol increasing properties

When rats were given intravenously the water-methanol extract of Olives at doses between 30 – 100 mg/kg, both systolic and diastolic blood pressure decreased in direct proportion to the given dose. At the dose of 100 mg/kg, the mean average blood pressure (MAP) decreased by 37.1%, compared to the control group (Gilani et.al. 2005).

When hyperlipidemic rats were given daily either the ethylacetate or water-methanol extract of either green or black Olives, at a dose of 5 mg/kg, for 16 weeks, total cholesterol and LDL-cholesterol decreased as follows: Green Olives, ethylacetate fraction, total cholesterol decreased by 24.2% and LDL-cholesterol decreased by 44.9%. Green Olives, water-methanol fraction, total cholesterol decreased by 20.5% and LDL-cholesterol decreased by 47.1%. Black Olives, ethylacetate fraction, total cholesterol decreased by 27.1% and LDL-cholesterol decreased by 68.8%, compared to controls. In all these parameters, $p < 0.05$. But HDL-cholesterol increased with every fraction, Black Olives water-methanol fractions increases HDL-cholesterol by 62.5% ($p < 0.05$), compared to the controls (Fki et.al. 2005).

Olive leaf

(Olea Europaea)

Olive tree has been cultivated for thousands of years all around the Mediterranian sea. Olives and Olive oil has been used for thousands of years as food. Olive tree leaves has been used for medicinal purposes, especially to decrease high blood pressure. The effective compounds are especially Oleuropin and Hydroxytyrosol.

Olive tree leaves have
- Blood pressure decreasing properties
- Total cholesterol decreasing properties
- LDL-cholesterol decreasing properties
- VLDL-cholesterol decreasing properties
- Triglycerides decreasing properties

– HDL-cholesterol increasing properties

When 40 pairs of twins were used as volunteers and given 1000 mg of Olive tree leaf extract EFLA943 daily, for 8 weeks, systolic blood pressure decreased 11 mmHg (137 mmHg → 126 mmHg) and diastolic blood pressure decreased 4 mmHg (80 mmHg → 76 mmHg) compared to the control group (Moccetti et.al. 2008).

When volunteers were given Olive tree leaf extract EFLA943 1000 mg daily, for 8 weeks, systolic blood pressure decreased by 11.5 mmHg and diastolic blood pressure decreased by 4.8 mmHg, compared to the control group (Susali et.al. 2011). This was a doubble blind experiment. Also triglycerides decreased significantly in the EFLA943 group.

When 30 volunteers were given Olive tree leaf extract daily for 3 months, blood pressure decreased significantly ($p < 0.01$), compared to the control group (Cherif et.al. 1996).

When rats were fed Olive tree leaf extract, blood pressure decreased significantly (Khayya et.al. 2002).

When rats were given either Oleuropin 8 mg/kg or Hydroxytyrosol 16 mg/kg daily, for 4 weeks, total cholesterol decreased significantly (Jemal et.al. 2009).

When rats were given 10% Olive tree leaves in their daily diet, for 2 months, total cholesterol decreased by 47% ($p < 0.01$), compared to the control group (Bennani-Kabchi et.al. 1999).

When hyperlipidemic rats were given Olive tree leaf extract daily, both total cholesterol, LDL-cholesterol and triglycerides decreased, but HDL-cholesterol increased (Jemal et.al. 2008).

Olive oil, Virgin

Olive oil is one of the most famous cooking- and salad oils, and it has been used around the Mediterranian sea for several thousands of years. Cold pressed Olive oil is called Virgin Olive oil. In Virgin Olive oil, all the healthy Polyphenols are left to the oil. Olive Oil has large amount of Oleic acid, up to 70 – 80%, depending on the Olive origin.

Virgin Olive oil has
– Blood pressure decreasing properties
– Total cholesterol decreasing properties
– LDL-cholesterol decreasing properties
– HDL-cholesterol increasing properties

When 64 elderly volunteers, of which 31 were hypertensive, were given 60 grams Virgin Olive oil daily, for 4 weeks, systolic blood pressure decreased 15 mmHg (150 mmHg → 135 mmHg; $p < 0.01$) in the hypertensive group, compared to the control group, which was given 60 grams Sunflower oil daily. In the normotensive group, Virgin Olive oil decreased total cholesterol by 10.8% (186.6 mg/dl → 166.6 mg/dl; $p < 0.01$) and LDL-cholesterol by 12.2% (113.0 mg/dl → 99.2 mg/dl; $p < 0.01$), compared to the Sunflower group (Perona et.al. 2004).

When 129 volunteers from Brazil, USA and Ghana, were given 30% of their daily energy need as Olive oil, for 8 weeks, systolic blood pressure decreased by 6.32 mmHg (p < 0.05) and diastolic blood pressure decreased by 2.68 mmHg (p < 0.05), compared to the control group (Sales et.al. 2008).

When 25 volunteers used daily either low-Phenolic, Medium-Phenolic or high-Phenolic Olive oil or placebo, LDL-cholesterol decreased by 6.4%, 8.8% and 12.2%, and HDL-cholesterol increased by 9.0%, 14.3% and 23.5%, compared to the placebo group. Systolic blood pressure decreased by 3.3%, 6.3% and 7.7%, and diastolic blood pressure decreased by 4.2%, 7.7% and 10.8%, compared to placebo group (Al-Rewashdeh 2010). In all these changes, p < 0.05.
Clearly: The more Olive oil has Phenolic compounds, the bigger are the changes.

The same kind of changes in systolic- and diastolic blood pressure has been verified in other experiments too (Ruiz-Gutierre et.al. 1996).

When hypertensive rats were given 2.0 g/kg Olive Oil daily, for 14 days, systolic blood pressure decreased by 26 mmHg (p < 0.001), compared to the control group (Teres et.al. 2008). When pure Oleic acid was given 2 g/kg daily, for 14 days, systolic blood pressuer decreased by 21 mmHg (p < 0.001). Both Virgin Olive oil and pure Oleic acid decreased blood pressure also acutely, Virgin Olive oil by 20 mmHg (p < 0.001) at a dose of 2 g/kg, and pure Oleic acid by 14 mmHg (p < 0.05), at a dose of 1.0 g/kg (Teres et.al. 2008).

Orange juice

(Citrus Sinensis)

Orange is one of the most often used fruit in the World, which has a very long history of cultivation. It contains very large amounts of Flavonoids, Hesperidin and others.

Orange juice has
- Blood pressure lowering properties
- Total cholesterol lowering properties
- LDL-cholesterol lowering properties
- Triglycerides lowering properties
- HDL-cholesterol increasing properties

When 24 healthy, overweight volunteers were given 5 dl Orange juice daily, for 4 weeks, diastolic blood pressure decreased (p < 0.02) significantly, compared to the control group (Morand et.al. 2011).

Diastolic blood pressure decreased also significantly in volunteers, when they were given control drink, which contained the Flavonoid Hesperidin (Morand et.al. 2011).

Hesperidin is known to decrease blood pressure in animal experiments. When hypertensive rats were given Hesperidin 30 mg/kg daily, for 15 weeks, both blood pressure and heart rate decreased (Ohtsuki et.al. 2002).

When 25 hyperlipidemic volunteers were given 7.5 dl Orange juice daily, for 4 weeks, HDL-cholesterol increased by 21% (p < 0.01), compared to the control group (Kurowska et.al. 2000).

When 45 hyperlipidemic volunteers were given 7.5 dl Orange juice daily for 60 days, LDL-cholesterol (160 mg/dl → 141 mg/dl; p < 0.01) decreased significantly, compared to the control group (Cesar et.al. 2010).

When 13 women were given 5 dl Orange juice daily, for 3 months, and at the same time they made 3 times per week 1 hour aerobic exercise, LDL-cholesterol decreased by 15% (p < 0.05) and HDL-cholesterol increased by 18% (p < 0.05), compared to the control group, which made the same amount of aerobic exercise (Aptekmann et.al. 2010).

When rats were given Orange juice 5 g/kg daily, for 15 days, total cholesterol decreased by 31%, LDL-cholesterol decreased by 44% and triglycerides decreased by 33%, but HDL-cholesterol increased significantly, compared to the control group (Trovato et.al. 1996).

Orange peel

(Citrus Sinensis)

Orange is a delicious fruit, which has been cultivated for thousands of years. Normally only the fruit pulp is used, but Orange peel contains very large amounts of Polymethoxylated Flavonoids, such as Nobiletin, Tangeretin, Hesperidin and Naringin, which have many pharmacological functions.

Orange peel has
- Blood pressure lowering properties
- Total cholesterol lowering properties
- LDL-cholesterol lowering properties
- VLDL-cholesterol lowering properties
- Triglycerides lowering properties
- HDL-cholesterol increasing properties

When rats were fed Orange peel Flavones 1.5% of their daily diet, for 49 days, total cholesterol decreased by 45%, LDL-cholesterol decreased by 69%, VLDL-cholesterol decreased by 30% and triglycerides decreased by 24%, but HDL-cholesterol increased by 45%, compared to the control group (Green et.al. 2011).

Same kind of results have been obtained also in many other experiments (Kurowska et.al. 2006; Parmar et.al. 2008; Magda et.al. 2008).

When 80 volunteers were given daily 1480 mg Orange peel and Phellodenron Amurense bark extract daily, for 8 weeks, total cholesterol decreased by 21.6% (p < 0.001), LDL-cholesterol decreased by 44.6% (p < 0.001) and triglycerides decreased by 18.1% (p < 0.05), systolic blood pressure decreased by 6.0% (p < 0.05), diastolic blood pressure decreased by 13.1% (p < 0.001), but HDL-cholesterol increased by 11.8% (p < 0.05), compared to the control group (Obern et.al. 2008). This was a double blind experiment. Phellodendron Amurense bark contains Berberine.

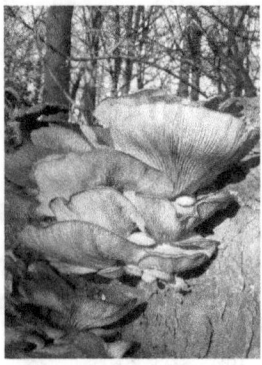

Oyster Mushroom

(Pleurotus Ostreatus)

Oyster mushroom is a very popular, eatable mushroom, which has many medicinal properties. It can be purchased either as raw or as pills in ordinary Supermarkets.

Oyster mushroom has
- Blood pressure lowering properties
- Total cholesterol lowering properties
- LDL-cholesterol lowering properties
- HDL cholesterol increasing properties
- Triglycerides lowering properties

When 89 diabetic volunteers were given Oyster mushroom daily, for 24 days, both systolic blood pressure ($p < 0.01$) and diastolic blood pressure ($p < 0.01$) decreased significantly. Also total cholesterol and triglycerides decreased significantly (Khatun et.al. 2007).

When 150 diabetic volunteers were given Oyster mushroom daily for 3 months, both blood pressure and total cholesterol decreased significntly (Agrawal et.al. 2010).

It is known, that Oyster mushroom extracts inhibit ACE (Chang 1996).

In experiments with rats, Oyster mushroom decrease both LDL-cholesterol and triglycerides, but increase HDL-cholesterol (Alam et.al. 2007; Alam et.al. 2011; Hossan et.al. 2003; Bobek et.al. 1993).

In animal experiments, Oyster mushroom decreases blood pressure (Tam et.al. 1986; Miyazawa et.al. 2008).

When 20 volunteers were given 30 grams of dried Oyster mushroom daily, for 3 weeks, both triglycerides ($p < 0.0015$) and total cholesterol ($p < 0.059$) decreased significantly, compared to the control group (Schneider et.al. 2011).

When rats were fed 5% Oyster mushroom in their daily diet, for 40 days, total cholesterol decreased by 37%, triglycerides decreased by 45% and LDL/HDL-cholesterol ratio decreased by 64% (Alam et.al. 2009).

Pangamic acid

Pangamic acid occurs generally in nature. It is called also as vitamin B-15.

Good sources for Pangamic acid are different seeds and beans, especially Apple seeds, Maize, Chickpea, Kidney bean and Mung bean.

Pangamic acid is sold as Calciumpangamate, which is the Calcium salt of Pangamic acid.

Pangamic acid has
- Total cholesterol lowering properties
- HDL-cholesterol increasing properties

When 60 sportsmen were given 160 mg Pangamic acid daily, for 4 weeks, the HDL-cholesterol increased (46.9 mg/dl $\rightarrow$ 54.4 mg/dl; $p < 0.001$) and total cholesterol decreased ($p < 0.01$), compared to control gorup (Almeida et.al. 1993). The HDL-cholesterol increased by 16.0%.

When rats were given pangamic acid at a dose between 50 – 250 mg/kg, for 4 – 7 days, the total cholesterol decreased by 15 – 36%. When Pangamic acid was given to hyperlipidemic rats at a dose between 12.5 – 50 mg/kg, the total cholesterol decreased by 40 – 69% (Atal et.al. 1980).

Also in other trials with arteriosclerosis patients the Pangamic acid has increased the HDL-cholesterol (Rastopchin 1984).

Pantethine

Pantethine is the natural metabolite of B5 vitamin Pantothenic acid in human body. From Pantethine the cells make Coenzyme A. Pantethine can be purchased as a food supplement in pill form. It has been known over 30 years, that Pantethine has strongly decreasing effect on cholesterol- and triglyceride values. It has been researched very much during the last 30 years. Pantethine is an ideal compound to lower high cholesterol- and triglyceride levels, and it has no known side effects. Pantethine increases the good HDL-cholesterol, but Statins decrease the good HDL-cholesterol.

Pantethine has
- Total cholesterol lowering properties
- LDL-cholesterol lowering properties
- Triglycerides lowering properties
- HDL-cholesterol increasing properties

In a meta-analysis with 28 different experiments and 646 hyperlipidemic volunteers, with daily Pantethine dose of 900 mg and test duration by average of 12.7 weeks, the following average changes were noticed:
- Total cholesterol decreased by 15.1%
- LDL-cholesterol decreased by 20.1%

- Triglycerides decreased by 32.9%
but
- HDL-cholesterol increased by 8.4% (McRae 2005).

These same results have been verified in a number of experiments with human volunteers (Rumberger et.al. 2011; Coronel et.al. 1991; Binaghi et.al. 1990; Eto et.al. 1987; Arsenio et.al. 1987; Arsenio et.al. 1986; Donati et.al. 1986; Murai et.al. 1985; Gaddi et.al. 1984; Arsenio et.al. 1984; Hiramatsu et.al. 1981).

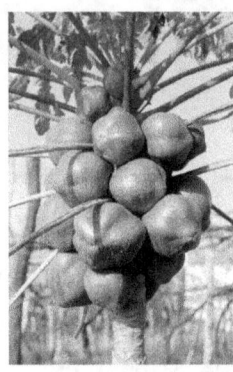

Papaya fruit

(Papaya Carica)

Papaya is a delicious tropical fruit, which can be purchased in every Supermarket.

Papaya has:
- Blood pressure lowering properties.
- Total cholesterol lowering properties.
- LDL-cholesterol lowering properties.
- Triglycerides lowering properties.
- HDL-cholesterol increasing properties.

Green Papaya fruit is used in many parts of the World in Folk medicine to lower high blood pressure (Lans 2006).

In rats the Papaya fruit extract decreases strongly blood pressure ($p < 0.01$), compared to controls (Eno et.al. 2000).

When rats were fed Papaya fruit extract, total cholesterol, LDL-cholesterol and triglycerides decreased significantly, but HDL-cholesterol increased (Lyer et.al. 2011).

Parsley

(Petroselinum Crispum)

Parsley is an ancient vegetable, which is cultivated all over the World. Parsley contains large amount of nutrients. All parts of parsley can be eaten: leaves, seeds and roots. Parsley is the best source of the Flavonoid Apigenin. Apigenin is a very strong antioxidant. Parsley leaves and seeds have been used hundreds of years also medicinally, especially as a diuretic and to lower high blood pressure.

Parsley has
- Blood pressure lowering properties
- Diuretic properties

In rats Parsley seeds water extract increases urine output by 110% ($p < 0.01$), compared to the control group (Kreydiyyh et.al. 2002).

When rats were given intravenously Parsley leaves ethanol extract at a dose between $0.33 - 10.0$ mg/kg, the mean average blood pressure (MAP) decreased by $6.54 - 42.34\%$ (Brankovic et.al. 2008). Parsley water extract decreased blood pressure by $3.16 - 25.26\%$.

When rats were given intravenously Parsley seeds water extract, blood pressure decreased by 30.2% ($p < 0.05$), compared to the control group (Campos et.al. 2009). Also a strong diuretic effect was noticed.

Parsley contains very large amouts of Apigenin.
Apigenin inhibits strongly ACE (Loizzo et.al. 2007; Sui et.al. 2010).

Passionfruit

(Passiflora Edulis, Passiflora Sp.)

Passionfruit is very popular fruit all over the World. There are tens of different Passionfruit species.

Passiofruit has
- Blood pressure lowering properties

The blood pressure lowering property of Passionfruit has been documented in several experiments. All parts of Passionfruits, pulp, skin, seeds and leaves decrease strongly blood pressure.

Passionfruit seeds are strongly vasorelaxant (Sano et.al. 2011).

When hypertensive rats were given Passionfruit skin methanolic extract 50 mg/kg orally, blood pressure decreased by 28 mmHg, one hour after the dose, compared to the control group (Ichimura et.al. 2006).

When hypertensive rats were given Passionfruit skin extract 50 mg/kg daily, for 8 weeks, systolic blood pressure decreased by 12.3 mmHg ($p < 0.01$), compared to the control group (Zibadi et.al. 2007).

When 30 volunteers were given Passionfruit skin extract 400 mg daily, for 4 weeks, systolic blood pressure decreased by 24.6 mmHg ($p < 0.001$), compared to the control group (Zibadi et.al. 2007). This was a doubble blind experiment.

When hypertensive volunteers were given dried Passionfruit juice extract 2 grams daily, systolic blood pressure decreased by 6.7 mmHg ($p < 0.05$) and diastolic blood pressure decreased by 5.3 mmHg (Rojas et.al. 2009). This was a doubble blind experiment.

Also in other experiments Passionfruit leaf extract and Passionfruit pulp decreased strongly both systolic and diastolic blood pressure (Rojas et.al. 2006; Patel et.al. 2011).

Peanut

(Arachis Hypogaea)

and Peanut oil

Peanuts are well known all over the World for the edible nuts and Peanut oil, which is much used as cooking oil, especially in Africa. Peanuts contain large amounts of L-Arginine and monounsaturated fatty acids.

Peanuts and Peanut oil have
- Blood pressure decreasing properties
- Total cholesterol decreasing properties
- LDL-cholesterol decreasing properties
- Triglycerides decreasing properties
- HDL-cholesterol increasing properties

When 54 hyperlipidemic volunteers were given Peanuts 77 grams daily, for 4 weeks, plasma total cholesterol/HDL-cholesterol ratio ($p = 0.001$) and LDL-cholesterol/HDL-cholesterol ratio ($p = 0.001$) decreased significantly, but HDL-cholesterol ($p < 0.001$) increased significantly, compared to the control group (Nouran et.al. 2010).

When 13 volunteers were given Peanuts daily, for 2 weeks, total cholesterol decreased by 7% ($p < 0.05$), compared to the control group (Trinidad et.al. 2010). This was a double blind experiment.

When 118 volunteers were given Peanuts 56 grams daily, for 4 weeks, total cholesterol, LDL-cholesterol and triglycerides decreased significantly, but HDL-cholesterol increased significantly in hyerlipidemic volunteers (McKiernan et.al. 2010).

When 15 volunteers were given daily Peanuts an amount, which corresponds to 1000 kcal energy intake, for 3 weeks, serum triglycerides decreased by 24% ($p < 0.05$), compared to the control group (Alper et.al. 2003).

When hamsters were fed with Peanuts, Peanut oil, defatted Peanuts or control diet daily, for 24 weeks, total cholesterol (p < 0.05), VLDL-cholesterol (p < 0.05) and LDL-cholesterol (p < 0.05) decreased significantly in all the Peanut groups, compared to the control group (Stephens et.al. 2010). The average decrease was 65% for total cholesterol, 77% for VLDL-cholesterol and 76% for LDL-cholesterol, compared to the control group.

When 129 volunteers, who were from Brazil, Ghana and USA, were given daily amount of Peanut oil, which corresonds to 30% of their daily energy intake, for 8 weeks, systolic blood pressure decreased by an average of 4.63 mmHg (p < 0.05) in the whole group, and 9.44 mmHg (p < 0.05) in the Ghanaian group, compared to the control values (Sales et.al. 2008).

Peanuts and especially Peanut skins have strong vasorelaxant property (Fitzpatrick et.al. 1995). Of all the 54 foodstuff studied, Peanut had the strongest vasolexant effect, together with Cinnamon.

In China the following methos is used to treat high blood pressure: Peanuts are put for 7 days in red Wine, and after this 10 Peanuts are taken in the morning and 10 Peanuts in the evening.

Peanut skins have very large amounts of dietary fiber and healthy Polyphenols. When Peanut skin was fed daily to rats, for 3 weeks, total cholesterol decresed by 40.8% (p < 0.05) and LDL-cholesterol decreased by 49.3% (p < 0.05), compared to the control group (Shimizu-Ibuka et.al. 2009).

Peppermint

(Mentha Piperita)

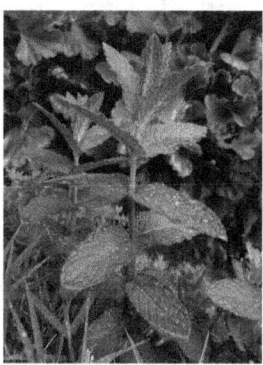

Peppermint is a very old spice, tea and medicinal plant.

Peppermint has
- Blood pressure lowering properties
- Total cholesterol lowering properties
- LDL-cholesterol lowering properties
- Triglycerides lowering properties

When 25 volunteers drank 2 times daily, 20 grams peppermint in 200 ml water, total cholesterol decreased in 66.9% of volunteers, LDL-cholesterol decreased in 52.3% of volunteers, triglycerides decreased in 58.5% of volunteers and blood pressure decreased in 52.5% of volunteers (Barbalho et.al. 2011).

When rats were fed with Peppermint water extract 100 mg/kg daily, for 3 weeks, total cholesterol (p < 0.05), LDL-cholesterol (p < 0.05) and triglycerides (p < 0.05) decreased significantly, but HDL-cholesterol (p < 0.05) increased significantly, compared to the control group (Badal et.al. 2011).

Other Mint species have also blood pressure and cholesterol lowering properties.

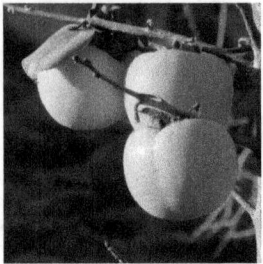

Persimmon

(Diospyros Kaki)

Persimmon, or Sharon, as it is also called, is a delicious fruit, which can be bought in every Supermarket.

Persimmon has
- Total cholesterol lowering properties
- LDL-cholesterol lowering properties
- Triglycerides lowering properties

When rats, which got 1% cholesterol in their daily food, were given 7% Persimmon added to the daily food, for 4 weeks, their total cholesterol decreased by 20% ($p < 0.001$), LDL-cholesterol decreased by 31% ($p < 0.001$) and triglycerides decreased by 19% ($p < 0.001$), compared to the control group (Gorinstein et.al. 1989).

The total cholesterol, LDL-cholesterol and triglycerides lowering properties of Persimmon has been verified in many experiments (Gorinstein et.al. 2000; Matsumoto et.al. 2010; Lee et.al. 2008).

Phosphorous

Phosphorous is an essential Macro mineral for Humans.

Phosphorous has:
- Blood pressure lowering properties.

In research made in Belgium concerning 4167 men and 3891 women, it was noticed, that serum phosphorous concentration and systolic blood pressure had a negative correlation between them (Kesteloot et.al. 1989).

When diet of 13444 volunteers was examined, it was noticed, that volunteers, who had higher intake of Phosphorous from food, had lower blood pressure (Alonso et.al. 2010).

When 4680 volunteers were examined in Japan, China, Great Britain and USA, it was noticed, that volunteers with higher intake of Phosphorous from food, had lower blood pressure (Elliott et.al. 2008).

When rats were fed Phosphorous in their water daily, for 16 weeks, systolic blood pressure decreased by 10.8% (222 mmHg → 198 mmHg) (Bindels et.al. 1987).

Pineapple Sage

(Salvia Elegans)

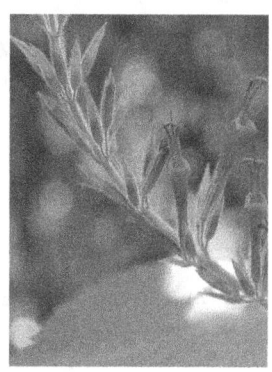

Pineapple Sage is a very beautiful, red flowering Sage species. Pineapple Sage is a salad- and medicinal plant. The leaves can be used in salads, and they are used as food in Mexico and Oginawa, Japan. Pineapple Sage is used medicinally in insomnia, high blood pressure and migraine. Its cultivation is very easy.

Pineapple Sage has
- Blood pressure lowering properties
- Fat reducing properties

Pineapple Sage inhibits strongly ACE (Jimenez-Ferrer et.al. 2010).

When mice were made hypertensive by Angiotensin II, and given Pineapple Sage water-ethanol extract at a dose of 10 mg/kg, systolic blood pressure decreased by 17.0% (204.1 mmHg → 169.4 mmHg; $p < 0.05$) and diastolic blood pressure decreased by 17.8% (137.0 mmHg → 112.6 mmHg; $p < 0.05$), compared to the control group (Jimenez-Ferrer et.al. 2010).

In Japan it has been noticed, that Pineapple Sage decreases adipogeneisis, which means, it has anti-obese properties (Niwano et.al. 2009).

Pinto bean

(Phaseolus Vulgaris)

Pinto bean is a common bean, which is consumed as a food all over the World.

Pinto bean has
- Total cholesterol lowering properties
- LDL-cholesterol lowering properties

When 16 volunteers were given ½ cup of Pinto beans daily together with normal food, for 8 weeks, total cholesterol decreased by 8.4% (218 mg/dl → 199 mg/dl; $p = 0.011$) and LDL-cholesterol decreased by 8.6% (138 mg/dl → 125 mg/dl; $p = 0.013$), compared to the control group (Winham et.al. 2007).

Also in another research it was verified, that Pinto beans decreased significantly both total cholesterol ($p < 0.05$) and LDL-cholesterol ($p < 0.05$) (Finlay et.al. 2007). The used amount of Pinto beans was 130 grams daily, for 12 weeks.

Pitahaya fruit

(Hylocereus Undatus, Hylocereus Sp.)

Pitahaya fruit originates from Mexico, but it is now cultivated in many tropical countries in Asia also. Pitahaya can be purchased from ordinary Supermarkets.

Pitahaya fruit has
- Blood pressure lowering properties
- Total cholesterol lowering properties
- LDL-cholesterol lowering properties
- Triglycerides lowering properties
- HDL-cholesterol increasing properties

The blood pressure, total cholesterol, LDL-cholesterol and triglyceride decreasing but HDL-cholesterol increasing effect of Pitahaya have been noticed in many experiment with humans (Anand et.al. 2010; Kow et.al. 2005; Chong et.al. 2006; Chong et.al. 2006; Fazila et.al. 2006; Marhazlina et.al. 2006; Jamatul et.al. 2005).

Pomegranate

(Punica Granatum)

Pomegranate is a very popular fruit all around the World, and it is cultivated especially around the Mediterranian countries. Pomegranate contains large amount of functionally healthy Tannins and Anthocyanides. Pomegranate can be purchased from Supermarkets all around the year.

Pomegranate has
- Blood pressure lowering properties
- Total cholesterol lowering properties
- LDL-cholesterol lowering properties
- HDL-cholesterol increasing properties

When 10 volunteers were given daily Pomegranate juice, for 12 months, systolic blood pressure decreased by 12% (Aviram et.al. 2004).

When rats were fed Pomegranate juice extract either 100 mg/kg or 300 mg/kg daily, for 4 weeks, the mean average blood pressure (MAP) decreased significantly, compared to the control group (Mohan et.al. 2010).

When 51 hyperlipidemic volunteers were given Pomegranate seed oil 400 mg daily, for 4 weeks, triglycerides decreased ($p < 0.009$) significantly, compared to the control group (Mirmiran et.al. 2010). This was a doubble blind experiment.

When 22 diabetic volunteers were given Pomegranate juice 40 grams daily, for 8 weeks, both total cholesterol (p < 0.006) and LDL-cholesterol (p < 0.006) decreased significantly, compared to the control group (Esmaillzadeh et.al. 2006).

Potassium

Potassium is an essential Macro mineral for human body. Potassium exists in large amounts in Banana and Potatoes.

Potassium has:
- Blood pressure lowering properties.

When 150 volunteers were given 60 mmol Potassium daily, for 12 weeks, systolic blood pressure decreased by 5.0 mmHg (p < 0.001), compared to the control group (Gu et.al. 2001).

When rats, which drank 1% Salt water, were given 0.2% or 1.0% Potassiumchloride at the same time daily, for 28 days, systolic blood pressure decreased from 177 mmHg (0% KCI) to 131 mmHg (0.2% KCI) and 120 mmHg (1.0% KCI) (Fujita et.al. 1983).

When 14 volunteers were given Potassiumchloride or Potassiumcitrate, 96 mmol daily, for 7 days, systolic blood pressure decreased to 140 mmHg and 138 mmHg, respectively, from initial value of 151 mmHg (Feng et.al. 2005). This was a doubble blind experiment.

When 11 volunteers were given food with very low amount of Potassium, systolic blood pressure increased by 5.0 mmHg (p < 0.02) (Coruzzi et.al. 2001).

Propolis

Propolis is a resinious material collected by honey bees. Honey bees use Propolis to block small holes. Propolis has been used hundreds of years also medicinally in different ailments. Propolis contains very large number of different Polyphenols, Flavonoids such as Galangin, CAPE (Caffeic acid phenethyl ester), Quercetin, Rutin etc. The composition of Propolis varies a lot all around the World.

Propolis has
- Blood pressure decreasing properties
- Total cholesterol decreasing properties
- LDL-cholesterol decreasing properties
- Triglycerides decreasing properties
- HDL-cholesterol increasing properties

There are many hypotensive compounds extracted from Propolis.

The CAPE extracted from Propolis decreased significantly blood pressure in experiments with rats (Iraz et.al. 2005).

The Isokunaretin, Dihydrokaempferide and Betuletol extracted from Brazilian Propolis are strongly hypotensive in experiments with rats (Maruyama et.al. 2009).

The Di- and Tri-Caffeoylquinic acids extracted from Brazilian Propolis are strongly hypotensive in experiments with rats (Mishima et.al. 2005).

When hypertensive rats were fed daily Propolis, for 4 weeks, systolic blood pressure decreased significantly, compared to the control group (Kubota et.al. 2004).

Propolis decreases significantly total cholesterol, LDL-cholesterol and triglycerides, but increases significantly HDL-cholesterol in experiments with rats, mice and rabbits (Klankaya et.al. 2002; Koya-Miyata et.al. 2009; Zhu et.al. 2011; Fuliang et.al. 2005; El-Sayed et.al. 2009; Abo-Selim et.al. 2009; Nader et.al. 2010).

In human experiments Propolis has reduced total cholesterol by 15.7% and LDL-cholesterol by 20.5% (Kasianenko et.al. 2010).

Proso Millet

(Panicum Miliaceum)

Proso Millet has been cultivated for a very long time, at least over 7000 years in China and East Europe. Nowadays it is also cultivated in Africa and North America. It can be grown in very dry lands, and it needs the least amount of water of any grain species. Proso Millet does not contain Glutein, so it is ideal grain for persons, who can not eat ordinary Glutein containing grains.

Proso Millet has
  − HDL-cholesterol increasing properties

The HDL-increasing property of Proso Millet is very strong.

When diabetic mice were fed 20% of Proso Millet protein in their daily diet, for 3 weeks, HDL-cholesterol increased by 51.8% (p < 0.05), compared to the control group, which were given the same amount of Casein protein (Park et.al. 2008).

When rats were given in their daily diet Proso millet, for 5 weeks, HDL-cholesterol increased by 21.5% (p < 0.05), compared to the control group, which was given ordinary food (Lee et.al. 2010).

When mice were given Proso Millet protein in their daily diet, for 3 weeks, HDL-cholesterol increased by 23.1% (p < 0.05), compared to the control group, which was given the same amount Casein protein (Nishizawa et.al. 1995).

The HDL-cholesterol increasing property of Proso Millet has been verified also in other animal experiments (Nishizawa et.al. 1996; Shimanuki et.al. 2006).

Prunes

(Prunus Domestica)

Prunes are dried Plums (Prunus Domestica). Prunes are used all around the World as food. Prunes contain extremely large amounts of Potassium, 745 mg/100 g. Prunes have also a great amount of functionally important Polyphenols, 184 mg/100 g. Most of these Polyphenols are Chlorogenic acid (Stacewicz-Sapountzakis et.al. 2001). Both Potassium and Chlorogenic acid decrease blood pressure.

Prunes have
- Blood pressue lowering properties
- Total cholesterol lowering properties
- LDL-cholesterol lowering properties

When 259 volunteers, with mild hypertension, were given 3 Prunes, about 12 grams daily, for 8 weeks, their systolic blood pressure (134.0 mmHg $\rightarrow$ 126.7 mmHg; $p < 0.004$), diastolic blood pressure (86.45 mmHg $\rightarrow$ 81.9 mmHg; $p < 0.056$), total cholesterol (189.4 mg/dl $\rightarrow$ 161.4 mg/dl; $p < 0.002$) and LDL-cholesterol (101.6 mg/dl $\rightarrow$ 82.1 mg/dl; $p < 0.017$) decreased significantly, compared to the control group (Ahmed et.al. 2010).

When 41 volunteers were given 12 Prunes, about 100 grams daily, for 4 weeks, their LDL-cholesterol (4.1 mmol/L $\rightarrow$ 3.9 mmol/L) decreased significantly, compared to the control group (Tinker et.al. 1991).

When mice were fed Prunes, either 4.75% or 9.8% of total food, for 5 months, both total cholesterol and triglycerides decreased significantly, compared to the control group (Gallaher et.al. 2009).

Pu-Erh tea

(Camellia Sinensis)

Pu-Erh tea is made by a fermentation process from Green tea. The duration of fermentation may be over 10 years. Most Pu-Erh tea comes from Yunnan province, in China. As a result of fermentation, Pu-Erh tea contains large amounts of Statins and GABA, which are known to decrease both cholesterol and high blood pressure (Jeng et.al. 2007). Pu-Erh can be purchased from ethnic Chinese supermarkets.

Pu-Erh tea has
- Total cholesterol lowering properties
- LDL-cholesterol lowering properties
- Triglycerides lowering properties
- HDL-cholesterol increasing properties
- Body weight decreasing properties

When 90 volunteers with metabolic syndrome were given Pu-Erh tea daily, for 3 months, total cholesterol (p < 0.05), LDL-cholesterol (p < 0.05), triglycerides (p < 0.05) and bodyweight (p < 0.05) decreased significantly, but HDL-cholesterol increased significantly, compared to the control group (Chu et.al. 2011). This was a double blind experiment.

When 47 volunteers were given Pu-Erh water extract 1.0 grams daily, for 3 months, total cholesterol (5.91 mmol/L → 5.62 mmol/L; p < 0.01), LDL-cholesterol (4.11 mmol/L → 3.81 mmol/L; p < 0.01), triglycerides (1.38 mmol/L → 1.33 mmol/L; p < 0.01) and bodyweight (60.1 kg → 59.2 kg; p < 0.05) decreased significantly, compared to the control group (Fujita et.al. 2008). This was a double blind experiment.

When 20 volunteers were given Pu-Erh tea extract daily, for 8 weeks, total cholesterol (p < 0.05), LDL-cholesterol (p < 0.05) and bodyweight (p < 0.05) decreased significantly, compared to the control group (Fujita et.al. 2008).

When rats were given in their daily diet either 1.5% or 4.0% Pu-Erh tea, for 30 weeks, bodyweight decreased by 13% (p < 0.0005), triglycerides decreased (p < 0.05 in 1.5% group; p < 0.0005 in 4.0% group), total cholesterol decreased by 23% (p < 0.0001 in 1.5% group), LDL-cholesterol decreased by 44% (p < 0.0001 in 1.5% group), but HDL-cholesterol increased (p < 0.05 in 4.0% group), compared to the control group (Kuo et.al. 2005). In the experiment Black tea, Pu-Erh tea, Green tea and Oolong tea were tested, but Pu-Erh showed the strongest effect.

The total cholesterol, LDL-cholesterol and triglycerides lowering effect, but HDL-cholesterol increasing effect of Pu-Erh tea has been verified also in other experiments (Hou et.al. 2009; Cao et.al. 2011).

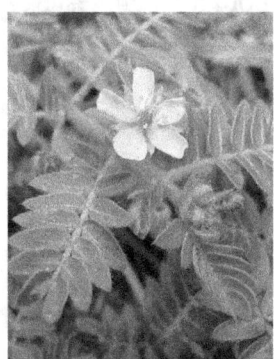

(Author: Forest & Kim Starr)

Puncture Vine

(Tribulus Terrestris)

Puncture Vine is a very old medicinal plant, which grows in Asia and Europe. It has many medicinal properties. Puncture Vine is used against high cholesterol values, high blood pressure and impotence. It is both cardiotonic and diuretic, and increases testosterone. It is used in cardiovascular diseases in Turkey, Iran, Indian and China. Its cultivation is very easy.

Puncture Vine has
- Blood pressure lowering properties
- Total cholesterol lowering properties
- LDL-cholesterol lowering properties
- Triglycerides lowering properties

–   Diuretic properties

Puncture Vine is strongly diuretic (Al-Ali et.al. 2003).

When hypertensive rats were given Puncture Vine water extract 10 mg/kg daily, for 4 weeks, systolic blood pressure decreased 60 mmHg (150 mmHg → 90 mmHg; $p < 0.001$), compared to the control group. Also Puncture Vine strongly inhibits ACE (Shariff et.al. 2003).

The strong blood pressure lowering effect of Puncture Vine has been noticed also in other experiments (Phillips et.al. 2006).

When rabbits were given Puncture Vine extract 5 mg/kg daily, for 8 weeks, total cholesterol decreased by 65% ($p < 0.001$), LDL-cholesterol decreased by 66% ($p < 0.001$) and triglycerides decreased by 55% ($p < 0.01$), compared to the control group (Tuncer et.al. 2009).

The same cholesterol lowering effect has been noticed also in other experiments with chickens (Grigorova et.al. 2008).

Purple Corn

(Zea Mays)

Purple Corn contains Anthocyanins in the grain. Purple Corn originates from South America. It has been cultivated for thousands of years by the South American Indians.

Purple Corn has
–   Blood pressure lowering properties

When rats with high blood pressure were fed Purple Corn for 5 – 15 weeks, the blood pressure decreased significantly (Toyoshi et.al. 2004; Shindo et.al. 2007; Amnueysit et.al. 2010).

The water-ethanol extract of Purple Corn is a vasodilator (Moreno-Loiza et.al. 2010).

Allready much earlier Corn was shown to be a vasodilator (Fitzpatrick et.al. 1995).

Purple Potato

(Solanum Tuberosum)

Potato originates from South-America, Peru, Ecuador and Chile. There are hundreds of different types of Potato cultivars. Dark red, dark blue and black potatoes contain very high levels of functionally healthy Anthocyanides, Phenolic acids and Carotenes. But the ordinary white Potatoes do not contain these compounds. Typical colored Potatoes are: Blue Kongo, Inca Red and Shetland Black. These potatoes have strong antioxidative properties.

Purple Potato has
- Blood pressure lowering properties

When 18 hypertensive volunteers were given 6 – 8 small Purple Potatoes, together with their skins, daily, for 4 weeks, systolic blood pressure decreased by 5 mmHg or 3.5%, and diastolic blood pressure decreased by 4 mmHg or 4.3%, compared to the control group (Vinson et.al. 2012).

Purple Potato contain up to 3 times more antioxidants, than ordinary Potato (Zhao et.al. 2009; Lachman et.al. 2005).

Potato hydrolysates contain compounds, which strongly inhibit ACE (Pihlanto et.al. 2008).

Potato is an excellent source of Potassium. In a typical Potato, the Potassium content varies between 300 – 450 mg/100 g (Burrowes et.al. 2008). Potassium is known to decrease blood pressure.

Purslane

(Portulaca Oleracea)

Purslane is very well known vegetable and salad plant. Purslane has extremely large amounts of Omega-3 fatty acids, Flavonoids, Polyphenols, Anthocyanides, beta-Carotene and vitamins C and E, and also Melatonin. It is easy to cultivate.

Purslane has
- Total cholesterol lowering properties
- LDL-cholesterol lowering properties
- VLDL-cholesterol lowering properties
- HDL-cholesterol increasing properties
- Triglycerides lowering properties

When 11 volunteers were given 6 grams of dried Purslane daily, for 4 weeks, total cholesterol decreased by 15.5% (266.4 mg/dl → 225.6 mg/dl; $p < 0.05$), LDL-cholesterol decreased by 27.6% (182.45 mg/dl → 132.09 mg/dl; $p < 0.05$) but HDL-cholesterol increased by 9.3% (49.46 mg/dl → 54.06 mg/dl; $p < 0.05$), compared to the control group (Besong et.al. 2011). Also Hematocrit increased by 15.7% (41.55 → 48.09).

When rats with high cholesterol values were given ethanol extract of Purslane at a dose of 150 mg/kg daily, for 8 weeks, triglycerides decreased by 12.5%, total cholesterol decreased by 26.2% ($p < 0.05$) and LDL-cholesterol decreased by 42.3% ($p < 0.05$), but HDL-cholesterol increased by 54.2%, compared to the control group (Hussein 2010).

When rabbits were given ethanol extract of Purslane at doses between 200 mg/kg – 800 mg/kg daily, for 8 weeks, total cholesterol ($p < 0.05$), LDL-cholesterol ($p < 0.05$) and VLDL-cholesterol ($p < 0.05$) decreased significantly, but HDL-cholesterol ($p < 0.05$) increased significantly, compared to the control group (Movahedian et.al. 2007).

Pygnogenol

Pygnogenol is a standardised water-ethanol extract of French Maritime Pine (Pinus Pinaster) bark. It contains large amounts of Flavonoids, Procyanides, Ferulic acid etc.

Pygnogenol has
- Blood pressure lowering properties
- Total cholesterol lowering properties
- LDL-cholesterol lowering properties

When 21 volunteers were given Pygnogenl 120 mg daily, for 3 months, total cholesterol decreased by 7.9% (5.41 mmol/L → 4.98 mmol/L; $p < 0.07$) and LDL-cholesterol decreased by 19.1% (3.44 ml/L → 2.78 mmol/L), compared to the control group (Durackova et.al. 2003). This was a doubble blind experiment.

When 11 volunteers were given Pygnogenol 200 mg daily, for 8 weeks, systolic blood pressure decreased (139.9 mmHg → 132.7 mmHg; $p < 0.05$) significantly, compared to the control group (Hosseini et.al. 2001). Diastolic blood pressure decreased by 1.8 mmHg. This was a doubble blind experiment.

The blood pressure lowering property of Pygnogenol has been noticed also in other experients Kwak et.al. 2009; Liu et.al. 2004).

Quercetin

Quercetin is a Flavonoid, which exists in many plants. Quercetin is one of the strongest antioxidants. The best natural sources for Quercetin are Apples, Green tea, Red Onion and Onion leaves.

Quercetin has
- Blood pressure lowering properties
- Total cholesterol lowering properties
- LDL-cholesterol lowering properties
- Triglycerides lowering properties
- HDL-cholesterol increasing properties

When 41 volunteers, of which 22 were hypertensive, were given Quercetin 730 mg daily, for 28 days, systolic blood pressure decreased by 7 mHg ($p < 0.01$) and diastolic blood pressure decreased by 5 mmHg ($p < 0.01$) in the hypertensive group (Edwards et.al. 2007). This was a doubble blind experiment.

When 93 volunteers were given Quercetin 1250 mg daily, for 6 weeks, systolic blood pressure decreased by 2.9 mmHg ($p < 0.01$) in the whole group (Egert et.al. 2009). This was a doubble blind experiment.

When 49 smoking volunteers were given Quercetin 100 mg daily, for 10 weeks, both systolic (p < 0.01) and diastolic (p < 0.01) decreased significantly. Also total cholesterol (p < 0.05) and LDL-cholesterol (p < 0.01) decreased, but HDL-cholesterol (p < 0.01) increased significantly (Lee et.al. 2011). This was a doubble blind experiment.

When 49 healthy men were given Quercetin 150 mg daily, for 8 weeks, systolic blood pressure (p < 0.044) decreased significantly. Also triglycerides (p < 0.025) decreased, but HDL-cholesterol (p < 0.025) increased significantly (Pfeuffer et.al. 2011). This was a doubble blind experiment.

When rats were given Quercetin 10 mg/kg daily, for 5 weeks, systolic blood pressure decreased by 18%, diastolic blood pressure decreased by 23% and heart rate decreased by 12% (Duarte et.al. 2009).

The blood pressure lowering effect of Quercetin has been noticed also in other experiments (Perez-Vizcaino et.al. 2009).

In research with Japanese women, the daily Quercetin from food, mainly from Onions, correlated negatively with total cholesterol (r = -0.261; p < 0.01) and LDL-cholesterol (r = -0.263; p < 0.01) (Arai et.al. 2000).

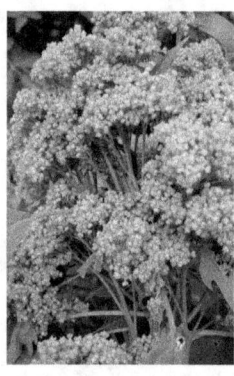

Quinoa

(Chenopodium Quinoa)

Quinoa has been cultivated in Peru for thousands of years. Quinoa seed contains large amount of nutrients. Quinoa seeds have Betaine up to 630 mg/100 g.

Quinoa seeds have
- Blood pressure lowering properties
- Total cholesterol lowering properties
- LDL-cholesterol lowering properties
- Triglycerides lowering properties

When mice were fed 2.5% Quinoa protein in their daily diet, for 4 weeks, total cholesterol decreased by 25.4% (268.2 mg/dl → 199.9 mg/dl; p < 0.005) and triglycerides decreased by 34.4% (84.5 mg/dl → 55.4 mg/dl; p < 0.05), compared to the control group (Takao et.al. 2005).

When rats were fed Quinoa seeds daily for 5 weeks, total cholesterol decreased by 26% (p < 0.05), LDL-cholesterol decreased by 57% (p < 0.008) and triglycerides decreased by 11% (p < 0.05), compared to the control group, which was fed with Corn (Pasko et.al. 2010).

When Quinoa flour was fed for hypertensive and hyperlipidemic rats daily for 5 weeks, systolic blood pressure decreased significantly, compared to the control group (Ogawa et.al. 2001).

Raisins

(Vitis Vinifera)

Raisins contain big amounts of dietary fiber and functionally important Polyphenols.

Raisins have
- Blood pressure lowering properties
- Total cholesterol lowering properties
- LDL-cholesterol lowering properties

When 34 volunteers were given 1 cup of Raisins daily, for 6 weeks, systolic blood pressure decreased 2.2% (124.1 mmHg → 121.8 mmHg; p = 0.008), total cholesterol decreased 9.4% (5.21 mmol/L → 4.82 mmol/L; p < 0.005) and LDL-cholesterol decreased 13.7% (3.21 mmol/L → 2.90 mmol/L; p < 0.0001), compared to the control group (Puglisi et.al. 2008).

Because red Grapes contain much higher amounts of Polyphenols, than green Grapes, it is better to use dark Raisins.

Ramsons, Wild Garlic

(Allium Ursinum)

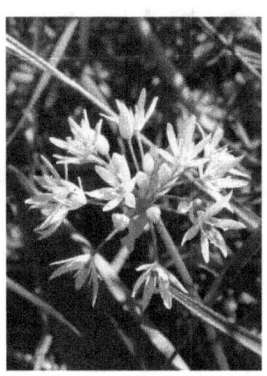

Wild Garlic is an Ancient food- and medicinal plant, which grows all over Europe, in moist and shadow places.

Wild Garlic has
- Blood pressure lowering properties
- Total cholesterol lowering properties
- HDL-cholesterol increasing properties

Wild Garlic inhibits strongly ACE (Rietz et.al. 1993), which possibly explains its blood pressure lowering property.

When rats were given Wild Garlic 1% in their daily diet, for 45 days, systolic blood pressure decreased significantly by 16 mmHg (189 mmHg → 173 mmHg), compared to the control group. Total cholesterol also decreased significantly by 12.0% (133 mg/dl → 117 mg/dl), but HDL-cholesterol increased, compared to the control group (Preuss et.al. 2001).

The Wild Garlic had stronger effect, than ordinary Garlic in this experiment, which also lowered significantly both blood pressure and total cholesterol, compared to the control group.

The Wild Garlic cholesterol decreasing property has been noticed also in other experiments (Sendl et.al. 1992).

Wild Garlic contains much higher amounts of Adenosine and Allicine, than Garlic. Adenosine is a very strong vasodilator.

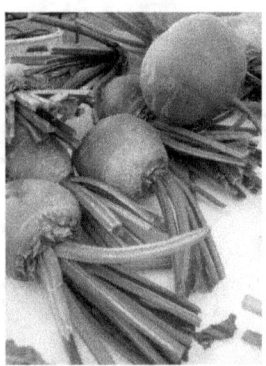

Red Beet

(Beta Vulgaris var Rubra)

Red Beet root is used as a food all around the World. Also the Red Beet leaves can be used as food. Red Beet has also much use as a medicinal plant, for example against cancer.

Red Beet has
- – Blood pressure lowering properties
- – Total cholesterol lowering properties
- – Triglycerides lowering properties

When 8 volunteers were given Red Beet juice 5 dl daily, for 15 days, and put on a steptest exercise, both their systolic and diastolic blood pressure were 4% (p <0.05) lower, than in the control group (Vanhatalo et.al. 2010).

When 9 volunteers were given 5 dl Red Beet juice daily, for 6 days, systolic blood pressure (129 mmHg → 124 mmHg; p < 0.01) decreased significantly, compared to the control group (Lansley et.al. 2011). This was a double blind experiment.

When rats with high cholesterol- and triglyceride levels were fed Red Beet 3% of their total food daily, both total cholesterol and triglycerides decreased significantly (Wroblewska et.al. 2011).

When horses were fed 25% Red Beet in their daily food, triglycerides decreased significantly (p < 0.058) (Hallebeek et.al. 2003).

When rats were fed Red Beet extract 1000 mg/kg – 4000 mg/kg daily, both total cholesterol and triglycerides decreased significantly, compared to the control group (Agarwal et.al. 2006).

Red Cabbage

(Brassica Oleracea var. Capitata var. Rubra)

Both white Cabbage and Red Cabbage are very important food plants. Red Cabbage has much more functionally healthy Anthocyanides and vitamin C, than does White Cabbage.

Red Cabbage has
- Total cholesterol lowering properties
- LDL-cholesterol lowering properties
- Triglycerides lowering properties
- HDL-cholesterol increasing properties

When rats were fed Cabbage ethanol extract, HDL-cholesterol increased significantly, compared to the control group (Jahodar et.al. 1995).

When Cabbage protein extract were fed to rats, both total cholesterol and triglycerides decreased significantly, compared to the control group, which was fed with Casein (Igarashi et.al. 1997).

When rats were fed Cabbage extract, total cholesterol decreased significantly, compared to the control group. Also the compound S-Methyl-L-Cysteine Sulfoxide extracted from Cabbage decreased total cholesterol significantly (Komatsu et.al. 1998).

When 77 volunteers were given daily 320 grams daily drink made from Cabbage and Broccoli, for 12 weeks, serum LDL-cholesterol decreased by 8.5% ($p < 0.05$), compared to the control group (Takai et.al. 2003). This was a doubble blind experiment.

When rats were fed Cabbage ethanol extract at a dose of 500 mg/kg daily, for 12 weeks, total cholesterol decreased by 23.2% ($p < 0.05$), compared to the control group (Waqar et.al. 2010).

Red Clover

(Trifolium Pratense)

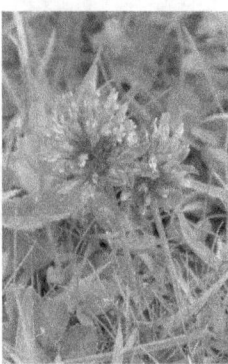

Red Clover is a very old cultivated plant, for animal food and medicinal uses. Its cultivation is very easy. Red Clover flower contains large amounts of Isoflavonoids, such as Genistein, Daidzein, Formonetin and Biochanin.

Red Clover has
- Blood pressure lowering properties
- Total cholesterol lowering properties
- LDL-cholesterol lowering properties
- Triglycerides lowering properties
- HDL-cholesterol increasing properties

When 16 diabetic volunteers were given 50 mg of Red Clover isoflavonoids daily, for 4 weeks, systolic blood pressure decreased 8.0 mmHg ($p < 0.05$) and diastolic blood pressure decreased 4.3 mmHg ($p < 0.05$), compared to the control group (Howes et.al. 2003). This was a doubble blind experiment.

When 22 volunteers were given Red Clover Isoflavonoids for 12 months, total cholesterol, LDL-cholesterol and triglycerides decreased, but HDL-cholesterol increased significantly, compared to the control group (Terzic et.al. 2009).

When 46 volunteers were given Red Clover Isoflavonoids 28.5 – 85.5 mg daily, for 6 months, HDL-cholesterol increased significantly by 15.7 – 28.6% ($p = 0.02$; $p = 0.027$), compared to the control group (Clifton-Bligh et.al. 2001). This was a doubble blind experiment.

Red Grapefruit

(Citrus Paradisi)

Red Grapefruit is a very popular fruit all around the World. Compared to the ordinary Yellow Grapefruit, Red Grapefruit has large amount of Lycopene, which is a very strong antioxidant.

Red Grapefruit has
- Blood pressure lowering properties
- Total cholesterol lowering properties
- LDL-cholesterol lowering properties
- Triglycerides lowering properties

In human volunteers, Red Grapefruit juice decreases both systolic and diastolic blood pressure. This happens in both normotensive and hypertensive persons (Diaz-Juarez et.al. 2009).

When 57 volunteers were given 1 Red Grapefruit daily within the normal food, for 30 days, total cholesterol decreased by 15.5%, LDL-cholesterol decreased by 20.3% and triglycerides decreased by 27.2% (Park et.al. 2009).

In experiments with rats, Grapefruit juice given daily, for 60 days, decreased significantly total cholesterol levels (Deyhim et.al. 2006).

Red Grape juice and red Grapes

(Vitis Vinifera)

Red Grapes and red Grape juice contain significantly more functionally healthy Polyphenols, than do white Grapes. Red Grapes can be purchased from supermarkets all around the year, and also there are red Grape juices, like BIOTTA available.

Red Grapes and red Grape juice have
  – Blood pressure lowering properties
  – Total cholesterol lowering properties
  – LDL-cholesterol lowering properties
  – Triglycerides lowering properties
  – HDL-cholesterol increasing properties

When 80 volunteers were given Concord Grape juice 3.4 dl daily, for 12 weeks, systolic blood pressure decreased by 5.7 mmHg (142.7 mmHg → 137.0 mmHg; $p < 0.05$) and diastolic blood pressure decreased by 5.8 mmHg (87.9 mmHg → 82.1 mmHg; $p < 0.05$), compared to the control group (Mark et.al. 2003).

When 40 volunteers were given 5.5 ml/kg (about 3.3 dl/60 kg) Concord Grape juice daily, for 8 weeks, systolic blood pressure decreased by 7.2 mmHg ($p = 0.005$) and diastolic blood pressure decreased by 6.2 mmHg ($p = 0.001$), compared to the control group (Park et.al. 2004). This was a double blind experiment.

When 10 volunteers were given dried red Grape flour 10 grams daily, for 3 weeks, triglycerides decreased by 23.0% (1.13 mmol/L → 0.87 mmol/L; $p = 0.005$), compared to the control group (Twait et.al. 2007).

When 32 volunteers were given 1.0 liter red Grape juice daily, for 2 weeks, total cholesterol (4.34 mmol/L → 4.01 mmol/L; $p < 0.001$) and LDL-cholesterol (2.69 mmol/L → 2.39 mmol/L; $p < 0.01$) decreased significantly, but HDL-cholesterol (0.70 mmol/L → 0.83 mmol/L; $p < 0.001$) increased significantly, compared to the control group (Castilla et.al. 2008).

When 26 volunteers were given 3.0 dl red Grape juice daily, for 4 weeks, HDL-cholesterol increased by 7.0% (41.44 mg/dl → 44.37 mg/dl; $p < 0.0001$), but Homocysteine decreased by 19.48% ($p < 0.001$), compared to the control group (Khadem-Ansari et.al. 2010).

When 41 volunteers were given red Grape juice 1.0 dl daily, for 2 weeks, total cholesterol decreased by an average of 0.405 mmol/L ($p < 0.001$), LDL-cholesteol decreased by 0.48 mmol/L ($p < 0.001$), but HDL-cholesterol increased by 0.357 mmol/L ($p < 0.001$), compared to the control group (Castilla et.al. 2006).

When 44 volunteers were given 36 grams red Grape flour daily, for 4 weeks, LDL-cholesterol decreased by an average of 6.9% ($p < 0.05$) and triglycerides decreased by an average of 10.0% ($p < 0.05$), compared to the control group (Zern et.al. 2005).

Red Onion

(Allium Cepa)

Red Onion has been used as a food and medicinal plant over 5000 years. It is used all over the World in folk medicine as a diuretic and to decrease high blood pressure and high cholesterol levels.

Red Onion has very high levels of the Flavonoid Quercetin, over 300 mg/kg, which is 6 times more than in Yellow Onion, which has about 50 mg/kg Quercetin. In the skin of Red Onion, the Quercetin content may be up to 6 – 8 grams/kg. Also Red Onion leaves contain Querceting more than 500 mg/kg. Querceting is known to lower high blood pressure and high cholesterol levels.

Red Onion has
- Blood pressure lowering properties
- Total Cholesterol lowering properties
- LDL-cholesterol lowering properties
- VLDL-cholesterol lowering properties
- Triglycerides lowering properties
- HDL-cholesterol increasing properties

The vasorelaxant property of Onion has been noticed in many experiments (Naseri et.al. 2007; Naseri et.al. 2008; Fitzpatrick et.al. 1995).

When volunteers were given 4 Onion-Olive oil capsules daily, for one week, both systolic and diastolic blood pressure decreased significantly (Kalus et.al. 2000). This was a doubble blind experiment.

The ethanol extracts of Red onion decreases blood pressure in rats (Brankovic et.al. 2011).

When rats were fed Red Onion 5% of their daily diet, for 4 weeks, systolic blood pressure decreased by an average of 20 mmHg, compared to the control group (Sakai et.al. 2003). This was a 10% decrease to the average blood pressure.

When diabetic volunteers were given Red Onion water extract daily, for 2 months, both triglycerides ($p < 0.05$) and VLDL-cholesterol ($p < 0.05$) decreased significantly, compared to the control group (Dineshkumar et.al. 2010).

When rats were fed Red Onion water extract 0.5 – 1.5 mg/kg daily, for 4 weeks, total cholesterol (p < 0.05), LDL-cholesterol (p < 0.05) and triglycerides (p < 0.05) decreased significantly, but HDL-cholesterol (p < 0.05) increased significantly, compared to the control group (Emmanuel et.al. 2011).

The same kind of results have been noticed also in other experiments (Bang et.al. 2009; Lata et.al. 1991; Ahluwalia et.al. 1989).

Red Raspberry

(Rubus Idaeus)

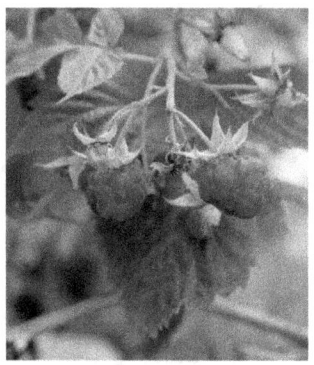

Red Raspberry is a very healthy berry, which contains large amounts of functionally healthy Polyphenols and Flavonoids.

Red Raspberry has
  – Blood pressure lowering properties

When hypertensive rats were given Red Raspberry ethanol extract either 100 mg/kg or 200 mg/kg daily, for 5 weeks, systolic blood pressure decreased by 13.1% (187.7 mmHg → 163.0 mmHg; p < 0.01) in the 100 mg/kg group, and 15.6% (187.7 mmHg → 158 mmHg; p < 0.01) in the 200 mg/kg group, compared to the control group (Jia et.al. 2011). Also the serum NO concentration increased by 87% (in the 100 mg/kg group; p < 0.01) and serum Endothelin-1 (ET-1) concentration decreased by 28.5% (in the 200 mg/kg group; p < 0.05).

Red Raspberry leaves contain very large amounts of Ellagic acid, 2.06% - 6.89% (Gudej et.al. 2004). Ellagic acid inhibits ACE and decreases blood pressure.

Red Rice

(Oryza Sativa + Monascus Purpureus)

Red Rice is Rice, which has been fermented by the micro fungus Monascus Purpureus. Red Rice originates from China. Red Rice has been in use in China, Korea and Japan for thousands of years as food and medicine.

Red Rice has
- Blood pressure lowering properties
- Total cholesterol lowering properties
- LDL-cholesterol lowering properties
- Triglycerides lowering properties

Red Rice has a strong inhibitory activity against ACE (Kuba et.al. 2009).

In experiments with rats, Red Rice decreases blood pressure in direct proportion to the dose used (Wang et.al. 2010).

When 79 volunteers were given Red Rice 600 mg, twice daily, for 8 weeks, total cholesterol decreased by 21.5%, LDL-cholesterol decreased by 27.7% and triglycerides decreased by 15.8%, compared to the control group (Lin et.al. 2005). This was a placebo controlled doubble blind experiment.

Red Wine

(Vitis Vinifera)

Red Wine is, along with Beer, one of the most often used alcohol beverage in the World. Grape Wine, Vitis Vinifera, has been cultivated for thousands of years in countries around the Mediterranian Sea. Both red and white Wine is made from grapes. Red Wine contains very large amounts of healthy Polyphenols, up to 1000 – 4000 mg/liter, which is much more than the 200 – 300 mg/liter in white Wines (Bravo et.al. 1998). This is the reason, that red Wine is regarded more healthy than white Wine.

The functional properties of red Wine are studied intensively at the moment. Red Wine increases strongly the healthy HDL-cholesterol, but its effects on blood pressure are biphasic: In some persons it may mildly increase blood pressure, but in other persons it decreased blood pressure. The ethanol in red Wine is known to increase blood pressure, but the red Wine Polyphenols are known to decrease blood pressure. On the other hand, small amounts of pure ethanol, 15 – 30 grams daily, have very positive effects on health, but large amounts of ethanol have clearly negative effects on health.

Red Wine has
- Blood pressure decreasing properties
- HDL-cholesterol increasing properties

- LDL-cholesterol decreasing properties
- Plasma viscosity decreasing properties
- Blood vessel elasticity increasing properties

When 44 volunteers were given red Wine 1.5 dl daily, for 90 days, LDL-cholesterol decreased by 0.30 mmol/L, compared to the control group (Kechagias et.al. 2011).

When 69 healthy volunteers were given red Wine 2.0 – 3.0 dl daily, for 4 weeks, HDL-cholesterol increased by 11 – 16% ($p < 0.05$), compared to the control group (Hansen et.al. 2005).

When 45 hyperlipidemic women were given red Wine 4.0 dl daily, for 6 weeks, LDL-cholesterol decreased by 8% ($p < 0.05$), LDL/HDL-cholesterol ratio decreased y 20% ($p < 0.01$) and total cholesterol/HDL-cholesterol ratio decreased by 14% ($p < 0.05$), but HDL-cholesterol increased by 17% ($p < 0.05$), compared to the control group (Naissides et.al. 2006).

When 10 healthy men were given red Wine 4.0 dl daily, for 2 weeks, HDL-cholesterol increased by 26% ($p < 0.01$), compared to the control group (Lavy et.al. 1994).

Ethanol generally increases blood pressure, about 1 mmHg for every 10 grams intake (Puddey et.al. 2006).

When 26 healthy volunteers were given red Wine 3.75 dl daily, systolic blood pressure increased by an average of 2.9 mmHg ($p < 0.05$), compared to the control group (Zilkens et.al. 2005). This amount of wine contains 39 grams of ethanol.

But when red Wine is given to either hypertensive or hyperlipidemic volunteers, it decreases blood pressure. When 13 middle aged, hypertensive volunteers were given red Wine 2.5 dl together with lunch, the mean average blood pressure (MAP) decreased by 5.3 mmHg ($p = 0.03$) and blood pressure was down the whole day, being lowest 3 hours after intake (8.0 mmHg; $p = 0.02$) (Foppa et.al. 2002). The amount of ethanol was 23 grams.

When 26 volunteers, of which 10 were hyperlipidemic, 9 hypertensive and 7 fully healthy, were given red Wine 2.5 dl daily, for 15 days, the mean average blood pressure (MAP) decreased in the whole group by 7 mmHg ($p < 0.01$). In the hypertensive group, systolic blood pressure decreased by 4 mmHg (153 mmHg $\rightarrow$ 147 mmHg; $p < 0.01$) and diastolic blood pressure decreased by 4 mmHg ($p < 0.01$), compared to the control group (Andrade et.al. 2009).

Red Wine inhibits ACE (Actis-Goretta et.al. 2006). The effect is stronger, than with white Wine.

Red Wine inhibits Endothelin-1 (ET-1), which is known to contract blood vessels. The inhibition has verified in 2 different experiments (Corder et.al. 2001; Khan et.al. 2002).

When healthy volunteers were given 1 glass of red Wine daily, for 3 weeks, plasma viscosity decreased by 7.7% ($p = 0.004$), compared to the control group. This effect lasted up to 3 weeks, after stopping the red Wine intake (Jensen et.al. 2006). When plasma viscosity decreases, it means a lower flow resistance in blood vessels.

With hypertensive rats, red Wine decreases significantly both systolic and diastolic blood pressure (Moura et.al. 2004).

When normotensive rats were given red Wine Polyphenols 20 mg/kg daily, for 7 days, systolic blood pressure decreased significantly (p < 0.01), compared to the control group. The effect was seen after 4 days from beginning of the experiment (Diebolt et.al. 2001).

In great many experiments with human volunteers and animals, it has been noticed, that red Wine is a strong vasodilator and increases the NO concentration in blood, and stimulates the eNOS activity (Leikert et.al. 2002; Zenebe et.al. 2003; Coimbra et.al. 2005; Porteri et.al. 2010; Sarr et.al. 2006).

At the moment, it seems to be, that 1 – 2 glass red Wine daily is very good for human health, and decreases cardiovascular risk factors very strongly.

Reishi

(Ganoderma Lucidum)

Reishi is one of the Worlds oldest medicinal mushrooms. It has been used in China, Korea and Japan over 2000 years against cancer, asthma, bronchitis, low immunity and high blood pressure. Reishi is very rare in nature, all over the Northern Hemisphere, but nowadays it is cultivated in large scale, especially in China. It is called Lingzhi in China.

Reishi has
- – Blood pressure lowering properties
- – Total cholesterol lowering properties
- – LDL-cholesterol lowering properties
- – Triglycerides lowering properties
- – HDL-cholesterol increasing properties

When hypertensive rats were given 5% Reishi in their daily diet, for 4 weeks, systolic blood pressure decreased significantly by 10 mmHg (p < 0.05), compared to the control group. Serum total cholesterol decreased by 20.6% (p < 0.01) and liver total cholesterol decreased by 55.7% (p < 0.01). Liver triglycerides decreased by 45.9% (p < 0.01), compared to the control group (Kabir et.al. 1988).

When 34 hypertensive volunteers were given Reishi extract 220 mg daily, for 14 days, systolic blood pressure decreased significantly in 82.5% of volunteers, compared to control group (Jin et.al. 1996). This was double blind experiment.

In many experiments it has been verified, that Reishi and compounds extracted from it, inhibit strongly ACE (Morogawa et.al. 1986; Abdullah et.al. 2012; Kim et.al. 2004).

When hypertensive rats were given Reishi water extract at a dose of 10 mg/kg, diastolic blood pressure decreased by 44.3% (Park et.al. 1987).

This blood pressure lowering effect has been verified also in other experiments (Lee et.al. 1990; Kanmatsuse et.al. 1985).

When 26 volunteers were given Reishi 1.44 grams daily, for 12 weeks, HDL-cholesterol increased but triglycerides decreased significantly, compared to the control group (Chu et.al. 2011). This was a double blind experiment. The used dose was significantly lower, than the Chinese recommended 6 grams daily (Teow et.al. 1996).

The total cholesterol, LDL-cholesterol and triglycerides decreasing, but HDL-cholesterol increasing properties of Reishi has been verified in great many experiments with mice, pigs, rats, hamsters and human cells (Khva et.al. 1989; Li et.al. 2011; Yang et.al. 2002; Hajjaj et.al. 2005; Chen et.al. 2005; Fenfangetal et.al. 2003; Feng et.al. 2008; Berger et.al. 2005; Tong et.al. 2008).

Resveratrol

Resveratrol is a Stilbenoid, a natural Phenolic compound, made by many plants, to prevent bacterial and fungal infections. Resveratrol exists especially in the skin of red Grapes and in the root of the medicinal plant Polygonum Cuspidatum. Resveratrol can be purchased from Supermarkets.

Resveratrol has
  – Blood pressure lowering properties
  – Total cholesterol lowering properties
  – LDL-cholesterol lowering properties
  – Triglycerides lowering properties
  – HDL-cholesterol increasing properties

The blood pressure lowering property of Resveratrol is well documented in animal experiments. When rats were given Resveratrol 5 mg/kg daily, for 3 weeks, systolic blood pressure decreased by 15%, compared to the control group (Mizyutani et.al. 2000). Same blood pressure lowering effect has been noticed in many other animal experiments (Bhatt et.al. 2001; Chan et.al. 2011; Rivera et.al. 2009; Inanaga et.al. 2009; Aubin et.al. 2008).

When 11 healthy, overweight volunteers were given 150 mg Resveratrol daily, for 30 days, both systolic blood pressure and triglycerides decreased significantly, compared to the control group (Timmers et.al. 2011). This was a doubble blind experiment.

The total cholesterol and LDL-cholesterol lowering properties of Resveratrol has been noticed in many animal experiments Do et.al. 2008; Robich et.al. 2010; Juhasz et.al. 2011; Seng et.al. 2011).

Rice bran

(Oryza Sativa)

Rice bran is a byproduct of Rice processing, when white rice is produced. Rice bran is the nutritionally most important part of rice. It contains large amounts of gamma-Oryzanol, Ferulic acid and Tocotrienols, which all have cholesterol- and blood pressure decreasing properties.

Rice bran has
- Blood pressure decreasing properties
- Total cholesterol decreasing properties
- LDL-cholesterol decreasing properties
- Triglycerides decreasing properties
- HDL-cholesterol increasing properties

When rats were given 60 g/kg Rice bran extract daily, for 8 weeks, both blood pressure ($p < 0.01$) and triglycerides ($p < 0.01$) decreased significantly, compared to the control group (Ardiansyah et.al. 2006). Also ACE activity was decreased significantly ($p < 0.01$).

When Ferulic acid, a component of Rice bran, was given daily to rats at a dose of 0.01 g/kg, for 8 weeks, blood pressure decreased ($p < 0.05$) significantly, compared to the control group (Ardiansyah et.al. 2007).

When 60 diabetic volunteers were given Rice bran 20 grams daily, triglycerides ($p < 0.01$) decreased significantly, but HDL-cholesterol ($p < 0.01$) increased significantly, compared to the control group (Tazakori et.al. 2006). Also LDL-cholesterol and total cholesterol decreased. This was a double blind experiment.

When 14 volunteers were given 84 grams Rice bran daily, for 6 weeks, total cholesterol (8.3%; $p < 0.05$) and LDL-cholesterol (13.7%; $p < 0.05$) decreased significantly, compared to the control group (Gerhardt et.al. 1998). This was a double blind experiment.

When mice were given in their daily diet either Rice bran or Ferulic acid, for 17 days, both total cholesterol and LDL-cholesterol decreased significantly in both groups, compared to the control group, which got normal diet (Jung et.al. 2007).

When 90 volunteers were given 100 mg of Rice bran Tocotrienols containing fraction daily, for 35 days, total cholesterol decreased by 20% ($p < 0.05$), LDL-cholesterol decreased by 25% ($p < 0.05$) and triglycerides decreased by 12%, compared to the control group (Qureshi et.al. 2002).

When 20 diabetic volunteers were given 20 grams Rice bran daily, for 3 months, total cholesterol decreased by 9.2% and LDL-cholesterol decreased by 13.7%, compared to the control group (Cheng et.al. 2010). The plasma free fatty acid concentration was 20% lower in Rice bran group, than in the control group.

When 45 diabetic volunteers were given different Rice bran products 20 grams daily, for 8 weeks, total cholesterol decreased by 11% ($p < 0.05$), LDL-cholesterol decreased by 15.5% ($p < 0.05$) and triglycerides decreased by an average of 7.5% ($p < 0.05$), compared to the control group

(Qureshi et.al. 2002). This was a double blind experiment.

Rice bran oil

(Oryza Sativa)

Rice bran oil is a by product of Rice processing. Rice bran oil is very popular as a cooking oil in China and Japan. Rice bran oil contains large amounts of gamma-Oryzanol and gamma-Tocotrienol, which lower both total cholesterol and blood pressure.

The cholesterol- and triglyceride lowering property of Rice bran oil has been verified in many experiments.

Rice bran oil has
- Total cholesterol lowering properties
- LDL-cholesterol lowering properties
- Triglycerides lowering properties

When 12 volunteers were given Rice bran oil daily, instead of normal cooking oils, for 30 days, total cholesterol decreased by 26.1% (247.3 mg/dl $\rightarrow$ 182.7 mg/dl; $p < 0.001$) and triglycerides decreased by 39.1% (349.8 mg/dl $\rightarrow$ 212.9 mg/dl; $p < 0.001$), compared to the control group (Raguram et.al. 1989).

When 73 volunteers were given daily an oil mixture of 80% Rice bran oil and 20% of Safflower oil, for 3 months, LDL-cholesterol decreased significantly, compared to the control group (Malve et.al. 2010). This was a double blind experiment,

When 80 volunteers were given daily 20 grams of Rice bran oil, for 4 weeks, total cholesterol decreased by 2.2% ($p = 0.045$) and LDL-cholesterol decreased by 3.5% ($p = 0.016$), compared to control group (Eady et.al. 2011). This was a double blind experiment.

When 14 volunteers were given daily 1/3 of their cooking oil as Rice bran oil, LDL-cholesterol decreased by 7% ($p < 0.0004$), compared to the control group (Marlene et.al. 2005). This was a double blind experiment.

When 14 volunteers took either Rice bran oil or Sunflower oil as their cooking oil daily, for 3 months, both LDL-cholesterol ($p < 0.05$) and triglycerides decreased significantly in the Rice bran oil group, compared to the Sunflower oil group (Kuriyan et.al. 2005).

In rats Rice bran oil increases HDL-cholesterol (Chou et.al. 2009).

Roman Chamomile

(Chamaemelum Nobile)

Roman Chamomile originates from North-Africa and Western Europe. It has been used for a long time as a medicinal plant, against Diabetes and also high blood pressure in Morocco. It is very easy to cultivate.

Roman Chamomile has
- Blood pressure lowering properties
- Diuretic properties

When hypertensive rats were given 140 mg/kg water extract of Roman Chamomile daily, for 20 days, systolic blood pressure decreased by 13.5 mmHg ($p < 0.01$). The extract decreased blood pressure also acutely. Allready a single dose decreased systolic blood pressure for 24 hours. Roman Chamomile has also a significant diuretic activity, which started 8 days after beginning of the experiment ($p < 0.01$) (Naoufel et.al. 2009).

The blood pressure lowering effect of Roman Chamomile has been noticed also in an other experiment with rats (Zeggwagh et.al. 2007).

Rooibos tea

(Aspalanthus Linearis)

Rooibos tea originates from South-Africa, Rooibos tea is very popular in the whole World, and can be purchased from ordinary supermarkets. Rooibos tea contains a lot of different Flavonoids.

Rooibos tea has
- Blood pressure lowering properties
- Total cholesterol lowering properties
- LDL-cholesterol lowering properties
- Triglycerides lowering properties
- HDL-cholesterol increasing properties

Rooibos tea inhibits ACE (Persson et.al. 2010).

In rats, Rooibos tea decreases blood pressure. The higher the dose, the higher the decrease in blood pressure (Khan et.al. 2006).

When 40 volunteers were give 6 cups of Rooibos tea daily, for 6 weeks, LDL-cholesterol decreased 9.3% (4.3 mmol/L → 3.9 mmol/L) and triglycerides decreased 29.4% (1.7 mmol/L → 1.2 mmol/L), but HDL-cholesterol increased 33.3% (0.9 mmol/L → 1.2 mmol/L), compared to the control group (Marnewick et.al. 2011).

In experiments with rats, Rooibos tea decreases significantly both total cholesterol and triglycerides (Iswaldi et.al. 2011; Ulicna et.al. 2010).

Rose hips

(Rose Canina, Rosa Sp.)

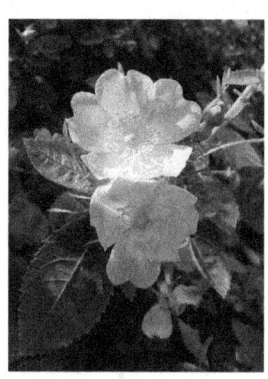

Rose hip is the berry of Roses. It is edible, and contains very large amount of different nutrients, especially vitamin C, beta-Carotene and Lycopene, Lycopene content varies between 10 – 80 mg/100 g fresh hips, depending on the Rose species. There are several tens of Wild Rose species all around the World, and especially in China. Rose hips can be purchased in Supermarkets as a dried flour.

Rose hips have
- Blood pressure lowering properties
- Total cholesterol lowering properties
- LDL-cholesterol lowering properties

When 31 overweight volunteers were given Rose hips 40 grams daily, for 6 weeks, systolic blood pressure decreased by 3.4% (4 mmHg; p = 0.021), total cholesterol decreased by 4.9% (p = 0.0018), LDL-cholesterol by 6.0% (p = 0.012) and LDL/HDL-cholesterol ratio by 6.5% (p = 0.041), compared to the control group (Andersson et.al. 2011). This was a double blind experiment.

The cholesterol lowering effect of Rose hips has been verified also in experiments with mice (Andersson et.al. 2011).

Rosmarin

(Rosmarinus Officinalis)

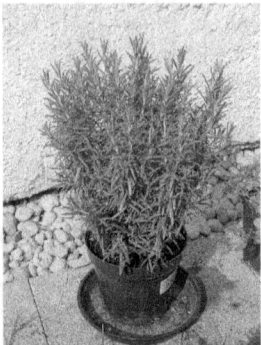

Rosmarin is a very popular, strong flavour spice. Rosmarin grows wild around the Mediterranian sea. It is strongly antioxidative, and it contains a lot of Flavonoids and also Rosmarinic acid.

Rosmarin has
- Blood pressure lowering properties
- Diuretic properties

The diuretic activity of Rosmarin has been verified in experiments with rats. Rats were given 8% strong Rosmarin water extract at a dose of 10 mg/kg daily, for 7 days. The urine output increased over 100% after the fifth day, compared to the control group (Haloui et.al. 2000).

The water extract of Rosmarin inhibits very strongly ACE (Kwon et.al. 2006).

When rats were fed fructose 60% of their daily diet, for 60 days, the rats became hypertensive. When rats were given Rosmaric acid 10 mg/kg daily, blood pressure decreased significantly, compared to the control group. Also in this experiment, Rosmarinic acid inhibited both ACE and Endothelin-1 (ET-1) (Karthik et.al. 2011).

Royal Jelly

Royal Jelly is the honey product, which is entirely fed by worker bees to the Bee Queen, as the only food. With the Royal Jelly, the Queen gets many times bigger and lives many times longer, than the ordinary worker bees. Royal Jelly has many medicinal properties, and there is a huge research activity around it.

Royal Jelly has
- Total cholesterol lowering properties
- LDL-cholesterol lowering properties
- VLDL-cholesterol lowering properties
- HDL-cholesterol increasing properties

In a meta-analysis, which looked after all the animal and human research around Royal Jelly and cholesterol, it was noticed, that when volunteers were given 50-100 mg Royal Jelly daily, LDL-cholesterol decreases by average of 14% and the serum total lipids decrease by average of 10% (Vittek 1995).

When 15 volunteers were given 6 grams of Royal Jelly daily, for 4 weeks, total cholesterol (p < 0.05), LDL-cholesterol (p < 0.05) and VLDL-cholesterol (p < 0.05) decreased significantly, compared to the control group (Guo et.al. 2007).

When rats were fed Royal Jelly 700 mg/kg daily, for 6 weeks, serum total cholesterol decreased (p < 0.01) significantly, but HDL-cholesterol (p < 0.05) increased significantly, compared to the control group (Shen et.al. 1995).

Rutin

Rutin is a Flavonoid, which exists in many plants. It has many pharmacological properties. Rutin is a cheap Flavonoid, and it can be purchased as 500 mg pills. Good dietary sources are especially Buckwheat, Tartary Buckwheat, Buckwheat sprouts and Red Onion.

Rutin has
- Blood pressure lowering properties
- Total cholesterol lowering properties
- LDL-cholesterol lowering properties
- Triglycerides lowering properties
- HDL-cholesterol increasing properties

When 40 diabetic volunteers were given 500 mg Rutin daily, for 4 months, systolic blood pressure decreased by 3.8 mmHg (130.2 mmHg → 126.4 mmHg), diastolic blood pressure decreased by 1.4 mmHg (85.1 mmHg → 83.7 mmHg), LDL-cholesterol decreased by 19.0% (78.74 mg/dl → 63.74 mg/dl), but HDL-cholesterol increased by 27.8% (37.4 mg/dl → 47.8 mg/dl), compared to the control group (Sattanathan et.al. 2011).

When 50 diabetic volunteers were given 500 mg Rutin daily, for 2 months, systolic blood pressure decreased by 4 mmHg (135 mmHg → 131 mmHg), diastolic blood pressure decreased by 1.9 mmHg (87.5 mmHg → 85.6 mmHg), LDL-cholesterol decreased by 11.3% (65.88 mg/dl → 59.6 mg/dl), but HDL-cholesterol increased by 10.2% (39.0 mg/dl → 43.0 mg/dl), compared to the control group (Sattanathan et.al. 2010).

Same kind of results have been obtained also in experiments with human volunteers (Sattanathan et.al. 2011) and rats (Fernandes et.al. 2010).

Sage

(Salvia Officinalis)

Sage is an ancient spice, herbal tea and medicinal plant, which has been used in Europe for thousands of years. Sage is used to increase memory, as an antibacterial and to reduce high blood pressure. The cultivation of Sage is very easy. The effective chemical compounds are Rosmarinic acid and Luteolin-7-Glucoside.

Sage has
- Blood pressure lowering properties
- Total cholesterol lowering properties
- LDL-cholesterol lowering properties
- Triglycerides lowering properties
- HDL-cholesterol increasing properties

When 6 healthy women were given Sage tea 3 dl, 2 times daily, for 4 weeks, systolic blood pressure decreased 5.4 mmHg (116.1 mmHg $\rightarrow$ 110.7 mmHg), diastolic lood pressure decreased 4.6 mmHg (68.2 mmHg $\rightarrow$ 63.6 mmHg), total cholesterol decreased by 16% ($p < 0.05$) and LDL-cholesterol decreased by 19.6% ($p < 0.05$), but HDL-cholesterol increased by 50.6% ($p < 0.05$), compared to control group (Sa et.al. 2009).

When 67 volunteers were given Sage leaf extract at a dose of 1500 mg daily, total cholesterol ($p < 0.001$), LDL-cholesterol ($p < 0.001$) and triglycerides ($p < 0.001$) decreased significantly, but HDL-cholesterol ($p < 0.001$) increased significantly, compared to the control group (Kianbakht et.al. 2011). This was a double blind experiment.

When diabetic rats were given Sage ethanol extract 0.4 g/kg daily, for 2 weeks, triglycerides decreased by 40% ($p < 0.001$) and total cholesterol decreased by 33% ($p < 0.001$), compared to the control group (Eidi et.al. 2009).

Sage water-ethanol extracts causes a long lasting hypotensive effect in cats (Todorov et.al. 1984).

Salt

(NaCl)

Salt is a molecule, which is a combination of chemical elements Sodium, Na and Chlorine, Cl. Both Sodium and Chlorine are essential elements in human nutrition. However, too much salt in daily diet causes hypertension.

Salt has
- Blood pressure increasing properties

The physiological need of salt in human diet is between 0.6 – 1.2 grams (10 – 20 mmol) daily (Brown et.al. 2009). But in almost every country around the World, too much salt is included in daily diet. In Europe, North-America and Asia, people get typically between 6 – 12 grams (100 – 200 mmo) salt daily (Brown et.al. 2009). In Europe and North-America up to 75% of salt comes from finished foods, fast foods, bread, cereals, Chips and Grilled products (Brown et.al. 2009).

In meta-analysis, which included 28 different experiments and 2954 volunteers, it was noticed, that decreasing the daily amount of salt by 6 grams, decreases systolic blood pressure by an average of 7.11 mmHg (p < 0.001) and diastolic blood pressure by an average of 3.88 mmHg (p < 0.05) in hypertensive volunteers (He et.al. 2002).

At the Brazilian Venezuelan border lives the Yanomami Indian tribe. Their daily salt intake is only 0.2 grams, by average. The total Sodium content of their urine is only 0.9 mmol, when it is typically 78 mmol (=4.6 grams salt) in persons living in Europe and North-America. The Yanomami average systolic blood pressure is 95.4 mmHg, and diastolic blood pressure is 61.4 mmHg. Overweight and alcohol is non-existent among Yanomami. Hypertension is totally non-existent among Yanomami (Mancilha-Carvalho et.al. 2002). This research is part of the International INTERSALT research.

Saffron

(Crocus Sativus)

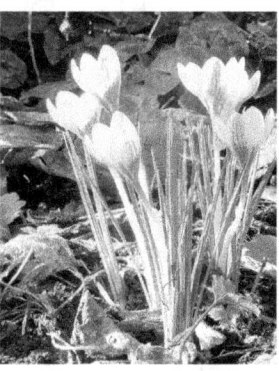

Saffron is the dried stigma of Crocus Sativus. Saffron is very popular but very expensive spice. Saffron is also used for many medical purposes.

Saffron has
- Blood pressure lowering properties
- Total cholesterol lowering properties
- LDL-cholesterol lowering properties
- Triglycerides lowering properties
- HDL-cholesterol increasing properties

The effective compounds in Saffron are Carotenoids Crocin, Crocetin and Safranal. These same compounds exist in fruits of Chinese Medicinal plant, Gardenia Jasminoides, which is used in China to lower high blood pressure.

When hypertensive rats were given either Saffron water extract, Crocetin or Safranal at different dosages, the mean average blood pressure (MAP) decreased significantly. For example, 1 mg/kg Saffron water extract, injected intavascularly, decreased MAP by 60 mmHg (Imenshadidi et.al. 2010).

When 10 volunteers were given Saffron 400 mg daily, for 7 days, both systolic and diastolic blood pressure decreased significantly, compared to the control group (Modaghegh et.al. 2008). This was a doubble bind experiment.

The total cholesterol, LDL-cholesterol and triglycerides lowering but HDL-cholesterol increasing property of Saffron, Crocin and Crocetin has been noticed in many experiments (Xu et.al. 2006; Sheng et.al. 2006; He et.al. 2008; In-Ah et.al. 2005).

Saturated fats

Saturated fats are fats, which do not contain carbon doubble bonds in their fatty acid chains. Typical saturated fats are butter, milk fat, cheese fat and generally the animal fats.

Saturated fats have
- Blood pressure increasing properties
- Total cholesterol increasing properties
- LDL-cholesterol increasing properties

In a meta-analysis with 395 experiments, of at least 1 month duration, it was noticed, that if part of saturated fats, corresponding to 10% of total daily energy, were replaced with complex carbohydrates, total cholesterol decreased by an average of 0.52 mmol/L, and LDL-cholesterol decreased by an average of 0.32 mmol/L (Clarke et.al. 1997). In the same research, it was noticed, that reducing the daily dietary amount of cholesterol by 200 mg, decreased further the total cholesterol by 0.13 mmol/L and LDL-cholesterol by 0.10 mmol/L.

Healthy young volunteers were given 2.5 weeks food containing 30 – 33% of their daily energy as saturated fats. After this they changed for 2.5 weeks on diet containing 30 – 33% of energy either as monounsaturated fats or Omega-6 polyunsaturated fats. Compared to the saturated fat group, total cholesterol decreased by 10%, LDL-cholesterol by 22% and HDL-cholesterol by 14%, in the Omega-6 group. In the monounsaturated group, total cholesterol decreased by 12%, LDL-cholesterol decreased by 15% and HDL-cholesterol decreased by 4%, compared to the saturated fat group (Hodson et.al. 2001).

When blood pressure and plasma fatty acid composition and fatty acid concentrations of 4033 healthy men were measured by Gas/Liquid chromatography, it was noticed, that blood pressure increased, when the concentration of saturated fatty acids increases in the plasma. Also blood pressure increased, when the total concentration of fatty acids increased in the plasma. Also blood pressure decreased, when the amount of Omega-6 fatty acids increased in the plasma (Grimsgaard et.al. 1999).

Schisandra Berry

(Schisandra Chinensis)

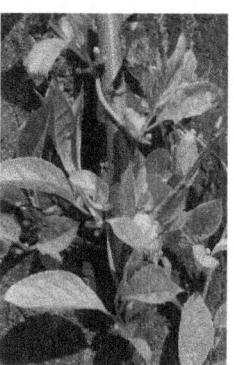

(Author: Doronenko)

Schisandra Berry originates from Russia and China. The berries are eatable, and they have Adaptogenic properties. Schisandra berries have been used in Russia already from 1940 as Adaptogenic plant, which increases working capacity and nonspecific stress capacity.

Schisandra Berries have
- Blood pressure lowering properties
- Total cholesterol lowering properties
- LDL-cholesterol lowering properties

In many experiments in Russia, when volunteers have taken a long time 1% Schisandra Berry extract, the blood pressure has decreased by 5 – 20 mmHg, depending of dose and the duration of the experiment (Panossian et.al. 2008).

Also Korean researchers have noticed, that Schisandra Berries have vasorelaxant properties (Rhyu et.al. 2006).

When rats were fed Schisandra Berry water extract either 0.2 mg/kg, 0.5 mg/kg, 2.0 mg/kg or 5.0 mg/kg daily, for 5 weeks, the systolic blood pressure, total cholesterol and LDL-cholesterol decreased significantly, compared to the control group (Kim et.al. 2011).

Schisandra vine is easily cultivated in Northern Hemisphere cold climates.

Scrambling Gynura

(Gynura Procumbens, Gynura Divaricata)

Scrambling Gynura is a fast growing plant, which is used in Indonesia, Singapore, Malaysia and Thailand against high blood pressure and high cholesterol levels. In Java and Singapore islands, Scrambling Gynura is used as a salad and vegetable. In Oginawa island in Japan Gynura Bicolor is grown as a vegetable. Its English name is Oginawa Spinach and Japanese call it Kinjiso.

Scrambling Gynura has
- Blood pressure decreasing properties
- Total cholesterol decreasing properties
- Triglycerides decreasing properties

When hypertensive rats were given Scrambling Gynura (Gynura Procumbens) water extract 500 mg/kg daily, for 4 weeks, systolic blood pressure decreased by 9.9% (191.7 mmHg → 172.7 mmHg; $p < 0.05$), compared to the control group. The serum NO level also increased by 60.7% ($p < 0.05$), compared to the control group (Kim et.al. 2006).

When rats were given purified water extract of the original ethanol extract of Scrambling Gynura (Gynura Procumbens) intravenously at doses between 0.625 – 10 mg/kg, the mean average blood pressure (MAP) decreased in direct proportion to the used dose, 20 – 80 mmHg ($p < 0.001$), compared to the control group. The extract also inhibited strongly ACE (Hoe et.al. 2007).

Also another Gynura, Gynura Divarica, inhibited strongly ACE (Wu et.al. 2011). This species is called BAI NBEI SAN QI by Chinese, and it has for a long time been used against high blood pressure.

The blood pressure decreasing properties of scrambling Gynura has been verified in many other experiments (Lam et.al. 1997; Lam et.al. 1998; Hoe et.al. 2011).

When diabetic rats were given ethanol extract of Scrambling Gynura, 150 mg/kg twice daily, for 7 days, total cholesterol decreased by 15.4% ($p < 0.01$) and triglycerides decreased y 27.8% ($p < 0.01$), compared to the control group (Zhang et.al. 2000).

Sesame oil

(Sesamum Indicum)

Sesame oil is pressed from Sesame (Sesamum Indicum) seeds. Sesame is generally used all around the World as cooking and salad oil.

Sesame oil has
- Blood pressure lowering properties
- Total cholesterol lowering properties
- LDL-cholesterol lowering properties

- Triglycerides lowering properties
- HDL-cholesterol increasing properties

When 50 hypertensive volunteers were given 35 grams of Sesame oil daily, for 45 days, systolic blood pressure (144.25 mmHg → 124.86 mmHg; $p < 0.001$) and diastolic blood pressure (97.9 mmHg → 83.8 mmHg; $p < 0.001$) decreased significantly, compared to the control group (Sankar et.al. 2006). Triglycerides decreased (194.8 mg/dl → 159.0 mg/dl; $p < 0.001$) also significantly.

When 18 diabetic volunteers were given 35 grams of Sesame oil daily, for 60 days, the plasma total cholesterol decreased by 20%, LDL-cholesterol decreased by 33.8% and triglycerides decreased by 14%, compared to the control group (Sankar et.al. 2011).

Shallot

(Allium Ascalonicum)

Shallot is a popular salad onion, which can be purchased from all Supermarkets. Shallot has very large amounts of Flavonoids, up to 681 mg/100 g, especially Myricetin, Quercetin, Rutin and Formonetin. The Quercetin content is very high, up to 398 mg/100 g (Vanitha et.al. 2009).

Shallot has
- Total cholesterol lowering properties
- LDL-cholesterol lowering properties
- Triglycerides lowering properties

When rats were fed ethanol extract of Shallot at a dose of 100 mg/kg daily, for 8 weeks, total cholesterol decreased by 47.1% ($p < 0.01$), LDL-cholesterol decreased by 42.8% ($p < 0.01$) and triglycerides decreased by 30.9% ($p < 0.05$), compared to the control group (Fallah et.al. 2010).

Shiitake

(Lentinus Edodes)

(Author: frankenstoen)

Shiitake is an Ancient food and medicinal mushroom, originally from East Asia, China, Japan and Korea. It is now cultivated all around the World.

Shiitake has
- – Blood pressure lowering properties
- – Total cholesterol lowering properties
- – LDL-cholesterol lowering properties
- – Triglycerides lowering properties

The cholesterol lowering property of Shiitake is known already 50 years ago (Kaneda et.al. 1966). The effective compound is Eritadenine.

When rats were fed Shiitake 5% of their daily diet, blood pressure decreased significantly (Kabir et.al. 1987).

The cholesterol- and triglycerides lowering property of Shiitake is well documentated, and depending of the daily dose and test duration, total cholesterol has decreased up to 25% and triglycerides have decreased up to 55% (Yang et.al. 2002; Handayani et.al. 2011; Kaneda et.al. 1966; Kabir et.al. 1989; Kabir et.al. 1987; Yamada et.al. 2002; Bisen et.al. 2010).

Slow Breathing Exercise

Slow Breathing decreases high blood pressure, when exercised both acutely and chronically.

When 20 hypertensive volunteers made controlled Slow Breathing exercise at a rhythm of 6 Breaths/Minute, both systolic blood pressure (149.7 mmHg → 141.4 mmHg; $p < 0.05$) and diastolic blood pressure (82.7 mmHg → 77.8 mmHg; $p < 0.05$) decreased significantly, compared to the control group (Chacko et.al. 2005).

When 18 volunteers exercised Slow Breathing 10 minutes daily, for 8 weeks, systolic blood pressure decreased by 7.5 mmHg ($p < 0.001$), compared to the control group (Grossman et.al. 2001).

Society Garlic

(Tulbaghia Vioolacea)

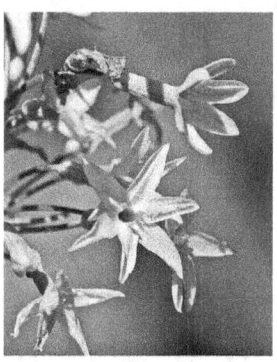

Society Garlic originates from South-Africa. It is also called Wild Garlic. It smells like ordinary Garlic. All parts of the plant can be eaten, and used in salads, especially leaves and flowers. It has a long time been used also as a medicinal plant, for high blood pressure. It is easy to cultivate and fast growing.

Society Garlic has
- Blood pressure lowering properties

This plant inhibits ACE very strongly. This has been verified in 2 different experiments (Ramesar et.al. 2008; Duncan et.al. 1999).

When Society Garlic water extract was fed to rats at a dose of 50 mg/kg daily, for 14 days, systolic blood pressure decreased by 9.12% ($p < 0.05$), compared to the control group. Also plasma Aldosteron concentration decreased significantly ($p < 0.05$) and Sodium in urine increased significantly, compared to the control group (Mackraj et.al. 2008).

When rats were given Society Garlic leaves ethanol extract intravenously at a dose between 5 – 150 mg/kg, both systolic and diastolic blood pressure decreased significantly ($p < 0.05$), compared to the control group (Raji et.al. 2012).

Soybean protein

(Glycine Max)

Soybean protein is used all around the World as a food for humans and animals. It can be purchased from every market as a Soybean flour. The Soybean flour can be easily added to all foods, drinks and bread.

Soybean protein has
- Blood pressure lowering properties
- Total cholesterol lowering properties
- LDL-cholesterol lowering properties
- Triglycerides lowering properties
- HDL-cholesterol increasing properties

When rats were given for 8 weeks with either Soybean protein or Casein in their food, the mean average blood pressure (MAP) in Soybean group (150 mmHg) was significantly lower than in the Casein group (164 mmHg) (Martin et.al. 2001).

In human trials, when participants ate Soybean protein 40 grams daily, for 12 weeks, the systolic blood pressure of hypertensive participants decreased 7.88 mmHg, and the diastolic blood pressure decreased 5.27 mmHg, compared to the control group. This was a double blind trial with 302 participants (He et.al. 2005).

In meta-analysis of human trials with 42 different studies, it was noticed, that the average drop in LDL-cholesterol was 5.5% and the average incerase in HDL-cholesterol was 3.2% in Soybean group, compared to the control group (Anderson et.al. 2011). The daily doses were between 15 – 65 grams, and the test time varied between 4 to 12 weeks.

In another meta-analysis with 38 studies, the average drop in total cholesterol was 9.3%, the average drop in LDL-cholesterol was 12.9% and the average drop in triglycerides was 10.5%, but the HDL-cholesterol increased by 2.4% (Anderson et.al. 1995) The daily Soybean protein intake was around 47 grams.

Soy Lecithin

Soy Lecithin is a popular functional food, which can be purchased from every Supermarket. It contains a lot of Phospholipids and Inositol.

Soy Lecithin has
- Total cholesterol lowering properties
- LDL-cholesterol lowering properties
- Triglycerides lowering properties
- HDL-cholesterol increasing properties

When volunteers with high cholesterol levels were given Soy Lecithin 500 mg daily, for 2 months, LDL-cholesterol decreased by 56.15% and total cholesterol decreased by 42.0% (Mourad et.al. 2010).

When volunteers with high cholesterol levels were given Soy Lecithin 12 grams daily, for 3 months, total cholesterol decreased by 15%, and triglycerides decreased by 23%, but HDL-cholesterol increased by 16% (Brook et.al. 1986).

When 65 volunteers with high cholesterol levels were given food, where animal protein was replaced with Soy protein, which included 6% Soy Lecithin, total cholesterol decreased by 18.6% (Sirtori et.al. 1985).

When diabetic volunteers with high cholesterol levels were given daily flour, which had 12% Soy Lecithin and 35% Soy protein, for 12 weeks, total cholesterol decreased by 12% ($p < 0.001$), triglycerides decreased by 22% ($p < 0.001$) and LDL-cholesterol decreased by 16% ($p < 0.001$), but HDL-cholesterol increased by 11% (Medic et.al. 2006).

When monkeys were fed with food containing 3.4% Soy Lecithin daily, for 8 weeks, total cholesterol decreased by 46% and LDL-cholesterol decreased by 55% (Wilson et.al. 1998).

In experiment with Hamsters, fed 3.4% Soy Lecithin daily, total cholesterol decreased by 38% and LDL-cholesterol decreased by 73% (Wilson et.al. 1998).

In experiments with rats, Soy Lecithin also decreased total- and LDL-cholesterol (Iwata et.al. 1992).

Soymilk

(Glycine Max)

Soymilk can nowadays be purchased from every Supermarket. Soymilk is extremely easy to use in cooking or to drink as such. Soymilk contains a lot of functionally healthy Isoflavonoids, Genistein and Daidzein.

Soymilk has
  – Blood pressure lowering properties
  – Total cholesterol lowering properties
  – LDL-cholesterol lowering properties

When 40 volunteers were given 2 times daily 5 deciliters of Soymilk, for 3 months, systolic blood pressure decreased by 18.4 mmHg and diastolic blood pressure decreased by 15.9 mmHg, compared to the control group (Rivas et.al. 2002). This was a doubble blind experiment.

When 42 volunteers were given Soymilk 5 deciliters daily, for 3 weeks, total cholesterol decreased by 11% ($p < 0.001$) and LDL-cholesterol decreased by 25% ($p < 0.001$), compared to the control group (Onuegbu et.al. 2011).

Allready relative small amounts of Soymilk makes significant changes to cholesterol- and blood pressure values.

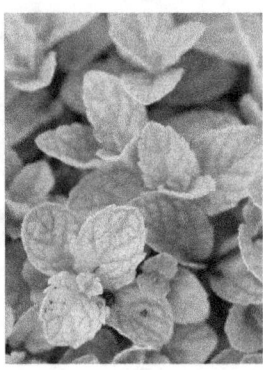

Spearmint

(Mentha Spicata var. Spicata,

Synonyme: *Mentha Cordifolia)*

Spearmint is a very popular vegetable, spice and medicinal plant, all over the World. Its cultivation is very easy. Spearmint is used medicinally in Asthma, Inflammation, stomach troubles etc.

Spearmint has
 — Blood pressure lowering properties

When hypertensive rats were given daily 200 mg/kg of Spearmint water extracct, for 3 weeks, systolic blood pressure decreased by 11.4% (199.1 mmHg → 176.4 mmHg; $p < 0.01$) and diastolic blood pressure decreased by 23.4% (129.1 mmHg → 98.8 mmHg; $p < 0.01$), compared to the control group (Pakdeechote et.al. 2011).

Spirulina

(Spirulina Platensis, Spirulina Sp.)

Spirulina is a single cell, dark green freshwater algae, which is very popular as a food supplement. It contains very large amounts of different nutrients.

Spirulina has
 — Blood pressure lowering properties
 — Total cholesterol lowering properties
 — LDL-cholesterol lowering properties
 — Triglycerides lowering properties
 — HDL-cholesterol increasing properties

When Spirulina was given 4.5 grams daily to 36 volunteers, for 6 weeks, triglycerides decreased (234 mg/dl → 168 mg/dl; $p < 0.001$), total cholesterol decreased (182 mg/dl → 163 mg/dl; $p < 0.001$) and LDL-cholesterol decreased (103 mg/dl → 86 mg/dl; $p < 0.013$) significantly, compared to the control group. But HDL-cholesterol increased (43 mg/dl → 50 mg/dl; $p < 0.01$) significantly. Both systolic blood pressure (120 mmHg → 109 mmHg; $p < 0.01$) and diastolic blood pressure (86 mmHg → 79 mmHg; $p < 0.05$) decreased significantly, compared to the control group (Torres-Duran et.al. 2007).

When 37 diabetic volunteers were given daily 8 grams Spirulina, for 12 weeks, triglycerides ($p < 0.05$) decreased significantly. Also total cholesterol, LDL-cholesterol and blood pressure decreased (Lee et.al. 2008).

When 23 hyperlipidemic volunteers were given Spirulina 1 gram daily, for 2 moths, triglycerides, total cholesterol and LDL-cholesterol decreased significantly, compared to the control group (Samuels et.al. 2002).

When 78 volunteers wer given 8 grams Spirulina daily, for 16 weeks, total cholesterol decreased significantly, compared to the control group (Park et.al. 2008). This was a double blind experiment.

In experiments with rats, Spirulina decreases blood pressure, triglycerides and LDL-cholesterol significantly (Juarez-Oropeza et.al. 2009).

When rabbits were fed in their daily diet either 1% or 5% Spirulina, for 8 weeks, LDL-cholesterol decreased by 26.4% in group, which got 1% Spirulina and 41.2% in group, which got 5% Spirulina, compared to the control group. Also HDL-cholesterol increased significantly (Cheong et.al. 2010).

Stevioside

(Stevia Rebaudiana)

The Stevioside glucoside is about 200 times more sweet than sugar. Stevioside is extracted from the plant Stevia Rebaudiana, which originates from Paraguay, South America. The Guarani Indians in Paraguay have used Stevia plant allready for hundreds of years as a sweetener. In Japan Stevioside has been used allready tens of years. In Paraguay it has been used for hundreds of years as a medicine, to decrease high blood pressure, in heart diseases and as a diuretic. Stevioside contain no calories at all.

Stevia and its Stevioside has
  – Blood pressure lowering properties
  – Diuretic properties

When 168 hypertensive volunteers were given 3 times per day 500 mg Stevioside, for 2 years, systolic blood pressure decreased by 10 mmHg (150 mmHg → 140 mmHg; $p < 0.05$) and diastolic blood pressure decreased by 6 mmHg (95 mmHg → 89 mmHg; $p < 0.05$) (Hsieh et.al. 2003). This was a double blind experiment. There was no side effects with Stevioside.

When 106 hypertensive volunteers were given 3 times per day 250 mg Stevioside, for 1 year, systolic blood pressure decreased by 13.4 mmHg (166.0 mmHg → 152.6 mmHg; $p < 0.05$) and diastolic blood pressure decreased by 10.4 mmHg (104.7 mmHg → 90.3 mmHg; $p < 0.05$) already after 3 months use (Chan et.al. 2000). This was a double blind experiment.

When rats were given intravenously 200 mg/kg Stevioside, systolic blood pressure decreased by 31% (200 mmHg → 137mmHg) and diastolic blood pressure decreased by 33% (149 mmHg → 100 mmHg) (Chan et.al. 1998).

In rats Stevia was strongly diuretic and increase Sodium output in urine (Melis et.al. 1995).

Stoneage diet

The early human beings, who lived 2 million years – 100 000 years ago, lived in so called Paleolithic time period. They were hunters and also gathered plant foods. Their daily diet was mostly lean meat, fish, birds, eggs, roots, wild vegetables, berries, fruits, nuts and honey. They drank water. There was no salt, no grains, no bread, no butter, no vegetable oils, no red wine. The fat content of daily food was low, because wild animal fat content is very low. About 65% of daily calories came from animals and 35% from plants.

This kind of diet is called "Stoneage diet" or "Paleolithic diet". It is now heavily researched, because it seems to be more healthy, than the famous Mediterranian diet.

Stoneage diet has
- Blood pressure decreasing properties
- Total cholesterol decreasing properties
- LDL-cholesterol decreasing properties
- VLDL-cholesterol decreasing properties
- Triglycerides decreasing properties
- HDL-cholesterol increasing properties
- Body weight and waist decreasing properties
- Insulin decreasing properties
- Blood sugar decreasing properties

When 9 volunteers lived on Stoneage diet for 9 days, systolic blood pressure decreased by 2.6 mmHg, diastolic blood pressure decreased by 3.4 mmHg ($p = 0.006$), total cholesterol decreased by 16% ($p = 0.007$), LDL-cholesterol decreased by 22% ($p = 0.003$), VLDL-cholesterol decreased by 35% ($p = 0.01$), triglycerides decreased by 35% ($p = 0.01$) and insulin decreased by huge 68% ($p = 0.07$) (Frasetto et.al. 2009).

When 13 diabetic volunteers were 3 months either on Stoneage diet or the normal Diabetic diet, the following properties decreased significantly on the Stoneage diet, compared to the diabetic diet: Diastolic blood pressure decreased by 4.0 mmHg ($p = 0.03$), systolic blood pressure decreased by 9.0 mmHg (149 mmHg → 140 mmHg), triglycerides decreased by 0.40 mmol/L ($p = 0.003$), body weight decreased by 3.0 kg ($p = 0.01$), Body Mass Index BMI decreased by 1.0kg/m2 ($p = 0.04$), and waist decreased by 4.0 cm ($p = 0.02$). But HDL-cholesterol increased by 0.08 mmol/L ($p = 0.08$) (Jönssön et.al. 2009).

When 10 Australian aboriginals in an experiment lived again 7 weeks in their original lands in Western Australia so, that they hunted and gathered all their food from nature, their body weight decreased by 8.0 kg (81.9 kg → 73.9 kg; 9.76% decrease), triglycerides decreased by huge 70% (4.0 mmol/L → 1.2 mmol/L), blood sugar decreased by 43.1% (11.6 mmol/L → 6.6 mmol/L), and Insulin decreased by 47.8%. The total energy per day was 1200 kcal, and about 64% came from animal protein. Fat content of diet was only 13%, because wild animals contain very little fat (O'Dea 1984).

When pigs were on daily Stoneage diet for 13 months, body weight decreased 22% (p = 0.0009), diastolic blood pressure decreased by 13% (123 mmHg → 110 mmHg; p = 0.007) and systolic blood pressure decreased by 6.6% (150 mmHg → 140 mmHg; p = 0.12), compared to the control group, which got normal grain food (Jönssön et.al. 2006).

Sugar beet fiber

(Beta Vulgaris var. Altissima)

From sugar beet processing to sugar there comes also a lot of sugar beet fiber, which is a popular functional food supplement.

Sugar beet fiber has
- Blood pressure lowering properties
- Total cholesterol lowering properties
- Triglycerides lowering properties
- HDL-cholesterol increasing properties

When 12 diabetic volunteers were given 40 grams of sugar beet fiber daily, for 8 weeks, systolic blood pressure decreased (p < 0.05) and HDL-cholesterol (p < 0.05) increased (Hagander et.al. 1989).

When rats were given in their daily diet 10% sugar beet fiber, for 28 days, both total cholesterol and triglycerides decreased significantly (Overton et.al. 1994).

When rats were fed wheat bread with sugar beet fiber, total cholesterol, LDL-cholesterol and triglycerides decreased significantly, compared to the conrtol group (Nakamura et.al. 2009).

Sweet Potato

(Ipomea Batatas)

Sweet Potato is a very common food plant, of which the root is used in cooking. Sweet Potatoes can be purchased from ordinary Supermarkets.

Sweet Potato has:
- Blood pressure lowering properties.

When hypertensive rats were fed Sweet Potato 1% of their daily diet, blood pressure decreased significantly, compared to the control group. Also heart rate decreased (Shindo et.al. 2007).

Sweet Potato inhibits ACE. Also, when volunteers drank Sweet Potato juice 1.2 dl daily, for 44 days, systolic blood pressure decreased significantly, in some volunteers even by 20 mmHg (Suda et.al. 2003).

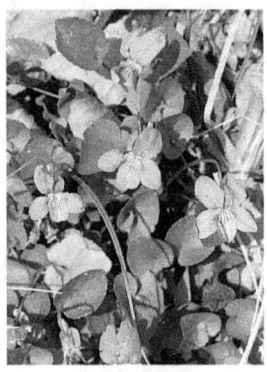

Sweet Violet

(Viola Odorata)

Sweet Violet is a very old medicinal plant, which has been in use at least 2500 years. Hippocrates mentioned its use against liver diseases, 2400 years ago. Also in India, Sweet Violet was used against cancer 2500 years ago. Sweet Violet contains Alkaloids, Saponins, Tannins, Polyphenols and Flavonoids. In Iran it is used against hypertension, asthma, bronchitis, insomnia, migraine, headache and skin disease (Ahvazi et.al. 2012).

Sweet Violet has
- Blood pressure decreasing properties
- Diuretic properties
- Total cholesterol decreasing properties
- LDL-cholesterol decreasing properties
- Body weight decreasing properties

When rats were given intravenously Sweet Violet water extract either 200 mg/kg or 400 mg/kg, urine volume increased by 40% and 89% ($p < 0.05$), compared to the control group (Vishal et.al. 2009). Furosemide at a dose of 4 mg/kg increased urine volume by 128% ($p < 0.01$), compared to the control group.

When rats were given intravenously Sweet Violet methanol-water extract at doses of 0.1 mg/kg, 0.3 mg/kg and 1.0 mg/kg, the mean average blood pressure (MAP) decreased by 15.4%, 27.8% ($p < 0.05$) and 48.6% ($p < 0.01$), compared to the control group (Siddiqi et.al. 2012).

When hyperlipidemic rats were given Sweet Violet methanol-water extract either 300 mg/kg or 600 mg/kg daily, for 6 weeks, total cholesterol decreased by 28.2% ($p < 0.05$) and 52.4% ($p < 0.01$), and LDL-cholesterol decreased by 30.4% ($p < 0.05$) and 61.6% ($p < 0.01$), compared to the control group. Body weight increased by 9.1% ($p < 0.05$) and 10.5% ($p < 0.01$) less, than in the control group (Siddiqi et.al. 2012).

Tamarind

(Tamarindus Indica)

Tamarind is a delicious fruit, originally from Asia and India. It is used in many different foods in Asia. Tamarind can be purchased from Ethnic Food Markets.

Tamarind pulp has
- Blood pressure lowering properties
- Total cholesterol lowering properties
- LDL-cholesterol lowering properties
- Triglycerides lowering properties
- HDL-cholesterol increasing properties

When Hamsters were fed Tamarind fruit 5% of their daily diet, for 10 weeks, total cholesterol decreased by 50%, LDL-cholesterol decreased by 73% and triglycerides decreased by 60%, but HDL-cholesterol increased by 61%, compared to the control group (Martinello et.al. 2006).

Same kind of results was also noticed in rat experiments by Azman (Azman et.al. 2011).

When 20 volunteers were given 30 mg/kg dried Tamarind fruit powder daily, for 4 weeks, systolic blood pressure decreased 3.4 mmHg ($p < 0.013$), total cholesterol decreased 11.3% (131.8 mg/dl $\rightarrow$ 118.4 mg/dl; $p < 0.031$) and LDL-cholesterol decreased 36.4% (78.2 mg/dl $\rightarrow$ 57.3 mg/dl; $p < 0.004$) (Iftekhar et.al. 2006).

Taurine

Taurine is a natural, Sulfur containing aminoacid, which exists in human body.

Taurine has
- Blood pressure lowering properties
- Total cholesterol lowering properties
- LDL-cholesterol lowering properties
- Triglycerides lowering properties

When young volunteers were give only 6 grams Taurine daily, for only 7 days, systolic blood pressure decreased 9.0 mmHg and diastolic blood pressure decreased 4.1 mmHg, compared to the control group (Fujita et.al. 1987). This was a double blind experiment.

In experiments with rats, Taurine decreased total cholesterol and LDL-cholesterol by 40%, and triglycerides by 53%, when rats were fed 1.5% Taurine in their food daily, for 5 weeks (Park et.al. 1999; Park et.al. 1998).

Thyme

(Thymus Vulgaris, Thymus Serpellym)

Thyme is a very old spice and medicinal plant, which is antibacterial and antiviral. Thyme is generally used against flu and influenza and high blood pressure.

Thyme has
- Blood pressure lowering properties

When hypertensive rats were given Thyme extract 100 mg/kg, systolic blood pressure decreased by 39.5% (243.6 mmHg → 147.3 mmHg; $p < 0.001$) and diastolic blood pressure decreased by 50.8% (161.5 mmHg → 79.4 mmHg; $p < 0.001$) (Miloradovic et.al. 2010). Thyme contains big amounts of Thymol, which is monoterpene.

In rats, Thymol, given in doses between 1 – 10 mg/kg, decreased blood pressure in direct relation with the dose used (Aftab et.al. 1995).

Tienchi Ginseng

(Panax Notoginseng)

Tienchi Ginseng, or Sanqi, is a close relative of the more common Panax Ginseng. Tienchi Ginseng is mostly cultivated in China, in Yunnan province. It can be purchased from Chinese supermarkets and Ethnic supermarkets. In China Sanqi is used to lower high blood pressure and high cholesterol levels.

Tienchi Ginseng has:
- Blood pressure lowering properties
- Total cholesterol lowering properties
- LDL-cholesterol lowering properties
- Triglycerides lowering properties
- HDL-cholesterol increasing properties

When rats were fed Tienchi Ginseng either 0.25%, 0.50% or 1.00% of their daily food, for 4 weeks, total cholesterol, LDL-cholesterol and triglycerides decreased significantly, but HDL-cholesterol increased significantly, compared to the control group (Xia et.al. 2011).

In great many animal experiments it has been noticed, that Tienchi Ginseng decreases total cholesterol, LDL-cholesterol and triglycerides ($p < 0.01$; $p < 0.05$) (Xu et.al. 1993; Ji et.al. 2007; Zhang et.al. 2008; Joo et.al. 2010; Xia et.al. 2011; Cicero et.al. 2003).

When 29 volunteers were given Tienchi Ginseng 1350 mg daily, for 30 days, their mean average blood pressure (MAP) in bicycle ergometer test was 109 mmHg, when it was 113 mmHg without Tienchi Ginseng (Liang et.al. 2005).

Both in experiments with rats and rabbits, it has been noticed that Tienchi Ginseng decreases blood pressure (Baek et.al. 2009; Lei et.al. 1986).

Tocotrienols

Tocotrienols are natural compounds, which exist in plants. Chemically they look like vitamin E. Tocotrienols are strong antioxidants. Good food sources are Palm oil, Rice Bran oil, Wheat germs, Rice etc.

Tocotrienols have
- Blood pressure lowering properties
- Total cholesterol lowering properties
- LDL-cholesterol lowering properties
- Triglycerides lowering properties

When 19 diabetic, hyperlipidemic volunteers were given Tocotrienols daily, for 60 days, total cholesterol decreased by 23%, triglycerides decreased by 30% and LDL-cholesterol decreased by 40%, compared to the control group (Baliarsingh et.al. 2005). This was a double blind experiment.

When 32 hyperlipidemic volunteers were given Tocotrienols 300 mg daily, for 6 months, both total cholesterol (10.8%; $p < 0.05$) and LDL-cholesterol (17.3%; $p < 0.05$) decreased significantly, compared to the control group (Yuen et.al. 2011). This was a double blind experiment.

When 120 hyperlipidemic volunteers were given 270 mg Citrus fruit Flavonoids and 30 mg Tocotrienols daily, for 12 weeks, total cholesterol decreased by 30% (293 mg/dl → 215 mg/dl; $p < 0.05$), LDL-cholesterol decreased by 27% (208 mg/dl → 156 mg/dl; $p < 0.05$) and triglycerides decreased by 34% (105 mg/dl → 73 mg/dl; $p < 0.05$), compared to the control group (Roza et.al. 2007). This was a doubble blind experiment.

When hypertensive rats were given Tocotrienols 15 mg/kg daily, for 3 months, systolic blood pressure decreased significantly (Newaz et.al. 2003).

When 36 healthy men were given Tocotrienols 80 mg, 160 mg or 320 mg daily, for 2 months, systolic blood pressure decreased significantly in the 160 mg group ($p < 0.024$) and in the 320 mg group ($p < 0.09$), compared to the control group (Rasool et.al. 2006). This was a doubble blind experiment.

Tomato

(Lycopersicum Esculentum)

Tomato is one of the Worlds most often used vegetable. Tomato contains large amounts of Lycopene and beta-Carotene.

Tomato has
- Blood pressure lowering properties
- Total cholesterol lowering properties
- LDL-cholesterol lowering properties
- HDL-cholesterol increasing properties

When 32 diabetic volunteers were give 200 grams raw Tomato daily, for 8 weeks, both systolic (p = 0.0001) and diastolic (p = 0.0001) blood pressure decreased sigificantly (Shidfar et.al. 2011).

When 50 hypertensive volunteers were given standardized Tomato extract daily, for 6 weeks, systolic blood pressure decreased by an average of 8.83% (143.1 mmHg → 130.5 mmHg; p < 0.001) and diastolic blood pressure decreased by an average of 6.22% (81.1 mmHg → 76.05 mmHg; p < 0.001), compared to the control group (Paran et.al. 2009). This was a double blind experiment.

When 98 volunteers were given 300 grams Tomato daily, for 4 weeks, HDL-cholesterol increased by 15.2% (p = 0.03), compared to the control group (Blum et.al. 2006).

When hamsters were fed Tomato 9% of their daily diet, for 8 weeks, total cholesterol decreased by 14.3% (p < 0.001), LDL-cholesterol decreased by 11.3% (p < 0.01) and triglycerides decreased by 14.3% (p < 0.001), but HDL-cholesterol increased by 28.8%, compared to the control group (Hsu et.al. 2008).

When hamsters were fed Tomatoes 53% of their daily diet, for 3 weeks, LDL-cholesterol decreased by 44%, VLDL-cholesterol decreased by 35% and triglycerides decreased by 31%, compared to the control group (Friedman et.al. 2000).

Tulsi, Holy Basil

(Ocinum Sanctum)

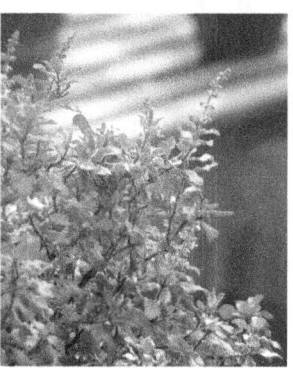

Tulsi, or Holy Basil, has been used for thousands of years as a medicinal plant in India. It is a close relative to our common Basil.

Tulsi has
- Blood pressure lowering properties
- Total cholesterol lowering properties
- Triglycerides lowering properties
- HDL-cholesterol increasing properties

When 90 diabetic patients were given Tulsi 2 grams daily, for 3 months, both systolic blood pressure (160 mmHg → 152 mmHg) and diastolic blood pressure (98 mmHg → 92 mmHg) decreased significantl, compared to the control group (Koechhar et.al. 2009).

In experiments with dogs, the oil extracted from Tulsi leaves decreased blood pressure significantly (Singh et.al. 2011).

The main component of oil extracted from Tulsi leaves is Eugenol (Prakash et.al. 2005).

With rabbits Tulsi decreases significantly total cholesterol and triglycerides, but increases HDL-cholesterol (Khanna et.al. 2010).

Ubiquinone

(Coenzyme Q10)

Ubiquinone is a natural compound found in every living cell. It has an extremely important role in the cell energy production.

Ubiquinone has
- Blood pressure lowering properties
- LDL-cholesterol lowering properties
- HDL-cholesterol increasing properties

When volunteers were given Ubiquinone 50 mg, 2 times daily, for 10 weeks, systolic blood pressure decreased by 11.9% (161.5 mmHg → 142.2 mmHg) and diastolic blood pressure decreased 15.6% (98.5 mmHg → 83.1 mmHg). LDL-cholesterol decreased by 14.7% (185 mg/dl → 157.8 mg/dl), but HDL-cholesterol increased by 9.2% (42 mg/dl → 45.9 mg/dl) (Digiesi et.al. 1992).

The blood pressure lowering property of Ubiquinone has been noticed also in other experiments with human volunteers (Yamagani et.al. 1975; Yamagani et.al. 1978; Folkers et.al. 1981; Digiesi et.al. 1990; Singh et.al. 1999; Langsjoen et.al. 1994).

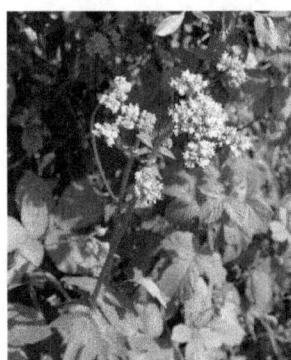

Valerian

(Valeriana Officinalis, Valeriana Wallichii)

Valerian is an ancient medicinal plant, which have been used hundreds of years as a relaxing and sleep inducing tea. It has also been used in cardiovascular diseases, such as high blood pressure and angina pectoris.

Valeriana root has
- Blood pressure decreasing properties

When rabbits were given intravenously Valerian root extract, both systolic and diastolic blood pressure and heart rate decreased, compared to the control group (Zhou et.al. 2009).

When rats were given intravenously Valerian (Valeriana Wallichii) root water extract at doses between 10 – 100 mg/kg, the mean average blood pressure (MAP) decreased in direct proportion to the dose used (Gilani et.al. 2005).

When guinea pigs were given orally Valerian root water- or ethanol extract, at doses between 50 – 200 mg/kg, blood pressure decreased by 5 – 26 mmHg ($p < 0.05$), depending on the dose. The effect of ethanol extract was stronger (Circosta et.al. 2007).

Also in human volunteers, Valerian root extract decreases ($p < 0.05$) significantly systolic blood pressure, compared to the control group (Cropley et.al. 2002).

In hyperlipidemic rats, Valerian root decreases both total cholesterol and LDL-cholesterol (Si et.al. 2003).

In patients with coronary heart disease, Valerian root extract decreased symptoms, attack frequency and duration in angina pectoris, at 87% of patients (Yang et.al. 1994).

Vegetarian diet

Vegans are know to have significantly lower blood pressure, cholesterol level and body weight, on average, than people who eat mixed food, containing animal products also. This has been verified many times.

Often dramatic changes can be seen already after 2 weeks in blood pressure and cholesterol levels, on vegetarian diet.

Vegetarian diet has
- Blood pressure lowering properties
- Total cholesterol lowering properties
- LDL-cholesterol lowering properties
- Body weight lowering properties

When 59 volunteers were put on a vegetarian diet for 14 days, systolic blood pressure decreased by 6 mmHg and diastolic blood pressure decreased by 3 mmHg, compared to the control group (Rouse et.al. 1983).

When 58 volunteers were put on a vegetarian diet for 6 weeks, systolic blood pressure decreased by 5 mmHg, compared to the control group (Margetts et.al. 1986).

When 10 healthy volunteers were 2 weeks on vegetarian diet with only vegetables, fruits and nuts as daily food, total cholesterol decreased by 24.6% ($p < 0.001$), LDL-cholesterol decreased by 33.3% ($p < 0.001$) and triglycerides decreased by 20.1% ($p = 0.005$), compared to the control group (Jenkins et.al. 1997).

15 hyperlipidemic men with normal blood pressure were put on vegetarian diet for 2 weeks with plant foods, and large amounts of fiber (40 g/100 kcal), little salt (5 g/day), little cholesterol (25 mg/day), milk daily and once a week 85 grams fish.
Results were as follows: Total cholesterol decreased by 21% (236 mg/dl → 210 mg/dl; $p < 0.05$), HDL-cholesterol decreased by 11% (46 mg/dl → 41 mg/dl; $p < 0.05$), triglycerides decreased by

44% (188 mg/dl → 105 mg/dl; p < 0.05) and bodyweight decreased by 2.9% (89.2 kg → 86.6 kg; p < 0.05), compared to the control group (Barnard et.al. 1987).

This means, that already within 2 – 6 weeks with controlled vegetarian diet plus little milk products, it is possible to dramatically decrease cholesterol, triglyceride and blood pressure values.

Veldt Grape

(Cissus Quadrangularis)

Veldt Grape is a vine, which originates from Africa and Asia. Especially in India, it has been used for hundreds of years as a vegetable and medicinal plant. It has been used to heal broken bones, against asthma and as a anti-inflammatory agent. The plant is edible, and is used in India as a vegetable salad, all around the year.

Veldt Grape has
- Total cholesterol decreasing properties
- LDL-cholesterol decreasing properties
- Triglycerides decreasing properties
- HDL-cholesterol increasing properties
- Body weight decrasing properties

When 62 obese volunteers were given standardized Veldt Grape extract 1000 mg daily, for 8 weeks, body weight decreased by 6.9% (p < 0.05) in the group with BMI higher than 30, and 4.8% in the group, with BMI lower than 30, compared to the placebo group. Fat-% decreased by 6.0% and 4.7% in these groups, compared to the placebo group. In the group, where BMI was higher than 30, total cholesterol decreased by 27.0% (p < 0.001), LDL-cholesterol decreased by 18.45 (p < 0.05) and triglycerides decreased by 36.8% (p < 0.001), but HDL-cholesterol increased by 50.5% (p < 0.01), compared to the placebo group. In the group with BMI lower than 30, total cholesterol decreased by 18.8% (p < 0.01), LDL-cholesterol decreased by 26.4% (p < 0.001) and triglycerides decreased by 15.0% (p < 0.05), but HDL-cholesterol increased by 19.6%, compared to the placebo group (Oben et.al. 2006). This was a double blind experiment.

When 24 volunteers were given Veldt grape extract 300 mg daily, for 10 weeks, body weight decreased by 8.7 kg (8.82%; p < 0.01), fat-% decreased by 4.73% (p < 0.05), total cholesterol decreased by 26.69% (150.34 mg/dl → 110.21 mg/dl; p < 0.05) and LDL-cholesterol decreased by 20.16% (80.41 mg/dl → 64.20 mg/dl; p < 0.001), compared to the placebo group (Oben et.al. 2008). This was a double blind experiment.

Vinegar

Vinegar can be made from Apples or Rice or other fruits or grains. Vinegar is generaly used all around the World in cooking and as a Functional healthy drink.

Vinegar has:
- Blood pressure lowering properties.

When rats were given vinegar or its main component, Acetic acid, in their daily food, for 13 weeks, blood pressure was 30 mmHg ($p < 0.05$) lower, than in the control group. Also plasma Aldosterone and Angiotensin II were significantly lower, than in the control group. Also plasma Renin and Angiotensin I activity were significantly lower, than in the control group (Kondo et.al. 2001).

Acetic acid decreases significantly ACE activity (Ogawa et.al. 2000).

Vinegar inhibits ACE in many other experiments (Ye et.al. 2004; Nishikawa et.al. 2001; Tsuzuki et.al. 1992).

Vitamin D

Vitamin D is essential to humans, and good sources are fatty fish and Sunlight on the skin. Many people lack of enough Vitamin D, especially at Winter time.

Vitamin D has
- Blood pressure lowering properties

In a meta-analysis, which consisted of 18 separate studies, there was shown to be a negative correlation between the blood Vitamin D content and blood pressure: The lower the Vitamin D level, the higher the blood pressure (Burgaz et.al. 2011).

When 148 women were given 800 IU Vitamin D daily, for 8 weeks, the systolic blood pressure decreased by 5.3% ($p < 0.05$), compared to the control group (Pfeifer et.al. 2001).

In a meta-analysis, which consisted of 8 separate studies, with volunteers having high blood pressure, extra Vitamin D given daily decreased, by average, the systolic blood pressure by 3.6 mmHg and the diastolic blood pressure by 3.1 mmHg (Witham et.al. 2009).

Wakame

(Undaria Pinnatifida)

Wakame is an edible seaweed, which is very popular food in Asia, especially in Japan, China and Korea, and nowadays all over the World. Wakame and other seaweeds have a long history as functional foods in Asia, and they have been used against high blood pressure, high cholesterol levels, obesity etc. Wakame contains large amounts of Fucoxanthines, Alginic Acid, Alginic acid Oligosaccharides etc.

Wakame has
- Blood pressure decreasing properties
- Total cholesterol decreasing properties
- Triglycerides decreasing properties

From the hot water extract of Wakame, 4 dipeptides, Tyrosine-Histidine, Lysine-Tyrosine, Phenylalanine-Tyrosine and Isoleucine-Tyrosine have been found, which strongly inhibit ACE and decrease blood pressure. When rats were given these dipeptides orally, 50 mg/kg, systolic blood pressure decreased 33 – 50 mmHg, within 3 – 6 hours after the dose. The blood pressure was down over 24 hours (Suetsuma et.al. 2004).

When 27 volunteers were given Wakame 6 grams daily, for 4 weeks, systolic blood pressure decreased y 10.5 mmHg (128.1 mmHg → 117.6 mmHg; p < 0.01), compared to the control group (Teas et.al. 2009). This was a double blind experiment.

When 73 volunteers were given 2.5 grams Sodium Alginate Oligosaccharides daily, for 4 weeks, diastolic blood pressure decreased by 8.3 mmHg (p < 0.01), compared to the control group (Takamitsu et.al. 2008). This was a double blind experiment.

When 36 volunteers were given 3.3 grams Wakame daily, for 8 weeks, systolic blood pressure decreased by 13 mmHg (p < 0.01) within 4 weeks, and diastolic blood pressure decreased by 9 mmHg (p < 0.01) in the same period, compared to the control group (Hata et.al. 2001).

When there was a reserch in Japan, concerning the correlation between blood pressure and daily Wakame intake of 456 small children, it was noticed, that girls with the highest daily Wakame intake, systolic blood pressure was 5.5 mmHg (p = 0.008) lower, than in the group of girls with the lowest daily Wakame intake.
In boys with highest daily Wakame intake, blood pressure was 3.2 mmHg (p = 0.038) lower, than in the boy group with the lowest daily Wakame input (Wada et.al. 2011).

When hypertensive volunteers were given 3.6 grams Wakame daily, for 4 weeks, systolic blood pressure decreased by 14 mmHg, compared to the control group (Nakato et.al. 1998).

The strong blood pressure decreasing property of Wakame was verified already 1960, by Dr. Kameda (Kameda 1960).

When 62 hypertensive volunteers were given Wakame fiber either 12 grams or 24 grams daily, for 4 weeks, the mean average blood pressure (MAP) decreased by 5.7 mmHg ($p < 0.05$, salt sensitive group) or 11.2 mmHg ($p < 0.001$; non salt sensitive group), compared to the control group (Krotkiewski et.al. 1991). This was a double blind experiment.

In experiments with rats, Wakame decreases significantly both total cholesterol (Choi et.al. 1992; Choi et.al. 1999; Iritani et.al. 1972) and triglycerides (Murata et.al. 1999).

Walnuts

(Juglans Regia)

Walnuts are familiar to everybody as a very healthy nut, which contain large amounts of polyunsaturated fats and protein.

Walnuts have
- Total cholesterol lowering properties
- LDL-cholesterol lowering properties

When 18 volunteers with high cholesterol levels were given Walnuts daily, corresponding to an amount of 32% of total daily calorific value or 40 – 65 grams daily, for 4 weeks, total cholesterol decreased by 4.4% ($p = 0.017$) and LDL-cholesterol decreased by 6.4% ($p = 0.010$), compared to the control group (Ros et.al. 2004).

When 56 volunteers were given Walnuts 41 – 56 grams daily, for 6 weeks, total cholesterol decreased by 4.1% ($p < 0.001$) and LDL-cholesterol decreased by 5.9% ($p < 0.001$), compared to the control group (Zambon et.al. 2000).

When 58 volunteers were given Walnuts 30 grams daily, for 6 months, LDL-cholesterol decreased by 10.1% ($p = 0.032$) (Tapsell et.al. 2004).

Water fast

Water is absolutely essential to all living organism. The recommended dose of water in humans is generally between 2 – 4 litres daily, in normal circumstances. Fast and especially water fast has many beneficial properties, such as correcting stomach problems and diarrhea, fast weight reduction and so on.

Water fast has
- Blood pressure lowering properties

The following experiment shows, how extremely large reductions in hypertensive patients can be achieved, with a very short term water- and juice fast.

In the experiment there were 174 hypertensive volunteers, with systolic blood pressure over 140 mmHg and diastolic blood pressure over 90 mmHg. The experiment was as follows: Firstly for 2 – 3 days the volunteers ate only fruits and vegetables. The following 10 days were water fast, during which only water was drank, and exercise and work was minimized. After this period, for 1 day, every 3 hour about 3.5 dl fresh juice was taken, and after this was a period of 6 – 7 days, during which vegetables, fruits, grains and beans were eaten.

The experiment lasted 16 days, and was strictly controlled.

Results: in the whole group the systolic blood pressure decreased by an average of 37.1 mmHg (159.1 mmHg → 121.9 mmHg) and diastolic blood pressure decreased by an average of 13.3 mmHg (89.2 mmHg → 75.9 mmHg).

In the group of 256 volunteers, with initial systolic blood pressure over 180 mmHg, there reduction in blood pressure were extremely large: Systolic blood pressure decreased by 59.6 mmHg (193.8 mmHg → 134.2 mmHg) and diastolic blood pressure decreased by 16.9 mmHg (96.4 mmHg → 79.4 mmHg) (Gooldhamer et.al. 2001).

All volunteers, who used before the experiment antihypertensive medication (Totally 6.3% of volunteers), STOPPED their medication after the experiment!

Watermelon

(Citrullus Vulgaris)

Watermelon is cultivated all around the World as a food. It can be purchased from ordinary Supermarkets all around the year. In China Watermelon has a long traditional use in lowering high blood pressure. The Chinese use the Watermelon skin for this purpose. Except the fruit pulp, also the seeds and skin parts are totally eatable.

Watermelon has
- Blood pressure lowering properties
- LDL-cholesterol lowering properties
- Triglycerides lowering properties
- HDL-cholesterol increasing properties

All parts of Watermelon, fruit pulp, skin parts and especially the seeds lower blood pressure and cholesterol.

Allready 1920 it was discovered, that Watermelon seeds contain a saponin, which strongly decreases blood pressure. This saponin was called Cucurbocitrin (Althausen et.al. 1926).

Also in other experiments researchers have noticed the blood pressure lowering properties of Watermelon seeds (Yadav et.al. 2011).

Watermelon has very large amounts of the amino acid Citrulline. Citrulline exists both in the fruit pulp and in the skin parts, typically between 1.3 – 1.9 mg/g fresh fruit (Rimando et.al. 2005).

In rats, Citrulline decreases strongly blood pressure, which lasts a long time (Koeners et.al. 2007).

The skin parts of Watermelon decreases both LDL-cholesterol and triglycerides in rat experiments (Parmar et.al. 2009).

Also in experiments with rats, Watermelon fruit pulp decreases LDL-cholesterol and increases HDL-cholesterol (Georgiana et.al. 2011).

Wax Gourd

(Benincasa Hispida)

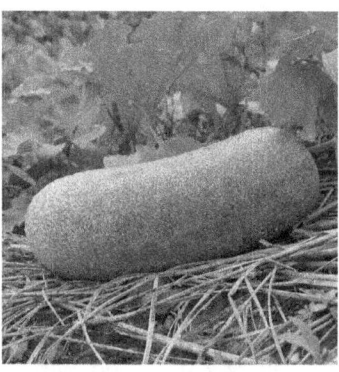

Wax Gourd is a well known food- and medicinal plant from Asia. In China and Japan Wax Gourd is used to lower high blood pressure.

Wax Gourd has
- Blood pressure lowering properties
- Total cholesterol lowering properties
- Triglycerides lowering properties
- Diuretic properties

Wax Gourd is known to inhibit ACE (Huang et.al. 2004),

Wax Gourd lowers high blood pressure in rats (Nakashima et.al. 2011).

Wax Gourd lowers very strongly the total cholesterol and triglycerides in rats (Yagnik et.al. 2009). During 1 week test trial the total cholesterol decreased 36.4% and the triglycerides decreased 53.1%, compared to the control group.

In many trials the Wax Gourd has been shown to have diuretic properties (Jayasree et.al. 2011; Dong et.al. 1995).

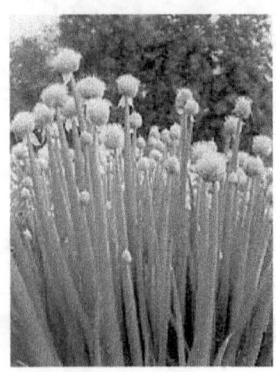

Welsh Onion

(Allium Fistulosum)

Welsh Onion has been cultivated for hundreds of years as a food, and it is very popular in China, Japan and Korea. Cultivation is very easy. All parts of the Welsh Onion can be used as food.

Welsh Onion has
- Blood pressure lowering properties
- Total cholesterol lowering properties
- LDL-cholesterol lowerin properties
- Triglycerides lowering properties
- HDL-cholesterol increasing properties

When rats were fed Welsh Onion 5% of their diet daily, for 4 weeks, systolic blood pressure decreased by 9.6%, total cholesterol decreased by 15.1% and HDL-cholesterol increased by 16.3%, compared to the control group (Aoyama et.al. 2008).

The blood pressure lowering property of Welsh Onion has been noticed also in nother experiments, after 4 weeks of daily feeding (Chen et.al. 2000; Yamamoto et.al. 2005).

When obese mice were fed 70% ethanol extract of Welsh Onion at a dose of 400 mg/kg daily, for 6.5 weeks, total cholesterol, LDL-cholesterol and triglycerides decreased significantly, compared to the control group (Sung et.al. 2011).

When rats were fed Welsh Onion daily, total cholesterol decreased significantly, compared to control group (Yamamoto et.al. 2010).

Wheat germs

(Tricium Aestivum)

Wheat germs are a very popular nutritional supplement. Wheat germs contain a lot of valuable nutrients, such as vitamin E, Betaine, Phosphorus, Octacosanol and so on.

Wheat germs have
- Total cholesterol lowering properties
- VLDL-cholesterol lowering properties

When volunteers, with high cholesterol levels between 6.58 – 9.50 mmol/L, were fed 30 grams Wheat germs daily, for 4 weeks, total cholesterol decreased by 8.3% and VLDL-cholesterol decreased by 40.6% (Cara et.al. 1991).

From the protein hydrolysate of Wheat germs, researchers have found a very strong ACE inhibitory tripeptide, Ile-Val-Tyr (Matsui et.al. 2000).

Wheat germs and their protein hydrolysates are suitable to treat both high cholesterol and high blood pressure levels.

Wheat grass

(Tricium Aestivum)

Wheat grass either as flour or frozen juice has a long time been a popular food supplement.

Wheat grass has
- Total cholesterol lowering properties
- LDL-cholesterol lowering properties
- VLDL-cholesterol lowering properties
- Triglycerides lowering properties
- HDL-cholesterol increasing properties

When rats were fed in their daily diet Wheat grass juice either 5 ml/kg or 10 ml/kg, for 3 weeks, total cholesterol decreased by 24% ($p < 0.05$), triglycerides decreased by 12% ($p < 0.05$), LDL-cholesterol decreased by 38% ($p < 0.05$) and VLDL-cholesterol decreased by 13% ($p < 0.05$), but HDL-cholesterol increased by 4%, in the 5 ml/kg group, compared to the control group. Total cholesterol decreased by 48% ($p < 0.001$), triglycerides decreased by 32% ($p < 0.001$), LDL-cholesterol decreased by 73% ($p < 0.001$) and VLDL-cholesterol decreased by 32% ($p < 0.001$), but HDL-cholesterol increased by 10% in the 10 ml/kg group, compared to the control group (Kothari et.al. 2008).

When hyperlipidemic rats were given in their daily diet either 5 ml/kg or 10 ml/kg Wheat grass juice, for 2 weeks, total cholesterol decreased by 50% ($p < 0.05$), triglycerides decreased by 22% ($p < 0..05$), LDL-cholesterol decreased by 56% ($p < 0.05$) and VLDL-cholesterol decreased by 22%

(p < 0.05), in the 5 ml/kg group, compared to the control group. Total cholesterol decreased by 60% (p < 0.05), triglycerides decreased by 38% (p < 0.05), LDL-cholesterol decreased by 69% (p < 0.05) and VLDL-cholesterol decreased by 38% (p < 0.05) in the 10 ml/kg group, compared to the control group (Kothari et.al. 2011).

When hyperlipidemic rabbits were given daily Wheat grass, total cholesterol decreased, but HDL-cholesterol increased, commpared to the control group (Sethi et.al. 2010).

Whey protein

Whey is a protein fraction of casein. Whey contains large amounts of BCAA amino acids, L-Leucine, L-Valine and L-Isovaline. Whey protein is very popular supplement among sportsmen.

Whey protein has
- Blood pressure lowering properties
- Total cholesterol lowering properties
- LDL-cholesterol lowering properties
- Triglycerides lowering properties
- HDL-cholesterol increasing properties

When 70 obese volunteers were given Whey protein 54 grams daily, for 12 weeks, systolic blood pressure decreased by 4% and diastolic blood pressure decreased by 3% (Pal et.al. 2010). In the same experiment, total cholesterol, LDL-cholesterol and triglycerides also decreased significantly.

In experiments with rats fed Whey protein daily for 2 weeks, total cholesterol decreased 51.6% and LDL-cholesterol decreased 74.7%, but HDL-cholesterol increased 26.4%, compared to the control group, which was fed Casein (Nagaoka et.al. 1992).

White Button mushroom

(Agaricus Bisporus)

White Button mushroom is known to everybody, and it is the most cultivated edible mushroom species in the World. It can be eaten raw, dried, fried or added into other foods.

White Button mushroom has
- Total cholesterol decreasing properties
- LDL-cholesterol decreasing properties
- Triglycerides decreasing properties

When hyperlipidemic rats were given in their daily food 1% fresh White Button mushroom, for 30 days, total cholesterol decreased significantly by 36.7% ($p < 0.05$), compared to the control group (Kaneda et.al. 1966).

When diabetic rats were given dried White Button mushroom 200 mg/kg daily, for 3 weeks, triglycerides decreased by 39.1% ($p < 0.05$), compared to the control group. Also, when hyperlipidemic rats were given dried White Button mushroom 200 mg/kg daily, for 4 weeks, total cholesterol decreased by 22.8% ($p < 0.05$) and LDL-cholesterol decreased by 33.1% ($p < 0.05$), compared to the control group (Jeong et.al. 2010).

The total cholesterol decreasing property of White Button mushroom has been verified also in another experiment (Fukushima et.al. 2000).

White Button mushroom contains up to 565 mg/kg dry weight Lovastatin, up to 125 mg/kg dry weight GABA and up to 932 mg/kg dry weight Ergothioneine (Chen et..al. 2012).

Lovastatin decreases cholesterol, GABA decreases blood pressure and Ergothioneine is a strong antioxidant.

White Button mushroom inhibits ACE (Ching et.al. 2011).

White Button mushroom should be eaten fresh, or dried or added at the last minute to other foods. Canned mushroom are of no medicinal value.

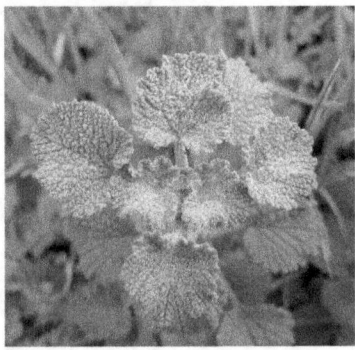

White Horehound

(Marrubium Vulgare)

White Horehound is an ancient medicinal plant, which grows naturally in Europe and North-Africa. White Horehound has been used for a long time in lung problems, in inflammation and in high blood pressure.

White Horehound has
- Blood pressure lowering properties
- Total cholesterol lowering properties
- LDL-cholesterol lowering properties
- Triglycerides lowering properties
- HDL-cholesterol increasing properties

White Horehound water extract is Vasorelaxant. The effective compounds are Marrubin and Marrubenol (Bardal et.al. 2003).

In rats White Horehound decreases significantly blood pressure and increases the volume of urine and Sodium in urine (Bardai et.al. 2001; Bardai et.al. 2004).

White Horehound water extract inhibits oxidation of humans LDL-cholesterol (Berrougui et.al. 2006).

When diabetic rats were given White Horehound water extract 500 mg/kg daily, for 4 weeks, total cholesterol decreased by 24.5% ($p < 0.05$), LDL-cholesterol decreased by 26.5% ($p < 0.05$) and triglycerides decreased by 4.0% ($p < 0.05$), but HDL-cholesterol increased by 104.9% ($p < 0.05$), compared to the control group (Elberry et.al. 2011).

References

Abdalla, Said E. The Biological Benefits of Blackmulberry *(Morus nigra)* Intake on Diabetic and non Diabetic Subjects. Research Journal of Agriculture and Biological Sciences 2006;2(6):349-357.

Abdalla S, Zarga MA, Sabri S. Effects of the flavone luteolin, isolated from *Colchicum richii,* on guinea-pig isolated smooth muscle and heart and on blood pressure and blood flow. Phytotherapy Research 1994 Aug;8(5):265-270.

Abdel-Moemin AR. Switching to black rice diets modulates low-density lipoprotein oxidation and lipid measurements in rabbits. Am J Med Sci 2011 Apr;341(4):318-24.

Abdul-Ghani A-S, Amin R, Suleiman MS. Hypotensive Effect of *Crataegus oxyacantha.* Int J. Crude Drug Res. 1987;25(4):216-220.

Abdul-Ghani A-S, Amin R. The vascular action of aqueous extracts of *Foeniculum vulgare* leaves. Journal of Ethnopharmacology 1988;24:213-218.

Abdullah N, Ismail SM, Aminudin N, Shuib AS, Lau BF. Evaluation of Selected Culinary-Medicinal Mushrooms for Antioxidant and ACE Inhibitory Activities. Evidence-Based Complementary and Alternative Medicine 2012:1-11.

Abo-Salem O, El-Edel RH, Harisa GEI, El-Halawany N, Ghonaim MM. Experimental diabetic nephropathy can be prevented by propolis: effect on metabolic disturbances and renal oxidative parameters. Pak. J. Pharm. Sci. 2009 Apr;22(2):205-210.

Achuthan CR, Padikkala J. Hypolipidemic effect of *Alpinia galanga* (Rasna) and *Kaempferia galanga* (Kachoori). Indian Journal of Clinical Biochemistry 1997;12(1):55-58.

Actis-Goretta L, Ottaviani JI, Fraga CG. Inhibition of angiotensin converting enzyme activity by flavanol-rich foods. J Agric Food Chem 2006 Jan 11;54(1):229-34.

Adachi K, Nanba H, Otsuka M, Kuroda H. Blood pressure-lowering activity present in the fruit body of Grifola frondosa (maitake). l. Chem Pharm Bull (Tokyo) 1988 Mar;36(3):1000-6.

Adegunloye BJ, Omoniyi JO, Owolabi OA, Ajagbona OP, Sofola OA, Coker HA. Mechanisms of blood pressure lowering effects of the calyx extract of *Hibiscus sabdariffa* in rats. African Journal of Medicine and Medical Sciences 1996;25:235-238.

Adeneye AA, Agbaje EO. Hypoglycemic and hypolipidemic effects of fresh leaf aqueous extract of *Cymbopogon citratus Stapf.* In rats. Journal of Ethnopharmacology 2007;112:440-444.

Adibelli Z, Dilek M, Akpolat T. Lemon juice as an alternative therapy in hypertension in Turkey. International Journal of Cardiology 2009;135:58-59.

Adisakwattana S, Moonrat J, Srichairat S, Chanasit C, Tirapongporn H, Chanathong B, Ngamukote S, Mäkynen K, Sapwarobol S. Lipid-Lowering mechanisms of grape seed extract *(Vitis vinifera* L) and its antihyperlidemic activity. Journal of Medicinal Plants Research 2010 Oct 18;4(20):2113-2120.

Adler AJ, Holub BJ. Effect of garlic and fish-oil supplementation on serum lipid and lipoprotein concentrations in hypercholesterolemic men. Am J Clin Nutr 1997 Feb;65(2):445-50.

Adnan F, Sadiq M, Jehangir A. Anti-hyperlipidemic effect of Acacia honey (Desi Kikar) in cholesterol – diet induced hyperlipidemia in rats. Biomedica 2011 Jan – Jun;27(13):62-67.

Aftab K, Atta-Ur-Rahman, Usmanghani K. Blood pressure lowering action of active principle from *Trachyspermum ammi* (L.) sprague. Phytomedicine 1995;2(1):35-40.

Aftab K. Doctorial Thesis: Pharmacological screening of natural products for their antihypertensive action. University of Karachi/Department of Pharmacology. Session: 1995. Subject: Pharmacy. No. of pages: 229.

Agarwal M, Srivastava VK, Saxena KK Kumar A. Hepatoprotective activity of *Beta vulgaris* against CCl_4-induced hepatic injury in rats. Fitoterapia 2006;77:91-93.

Aggarwal S, Singh K, Nagpal M, Kaur A, Ahluwalia P. Studies on the effect of lycored supplementation (Lycopene) on lipid per-oxidation and reduced glutathione in pregnancy induced hypertensive patients. Biomedical Research 2009;20(1):51-54.

Agil A, Navarro-Alarcón M, Ruiz R, Abuhamadah S, El-Mir MY, Vázquez GF. Beneficial effects of melatonin on obesity and lipid profile in young Zucker diabetic fatty rats. J Pineal Res. 2011 Mar;50(2):207-12.

Agrawal P, Rai V, Singh RB. Randomized placebo-controlled, single blind trial of holy basil leaves in patients with noninsulin-dependent diabetes mellitus. Int J Clin Pharmacol Ther. 1996 Sep;34(9):406-9.

Agrawal RP, Chopra A, Lavekar GS, Padhi MM, Srikanth N, Ota S, Jain S. Effect of oyster mushroom on glycemia, lipid profile and quality of life in type 2 diabetic patients. Australian Journal of Medical Herbalism 2010;22(2):50-54.

Agrewala JN, Pant MC. Effect of feeding *Carum copticum* seeds on serum lipids, high density lipoproteins & serum cholesterol binding reserve in the albino rabbits. Indian J Med Res 1986 Jan;83:93-95.

Agte VV, Jahagirdar MU, Tarwadi KV. The effects of Sudarshan Kriya Yoga on some physiological and biochemical parameters in mild hypertensive patients. Indian J Physiol Pharmacol 2011 Apr-Jun;55(2):183-7.

Ahirwar A, Singhai AK, Dixit VK. Effect of *Terminalia chebula* fruits on lipid profiles of rats. Journal of Natural Remedies 2003;3(1):31.

Ahluwalia P, Mohindroo A. Effect of oral ingestion of different fractions of Allium cepa on the blood and erythrocyte membrane-bound enzymes in rats. J Nutr Sci Vitaminol (Tokyo) 1989 Apr;35(2):155-61.

Ahmed T, Sadia H, Batool S, Janjua A, Shuja F. Use of Prunes as a control of hypertension. J Ayub Med Coll Abbottabad 2010;22(1):28-31.

Ahvazi M, Khalighi-Sigaroodi F, Charkhchiyan MM, Mojab F, Mozaffarian VA, Zakeri H. Introduction of Medicinal Plants Species with the Most Traditional Usage in Alamut Region. Iranian Journal of Pharmaceutical Research 2012;11(1):185-194.

Aihara K, Kajimoto O, Hirata H, Takahashi R, Nakamura Y. Effect of powdered fermented milk with *Lactobacillus helveticus* on subjects with high-normal blood pressure or milk hypertension. J. Am. Col. Nutr. 2005;4:257-265.

Aissaoui A, Zizi S, Israili ZH, Lyoussi B. Hypoglycemic and hypolipidemic effects of Coriandrum sativum L. in Meriones shawi rats. J Ethnopharmacol 2011 Sep 1;137(1):652-61.

Ait-Yahia D, Madani S, Savelli JL, Prost J, Bouchenak M, Belleville J. Dietary Fish Protein Lowers Blood Pressure and Alters Tissue Polyunsaturated Fatty Acid Composition in Spontaneously Hypertensive Rats. Nutrition 2003;19:342-346.

Aiyeloja AA, Bello OA. Ethnobotanical potentials of common herbs in Nigeria: A case study of Enugu state. Educational Research and Review 2006 April;Vol. 1 (1):16-22.

Ajay M, Chai J, Mustafa AM, Gilani AH, Mustafa MR. Mechanisms of the anti-hypertensive effect of *Hibiscus sabdariffa* L. calyces. Journal of Ethnopharmacology 2007;109:388-393.

Akasaka Y, Takahashi E, Miyate Y, Kudo K, Ikeda M, Shimizu C, Tachikawa E, Kashimoto T. Effect of red ginseng on bood pressure, heart rate and sympathetic activity in 5-hydroxydopamine treated rats. Eur J Pharmacol 1990;183:1004.

Akhtar MS, Ramzan A, Ali A, Ahmad M. Effect of Amla fruit (Emblica officinalis Gaertn.) on blood glucose and lipid profile of normal subjets and type 2 diabetic patients. Int J Food Sci Nutr. 2011 Sep;62(6):609-16.

Akila K, Ananthi T. Hypolipidaemic effect of *Brassica oleracea (L.)* and *Carum copticum seeds (L.)* on fructose and butter induced hyperlipidaemia in swiss albino rats. Adv. Pharmacol. Toxicol. 2010;11(3):145-149.

Akilen R, Tsiami A, Devendra D, Robinson N. Glycated haemoglobin and blood pressure-lowering effect of cinnamon in multi-ethnic Type 2 diabetic patients in the UK: a randomized, placebo-controlled, double-blind clinical trial. Diabet Med. 2010 Oct;27(10):1159-67.

Al-Ali M, Wahbi S, Twaij H, Al-Badr A. *Tribulus terrestris:* preliminary study of its diuretic and contractile effects and comparison with *Zea mays.* Journal of Ethnopharmacology 2003;85:257-260.

Al-Jaff FK. Effect of Coriander Seeds as Diet Ingredient on Blood Parameters of Broiler Chicks Raised under High Ambient Temperature. International Journal of Poultry Science 2011;10(2):82-86.

Al-Kassi GAM. Effect of Feeding Cumin *(Cuminum cyminum)* on the Performane and Some Blood Traits of Broiler Chicks. Pakistan Journal of Nutrition 2010;9(1):72-75.

Al-Rewashdeh AYA. Blood Lipid Profile, Oxidation and Pressure of Men and Women Consumed Olive Oil. Pakistan Journal of Nutrition 2010;9(1):15-26.

Al-Waili NS. Natural honey lowers plasma glucose, C-reactive protein, homocysteine, and blood lipids in healthy, diabetic, and hyperlipidemic subjets: comparison with dextrose and sucrose. J Med Food 2004;7(1):100-7.

Al-Zuhair H, El-Fattah AAA, el Latif HAA. Efficacy of simvastatin and pumpkin-seed oil in the management of dietary-induced hypercholesterolemia. Pharmacological Research 1997;35(5):403-408.

Al-Zuhair H, El-Fattah AAA, El-sayed MI. Pumpkin-seed oil modulates the effect of felodipine and captopril in spontaneously hypertensive rats. Pharmacological Research 2000;41(5):555-563.

Alam N, Hossain S, Khair A, Amin R, Asaduzzaman K. Comparative effects of oyster mushrooms on plasma lipid profile of hypercholesterolaemic rats. Bangladesh J. Mushroom. 2007;1:15-22.

Alam N, Amin R, Khan A, Ara I, Shim MJ, Lee MW, Lee UY, Lee TS. Comparative Effects of Oyster Mushrooms on Lipid Profile, Liver and Kidney Function in Hypercholesterolemic Rats. Mycobiology 2009;37(1):37-42.

Alam N, Yoon KN, Lee TS. Antihyperlipidemic activities of Pleurotus ferulae on biochemical and histological function in hypercholesterolemic rats. J Res Med Sci. 2011 Jun;16(6):776-86.

Albarracin C, Fuqua B, Geohas J, Juturu V, Finch MR, Komorowski JR. Comination of chromium and biotin improves coronary risk factors in hypercholesterolemic type 2 diabetes mellitus: a placebo-controlled, double-blind randomized clinical trial. J Cardiometab Syndr. 2007;2(2):91-7.

Algerholm-Larsen L, Raben A, Haulrik N, Hansen AS, Manders M, Astrup A, Effect of 8 week intake of probiotic milk products on risk factors for cardiovascular diseases. Eur. J. Clin. Nutr. 2000;54:288-297.

Allers NJ, Hay L, Schutte PJ, Steinmann CML, du Plooy SH, Böhmer LH. Long-term effects of a low dosage of grape seed proanthocyanidin extract on blood pressure in spontaneously hypertensive rats. South African Journal of Science 2008;104,

Almeida JP, Levy L, Graça R, Ferreira AS, Diogo N, Silva JR, Silva e Costa JM. Comparative double-blind study of the antiasthenic agent DMGG and placebo for assessing physical and biochemical performance in 60 athletes. Current Therapeutic Research 1993 Sep;54(3):339-357.

Alper CM, Mattes RD. Peanut Consumtion Improves Indices of Cardiovascular Disease Risk i Healthy Adults. Journal of the American College of Nutrition 2003;22(2):133-141.

Alonso A, Nettleton JA, Ix JH, de Boer IH, Folsom AR, Bidulescu A, Kestenbaum BR, Chambless LE, Jacobs DR Jr. Dietary phosphorus, blood pressure, and incidence of hypertension in the atjerosclerosis risk in communities study and the multi-ethnic study of atherosclerosis. Hypertension 2010 Mar;55(3):776-84.

Althausen TL, Kerr J. Watermelon-seed extract in the treatment of hypertension. American Journal of the Medical Sciences 1929 Oct;178(4):470-489.

Amalia L, Sukandar EY, Roesli RMA, Sigit JI. The Effect of Ethanol Extract of *Kucai (Allium schoenoprasum* L.) Bulbs on Serum Nitric Oxide Level in Male Wistar Rats. International Journal of Pharmacology 2008;4(6):487-491.

Amnueysit P, Tatakul T, Chalermsan N, Amnueysit K. Effects of purple field corn anthocyanins on broiler heart weight. Asian Journal of Food and Agro-Industry 2010;3(3):319-327.

Amrani S, Harnafi H, Bouanani Nel H, Aziz M, Caid HS, Manfredini S, Besco E. Hypolipidaemic activity of aqueous Ocimum basilicum extract in acute hyperlipidaemia induced by triton WR-1339 in rats and its antioxidant property. Phytother Res. 2006 Dec;20(12):1040-5.

Amrani S, Harnafi H, Gadi D, Mekhfi H, Legssyer A, Aziz M, Martin-Nizard F, Bosca L. Vasorelaxant and anti-platelet aggregation effects of aqueous Ocimum basilicum extract. J Ethnopharmacol 2009 Aug 17;125(1):157-62.

Anand SKR, Sattar MA, Abdullah NA, Abdullah MH, Salman IM, Rathore HA, Johns EJ. Effect of dragon fruit extract on oxidative stress and aortic stiffness in streptozotocin-induced diabetes in rats. Pharmacognosy Res. 2010 Jan;2(1):31-5.

Anderson JW, Gilliland SE. Effect of fermented milk (yogurt) containing Lactobacillus acidophilus L1 on serum cholesterol in hypercholesterolemic humans. Am Coll Nutr 1999 Feb;18(1):43-50.

Anderson JW, Bush HM. Soy protein effects on serum lipoproteins: a quality assessment and meta-analysis of randomized, controlled studies. J Am Coll Nutr. 2011 Apr;30(2):79-91.

Andersson U, Berger K, Högberg A, Landin-Olsson M, Holm C. Effects of rose hip intake on risk markers of type 2 diabetes and cardiovascular disease: a randomized, double-blind, cross-over investigation in obese persons. European Journal of Clinical

Nutrition 2011:1-6.

Andersson U, Henriksson E, Ström K, Alenfall J, Göransson O, Holm C. Rose hip exerts antidiabetic effects via a mechanism involving downregulation of the hepatic lipogenic program. Am J Physiol Endocrinol Metab 2011;300:111-121.

Andrade ACM, Cesena FHY, Consolim-Colombo FMC, Coimbra SR, Benjó AM, Krieger EM, da Luz PL. Short-term red wine consumption promotes differential effects on plasma levels of high-density lipoprotein cholesterol, sympathetic activity, and endothelial function in hypercholesterolemic, hypertensive, and healthy subjects. Clinics 2009;64(5):435-42.

Anila L, Vijayalakshmi NR. Flavonoids from *Emblica officinalis* and *Mangifera indica* – effectiveness for dyslipidemia. Journal of Ethnopharmacology 2002;79:81-87.

Anshelevich IuV, Merson MA, Afanas'eva GA. Serum aldosterone level in patients with hypertension during treatment by acupuncture. Ter Arkh 1985;57(10):42-5.

Aoyama S, Hiraike T, Yamamoto Y. Antioxidant, Lipid-Lowering and Antihypertensive Effects of Red Welsh Onion *(Allium fistulosum)* in Spontaneously Hypertensive Rats. Food Sci. Technol. Res. 2008;14(1):99-103.

Aptekmann NP, Cesar TB. Orange juice improved lipid profile and blood lactate of overweight middle-aged women subjected to aerobic training. Maturitas 2010 Dec;67(4):343-7.

Arai Y, Watanabe S, Kimira M, Shimoi K, Mochizuki R, Kinae N. Dietary intakes of flavonols, flavones and isoflavones by Japanese women and the inverse correlation between quercetin intake and plasma LDL cholesterol concentration. J Nutr. 2000 Sep;130(9):2243-50.

Arcari DP, Bartchewsky W, dos Santos TW, Oliveira KA, Funck A, Pedrazzoli , de Souza MF, Saad MJ, Bastos DH, Gambero A, Carvalho Pde O, Ribeiro ML. Antiobesity effects of yerba maté (Iles paraguariensis) in high-fat diet-induced obese mice. Obesity (Silver Spring) 2009 Dec;17(12):2127-33.

Ardiansyah, Shirakawa H, Koseki T, Ohinata K, Hashizume K, Komai M. Rice Bran Fractions Improve Blood Pressure, Lipid Profile, and Glucose Metabolism in Stroke-Prone Spontaneously Hypertensive Rats. J. Agric. Food Chem. 2006;54(5):1914-1920.

Ardiansyah, Shirakawa H, Koseki T, Hashizume K, Komai M. The Driselase-treated fraction of rice bran is more effective dietary factor to improve hypertenson, glucose and lipid metabolism in stroke-prone spontaneously hypertensive rats compared to ferulic acid. Br J Nutr. 2007 Jan;97(1):67-76.

Ardiansyah, Ohsaki Y, Shirakawa H, Koseki T, Komai M. Novel effects of a single administration of ferulic acid on the regulation of blood pressure and the hepatic lipid metabolic profile in stroke-prone spontaneously hypertensive rats. J Agric Food Chem. 2008 Apr 23;56(8):2825-30.

Ardiansyah, Shirakawa H, Inagawa Y, Koseki T, Komai M. Regulation of blood pressure and glucose metabolism induced by L-tryptophan in stroke-prone spontaneously hypertensive rats. Nutr Metab (Lond) 2011 Jun 28;8(1):45.

Argani H, Rahbaninoubar M, Ghorbanihagjo A, Golmohammadi Z, Rashtchizadeh N. Effect of L-carnitine on the serum lipoproteins and HDL-C subclasses in hemodialysis patients. Nephron Clin Pract. 2005;101(4):174-9.

Arokiyaraj S, Balamurugan R, Augustian P. Antihyperglycemic effect of *Hypericum perforatum* ethyl acetate extract on streptozotocin – induced diabetic rats. Asian Pasific Journal of Tropical Biomedicine 2011:386-390.

Arsenio L, Caronna S, Lateana M, Magnati G, Strata A, Zammarchi G. Hyperlipidemia, diabetes and atherosclerosis: efficacy of treatment with pantethine. Acta Biomed Ateneo Parmense 1984;55(1).25-42.

Arsenio L, Bodria P, Magnati G, Strata A, Trovato R. Effectiveness of long-term treatment with pantethine in patients with dyslipidemia. Clin Ther 1986;8(5):537-45.

Arsenio L, Bodria P, Bossi S, Lateana M, Strata A. Clinical use of pantethine by parenteral route in the treatment of hyperlipidemia. Acta Biomed Ateneo Parmense 1987;58(5-6):143-52.

Asaolu, Fiasyo M, Asaolu, Sunday S, Olugbenga OA, Aluko, Tola B. Hypolipemic effects of methanolic extract of *persea americana seeds* in hypercholestrolemic rats. Journal of Medicine and Medical Sciences 2010 May;1(4):126-128.

Asgary S, Naderi GH, Sarrafzadegan N, Mohammadifard N, Mostafavi S, Vakili R. Antihypertensive and antihyperlipidemic effects of Achillea wilhelmsii. Drugs Exp Clin Res 2000;26 (3):89-93.

Asgary S, Moshtaghian J, Naderi G, Fatahi Z, Hosseini M, Dashti G, Adibi S. Effects of dietary red clover on blood factors and cardiovascular fatty streak formation in hypercholesterolemic rabbits. Phytother Res. 2007 Aug;21(8):768-70.

Asha S, Taju G. Cardioprotective effect of *Terminalia arjuna* on caffeine induced coronary heart disease. IJPSR 2012;3(1):150-153.

Atal CK, Singh B, Gupta OP. Vitamin B$_{15}$ - for physical vigour, treatment of cardiovascular disorders and other disease conditions. Indian Drugs 1980 March;:187-188.

Aubin MC,Lajoie C, Clément R, Gosselin H, Calderone A, Perrault LP. Female rats fed a high-fat diet were associated with vascular dysfunction and cardiac fibrosis in the absence of overt obesity and hyperlipidemia: therapeutic potential of resveratrol. J Pharmacol Exp Ther 2008 Jun;325(3):961-8.

Avci G, Kupeli E, Eryavuz A, Yesilada E, Kucukkurt I. Antihypercholesterolaemic and antioxidant activity assessment of some plants used as remedy in Turkish folk medicine. J Ethnopharmacol 2006 Oct 11;107(3):418-23.

Aviram M, Rosenblat M, Gaitini D, Nitecki S, Hoffman A, Dornfeld L, Volkova N, Presser D, Attias J, Liker H, Hayek T. Pomegranate juice consumption for 3 years by patients with carotid artery stenosis reduces common arotid intima-media thickness, blood pressure and LDL oxidation. Clin Nutr 2004 Jun;23(3):423-33.

Azman KF, Amom Z, Azian A, Esa NM, Ali RM, Shah M, Kadir KK. Antiobesity effect of Tamarindus indica L. pulp aqueous extract in high-fat diet-induced obese rats. J Nat. Med. 2011 Oct 12.

Azmat A, Ahmed M, Zafar N, Ahmad SI. Hypotensive activity of methanolic extract of *Berberis Vulgaris* (root pulp and bark). Pakistan Journal of Pharmacology 2009 Jul.;26(2):41-47.

Badal RM, Badal D, Badal P, Khare A, Shrivastava J, Kumar V. Pharmacological Action of *Mentha piperita* on Lipid Profile in Fructose-Fed Rats. Iranian Journal of Pharmaceutical Research 2011;10(4):843-848.

Baek EB, Yoo HY, Park SJ, Chung YS, Hong EK, Kim SJ. Inhibition of Arterial Myogenic Responses by a Mixed Aqueous Extract of Salvia Miltiorrhiza and Panax Notoginseng (PASEL) Showing Antihypertensive Effects. Korean J Physiol Pharmacol 2009 Aug;13(4):287-93.

Bahrami M, Ataie-Jafari A, Hosseini S, Foruzanfar MH, Rahmani M, Pajouhi M. Effects of natural honey consumption in diabetic patients: and 8-week randomized clinical trial. International Journal of Food Sciences and Nutrition 2009;60(7):618-626.

Balaraman R, Dangwal S, Mohan M. Antihypertensive Effect of *Trigonella foenum-greacum*. Seeds in Experimentally Induced Hypertension in Rats. Pharmaceutical Biology 2006;44(8):568-575.

Balasuriya BWN, Rupasinghe HPV. Plant flavonoids as angiotensin converting enzyme inhibitors in regulation of hypertension. Functional Foods in Health and Disease 2011;5:172-188.

Baliarsingh S, Beg ZH, Ahmad J. The therapeutic impacts of tocotrienols in type 2 diabetic patients with hyperlipidemi. Atherosclerosis 2005 Oct;182(2):367-74.

Banappa SU, Basangouda MP. Apocynin improves endothelial function and prevents the development of hypertension in fructose fed rat. Indian J Pharmacol 2009 Oct;41(5):208-212.

Bang MA, Kim HA, Cho YJ. Alterations in the blood glucose, serum lipids and renal oxidative stress in diabetic rats by supplementation of onion (Allium cepa. Linn). Nutr Res Pract. 2009;3(3):242-6.

Bannan LT, Potter JF, Beevers DG, Saunders JB, Walters JRF, Ingram MC. Effect of alcohol withdrawal on blood pressure, plasma renin activity, aldosterone, cortisol and dopamine B-hydroxylase. Clinical Science 1984;66:659-663.

Bao DQ, Mori TA, Burke V, Puddey IB, Beilin LJ. Effects of dietary fish and weight reduction on ambulatory blood pressure in overweight hypertensives. Hypertension 1998 Oct;32(4):710-7.

Barbalho SM, Machado FMVF, Oshiiwa M, Abreu M, Guiger EL, Tomazela P, Goulart RA. Investigation of the effects of peppermint *(Mentha piperita)* on the biochemical and anthropometrc profile of university students. Cienc. Tecnol. Aliment. Campinas 2011;31(3):584-588.

Barnard RJ, Chaudhari JAHA, Miller JE, Kirschenbaum A. Effects of low-fat, low-cholesterol diet on serum lipids, platelet aggregation and thromboxane formation. Prostaglandis Leukotrienes and Medicine 1987;26:241-252.

Bastos JF, Moreira IJ, Ribeiro TP, Medeiros IA, Antoniolli AR, De Sousa DP, Santos MR. Hypotensive and vasorelaxant effects of citronellol, a monoterpene alcohol, in rats. Basic Clin Pharmacol Toxicol 2010 Apr;106(4):331-7.

Basu A, Du M, Leyva MJ, Sanchez K, Betts NM, Wu M, Aston CE, Lyons TJ. Blueberries Decrease Cardiovascular Risk Factors in Obese Men and Women with Metabolic Syndrome. The Journal of Nutrition 2010;140(9):1582-1587.

Behall KM, Scholfield DJ, Hallfrisch J. Diets containing barley significantly reduce lipids in mildly hypercholesterolemic men and women. Am J Clin Nutr 2004;80:1185-93.

Behall KM, Scholfield DJ, Hallfrisch J. Lipids Significantly Reduced by Diets Containing Barley in Moderately Hypercholesterolemic Men. Journal of the American College of Nutrition 2004;23(1):55-62.

Belguith-Hadriche O, Bouaziz M, Jamoussi K, El Feki A, Sayadi S, Makni-Ayedi F. Lipid-lowering and antioxidant effects of an ethyl acetate extract of fenugreek seeds in high-cholesterol-fed rats. J Agric Food Chem. 2010 Feb 24;58(4):2116-22.

Ben EE, Eno AE, Ofem OE, Aidem U, Itam EH. Increased plasma total cholesterol and high density lipoprotein levels produced by the crude extract from the leaves of *Viscum album* (Mistletoe). Nigerian Journal Of Physiological Sciences 2006;21(1-2):55-60.

Bennani-Kabchi N, Fdhil H, Cherrah Y, Kehel L, el Bouayadi F, Amarti A, Saidi M, Marquié G. Effects of Olea europea var, oleaster leaves in hypercholesterolemic insulin-resistant sand rats. Therapie. 1999 Nov – Dec;54(6):717-23.

Berger A, Rein D, Kratky E, Monnard I, Hajjaj H, Meirim I, Piguet-Welsch C, Hauser J, Mace K, Niederberger P. Cholesterol-lowering properties of Ganoderma lucidum in vitro, ex vivo, and in hamsters and minipigs. Lipids Health Dis. 2004 Feb 18;3(2): 1-12.

Berrougui H, Isabelle M, Cherki M, Khalil A. *Marrubium vulgare* extract inhibits human-LDL oxidation and enhances HDL-mediated cholesterol efflux in THP-1 macrophage. Life Sciences 2006;80:105-112.

Bertolami MC, Faludi AA, Batlouni M. Evaluation of the effects of a new fermented milk product (Gaio) on primary hypercholesterolemia. Eur J Clin Nutr 1999 Feb;53(2):97-101.

Besong SA, Ezekwe MO, Ezekwe EI. Evaluating the effects of freeze-dried supplements of purslane *(Portulaca oleracea)* on blood lipids in hypercholesterolemic adults. International Journal of Nutrition and Metabolism 2011 May;3(4):43-49.

Bhargava UC, Westfall BA, Siehr DJ. Preliminary pharmacology of ellagic acid from *Juglans nigra* (black walnut). Journal of Pharmaceutical Sciences 1968 Oct;57(10):1728-1732.

Bhargava UC, Westfall BA. The Mechanism of Blood Pressure Depression by Ellagic Acid. Exp Biol Med 1969 Nov;132(2): 754-756.

Bhatia J, Tabassum F, Sharma AK, Bharti S, Golechha M, Joshi S, Sayeed Akhatar M, Srivastava AK, Arya DS. Emblica officinalis exerts antihypertensive effect in a rat model of DOCA-salt-induced hypertension: role of (p) eNOS, NO and oxidative stress. Cardiovasc Toxicol 2011 Sep;11(3):272-9.

Bhatt SR, Lokhandwala MF, Banday AA. Resveratrol prevents endothelial nitric oxide synthase uncoupling and attenuates development of hypertension in spontaneously hypertensive rats. Eur J Pharmacol 2011 Sep 30;667(1-3):258-64.

Bhatti IU, Rehman FU, Khan MA, Marwat SK. Effect of Prophetic Medicine *Kalonji (Nigella sativa* L.) On Lipid Profile of Human Beings: An *In Vivo* Approach. World Applied Sciences Journal 2009;6(8):1053-1057.

Bhutkar PM, Bhutkar MV, Taware GB, Doijad V, Doddamani BR. Effect of Suryanamaskar Practice on Cardio-respiratory Fitness Parameters: A Pilot Study. Al Ameen J Med Sci 2008;1(2):126-129.

Binaghi P, Cellina G, Lo Cicero G, Bruschi F, Porcaro E, Penotti M. Evaluation of the cholesterol-lowering effectiveness of pantethine in women in perimenopausal age. Minerva medica 1990;81(6).475-9.

Bindels RJ, van den Broek LA, Hillebrand SJ, Wokke JM. A high phosphate diet lowers blood pressure in spontaneously hypertensive rats. Hypertension 1987 Jan;9(1):96-102.

Birari R, Javia V, Bhutani KK. Antiobesity and lipid lowering effects of Murraya koenigii (L) Spreng leaves extracts and mahanimbine on high fat diet induced obese rats. Fitoterapia 2010 Dec;81(8):1129-33.

Bisen PS, Baghel RK, Sanodiya BS, Thakur GS, Prasad GB. Lentinus edodes: a macrofungus with pharmacological activities. Curr Med Chem 2010;17(22):2419-30.

Biswas A, Dhar P, Ghosh S. Antihyperlipidemic effect of sesame (Sesamum indicum L.) protein isolate in rats fed a normal and high cholesterol diet. J Food Sci. 2010 Nov-Dec;75 (9);274-9.

Blum A, Merei M, Karem A, Blum N, Ben-Arzi S, Wirsansky I, Khazim K. Effects of tomatoes on the lipid profile. Clin Invest Med. 2006 Oct;29(5):298-300.

Bobek P, Galbavý S. Hypocholesterolemic and antiatherogenic effect of oyster mushroom (Pleurotus ostreatus) in rabbits. Nahrung 1999 Oct;43(5):339-42.

Bolkent S, Yanardag R, Karabulut-Bulan O, Yesilyaprak B. Protective role of *Melissa officinalis* L. extract on liver of hyperlipidemic rats A morphological and biochemical study. Journal of Ethnopharmacology 2005;99:391-398.

Bordia A, Verma SK, Srivastava KC. Effect of garlic *(Allium sativum)* on blood lipids, blood sugar, fibrinogen and fibrinolytic activity in patients with coronary artery disease. Prostaglandis, Leukotrienes and Essential Fatty Acids 1998;58(4):257-263.

Boyd SG, Boone BE, Smith AR, Conners J, Dohm GL. Combined dietary chromium picolinate supplementation and an exercise program leads to a reduction of serum cholesterol and insulin in college-aged subjects. J. Nutr. Biochem. 1998;9:471-475.

Branković S, Djosev S, Kitić D, Radenković M, Veljković S, Nesic M, Pavlović D. Hypotensive and negative chronotropic and inotropic effects of the aqueous and ethanol extract from parsley leaves (Petroselinum crispum). Journal of Clinical Lipidology 2008 Oct;2(55):191.

Branković S, Kitić D, Radenković M, Veljković S, Kostić M, Miladinović B, Pavlović D. Hypertensive and Cardioinhibotory effects of the Aqueous and Ethanol extracts of Celery (*Apium Graveolens,Apiaceae).* Acta Medica Medianae 2010; Vol. 49 (1):13-16.

Brankovic S, Radenkovic M, Kitic D, Veljkovic S, Ivetic V, Pavlovic D, Miladinovic B. Comparison of the hypotensive and bradycardic activity of ginkgo, garlic, and onion extracts. Clin Exp Hypertens 2011;33(2):95-9.

Bravo E, Amrani S, Aziz M, Harnafi H, Napolitano M. *Ocimum basilicum* ethanolic extract decreases cholesterol synthesis and lipid accumulation in human macrophages. Fitoterapia 2008;79:515-523.

Bravo L. Polyphenols: Chemistry, Dietary Sources, Metabolism, and Nutritional Significance. Nutrition Reviews 19998 Nov;56(11):317-333.

Brevik A, Gaivão I, Medin T, Jørgenesen A, Piasek A, Elilasson J, Karlsen A, Blomhoff R, Veggan T, Duttaroy AK, Collins AR. Supplementation of a western diet with golden kiwifruits (*Actinidia chinensis var.* 'Hort 16A':) effects on biomarkers of oxidation damage and antioxidant protection. Nutrition Journal 2011;10(54).1-9.

Brien SE, Ronksley PE, Turner BJ, Mukamal KJ, Ghali WA. Effect of alcohol consumption on biological markers associated with risk of coronary heart disease: systematic review and meta-analysis of interventional studies. BMJ 2011 Feb 22;342:1-15.

Broncel M, Kozirog M, Duchnowicz P, Koter-Michalak M, Sikora J, Chojnowska-Jezierska J. Aronia melanocarpa extract reduces blood pressure, serum endothelin, lipid, and oxidative stress marker levels in patients with metabolic syndrome. Med Sci Monit 2010 Jan;16(1):28-34.

Brook JG, Linn S, Aviram M. Dietary soya lecithin decreases plasma triglyceride levels and inhibits collagen- and ADP-induced platelet aggregation. Biochem Med Metab Biol 1986 Feb;35(1):31-9.

Brown IJ, Tzoulaki I, Candeias V, Elliott P. Salt intakes around the world: implications for public health. International Journal of Epidemiology 2009;38:791-813.

Brown L, Rosner B, Willett WW, Sacks FM. Cholesterol-lowering effects of dietary fiber: a meta-analysis. Am J Clin Nutr 1999;69:30-42.

Bruckert E, Giral P, Heshmati HM, Turpin G. Men treated with hypolipidaemic drugs complain more frequently of erectile dysfunction. J Clin Pharm Ther. 1996 Apr;21(2):89-94.

Burgaz A, Orsini N, Larsson SC, Wolk A. Blood 25-hydroxyvitamin D concentration and hypertenson: a meta-analysis. J Hypertens. 2011 Apr;29(4):636-45.

Burke V, Hodgson JM, Beilin LJ, Giangiulioi N, Rogers P, Puddey IB. Dietary Protein and Soluble Fiber Reduce Ambulatory Blood Pressure in Treated Hypertensives. Hypertenson 2001;38:821-826.

Burrowes JD, Ramer NJ. Changes in Potassium Content of Different Potato Varieties After Cooking. Journal of Renal Nutrition 2008;18(6):530-534.

Busserolles J, Gueux E, Rock E, Mazur A, Rayssiguier Y. Substituting Honey for Refined Carbohydrates Protects Rats from Hypertriglyceridemic and Prooxidative Effects of Fructose. J. Nutr. 2002;132:3379-3382.

Byun JS, Han YS, Lee SS. The effects of yellow soybean, black soybean, and sword bean on lipid levels and oxidative stress in ovariectomized rats. Int J Vitamin Nutr Res 2010 Apr;80(2):97-106.

Bättig K. Cardiovascular effects of everyday coffee consumption. Schweiz Med Wochenschr. 1992 Oct 10;122(41):1536-43.

Bäumer AT, Krüger CA, Falkenberg J, Freyhaus HT, Rösen R, Fink K, Rosenkranz S. The NAD(P)H oxidase inhibitor apocynin improves endothelial NO/superoxide balance and lowers effectively blood pressure in spontaneously hypertensive rats: comparison to calcium channel blockade. Clin Exp Hypertens 2007 Jul;29(5):287-99.

Cabassi A, Dumont EC, Girouard H, Bouchard JF, Le Jossec M, Lamontagne D, Besner JG, de Champlain J. Effects of chronic N-acetylcysteine treatment on the actions of peroxynitrite on aortic vascular reactivity in hypertensive rats. J Hypertens 2001 Jul;19(7):1233-44.

Cao X-G, Yu G, Ye X-L, Wang L-J, Li X-G. Research on Inhibition of Traditional Chinese Medicine Extrcts and Active Fraction on Angiotensin Converting Enzyme. Food and Drug 2009.

Cao Z-H, Gu D-H, Lin Q-Y, Xu Z-Q, Huang Q-C, Rao H, Liu E-W, Jia J-J, Ge C-R. Effect of pu-erth tea on body fat and lipid profiles in rats with diet-induced obesity. Phytotherapy Research 2011 Feb;25(2):234-238.

Campos KE, Balbi APC, Alves MJQF. Diuretic and hipotensive activity of aqueous extract of parsley seeds *(Petroselinum sativum* Hoffm.) in rats. Revista Brasileira de Farmacognosia Brazilian Journal of Pharmacognosy 2009 Mar;19(1A):41-45.

Cara L, Borl P, Armand M, Senft M, Lafont H, Portugal H, Pauli AM, Boulze D, Lacombe C, Lairon D. Plasma lipid lowering effects of wheat germ in hypercholesterolemic subjects. Plant Foods for Human Nutrition 1991;41;135-150.

Carbajal D, Casaco A, Arruzazabala L, Gonzalez R, Tolon Z. Pharmacological study of *Cymbopogon citratus* leaves. Journal of Ethnopharmacology 1989;25:103-107.

Caron MF, Hotsko AL, Robertson S, Mandybur L, Kluger J, White CM. Electrocardiographic hemodynamic effects of Panax ginseng. Ann Pharmacother 2002 May 1;36(5):758-763

Carranza J, Alvizouri M, Alvarado MR, Chávez F, Gómez M, Herrera JE. Effects of avocado on the level of blood lipids in patients with phenotype II and IV dyslipidemias. Arch Inst Cardiol Mex. 1995 Jul – Aug;65(4):342-8.

Carranza-Madrigal J, Herrera-Abarca JE, Alvizouri-Muñoz M, Alvarado-Jimenez MR, Chavez-Carbajal F. Effects of a Vegetarian Diet vs. A Vegetarian Diet Enriched with Avocado in Hypercholesterolemic Patients. Archives of Medical Research 1997;28(4):537-541.

Castilla P, Echarri R, Dávalos A, Cerrato F, Ortega H, Teruel JL, Lucas MF, Gómez-Coronado D, Ortuño J, Lasunción MA. Concentrated red grape juice exerts antioxidant, hypolipidemic, and antiinflammatory effects in both hemodialysis patients and healthy subjects. Am J Clin Nutr 2006;84:252-62.

Castilla P, Dávalos A, Teruel JL, Cerrato F, Fernández-Lucas M, Merino JL, Sánchez-Martin CC, Ortuño J, Lasunción MA. Comparative effects of dietary supplementation with red grape juice and vitamin E on production of superoxide by circulating neutrophil NADPH oxidase in hemodialysis patients. Am J Clin Nutr. 2008 Apr;87(4):1053-61.

Cesar TB, Aptekmann NP, Araujo MP, Vinagre CC, Maranhão RC. Orange juice decreases low-density lipoprotein cholesterol in hypercholesterolemic subjects and improves lipid transfer to high-density lipoprotein in normal and hypercholesterolemic subjects. Nutr Res. 2010 Oct;30(10):689-94.

Chacko NJ, Cesare P, Gaia C, Nadia C. Slow Breathing Improves Arterial Baroreflex Sensitivity and Decreases Blood Pressure in Essential Hypertension. Hypertension 2005;46:714-718.

Chan P, Xu D-Y, Liu J-C, Chen Y-J, Tomlinson B, Huang W-P, Cheng J-T. The effect of stevioside on blood pressure and plasma catecholamines in spontaneously hypertensive rats. Life Sciences 1998;63(19):1679-1684.

Chan P, Tomlinson B, Chen YJ, Liu JC, Hsieh MH, Cheng JT. A double-blind placebo-controlled study of the effectiveness and tolerability of oral stevioside in human hypertension. Br J Clin Pharmacol 2000 Sep;50(3):215-20.

Chan V, Fenning A, Iyer A, Hoey A, Brown L. Resveratrol improves cardiovascular function in DOCA-salt hypertensive rats. Curr Pharm Biotechnol 2011 Mar 1;12(3):429-36.

Chander R, Singh K, Khanna AK, Kaul SM, Puri A, Saxena R, Bhatia G, Rizvi F, Rastogi AK. Antidyslipidemic and antioxidant activities of different fractions of *Terminalia arjuna* stem bark. Indian Journal of Clinical Biochemistry 2004;19(2):141-148.

Chang R. Functional properties of mushrooms. Nutr. Rev. 1996;54:91-93.

Chang WH, Liu JF. Effects of kiwifruit consumption on serum lipid profiles and antioxidative status in hyperlipidemic subjects. Int J Food Sci Nutr. 2009 Dec;60(8):709-16.

Chatterjee TK, Chakraborty A, Pathak M, Sengupta GC. Effects of plant extract Centella asiatica (Linn.) on cold restraint stress ulcer in rats. Indian J Exp Biol 1992 Oct;30(10):889-91.

Chaturvedi A, Sarojini G, Devi NL. Hypocholeateromic effect of amaranth seeds (*Amaranthus esculantus*). Plant Foods for Human Nutrition 1993 Jul;44(1):63-70.

Chen CC, Hsu JD, Wang SF, Chiang HC, Yang MY, Kao ES. *Hibiscus sabdarriffa* extract inhibits the development of atherosclerosis in cholesterol-fed rabbits. J Agric Food Chem 2003;51:5472-7.

Chen CC, Chou FP, Ho YC, Lin WL, Wang CP, Hao ES. Inhibitory effects of *Hibiscus sabdarriffa* L. extract on low-density lipoprotein oxidation and anti-hyperlipidemia in fructose-fed and cholesterol-fed rats. J Sci Food Agric 2004;84:1989-96.

Chen CC, Liu LK, Hsu JD, Huang HP, Yang MY, Wang CJ. *Mulberry* extract inhibits the development of atherosclerosis in cholesterol-fed rabbits. Food Chemisty 2005;91:601-607.

Chen G, Luo YC, Li BP, Li B, Guo Y, Li Y, Su W, Xiao ZL. Effect of polysaccharide from Auricularia auricula on blood lipid metabolism and lipoprotein lipase activity of ICR mice fed a cholesterol-enriched diet. J Food Sci. 2008 Aug;73(6):103-8.

Chen G, Luo YC, Ji BP, Li B, Su W, Xiao ZL, Zhang GZ. Hypocholesterolemic effects of *Auricularia auricula* ethanol extract in ICR mice fed a cholesterol-enriched diet. J Food Sci. Technol 2011;48(6):692-698.

Chen HW, Wang SL, Chen XY. Preliminary study on effects of sodium ferulate in treating diabetic nephropathy. Zhongguo Zhong Xi Yi Jie He Za Zhi. 2006 Sep;26(9):803-6.

Chen JH, Chen HI, Tsai SJ, Jen CJ. Chronic consumption of raw but not boiled Welsh onion juice inhibits rat platelet function. J Nutr. 2000 Jan;130(1):34-7.

Chen PR, Chien KL, Su TC, Chang CJ, Liu T-L, Cheng H, Tsai C. Dietary sesame reduces serum cholesterol and enhances antioxidant capacity in hypercholesterolemia. Nutrition Research 2005;25:559-567.

Chen S, Ly G, Zhang X, Liu X, Zhang H, Zhu Y, Wu Y, Liu S, Ni Z. Anti-hypertensive effects of laiju extract in two different rat models. Asia Pac J Clin Nutr 2007;16(1):309-312.

Chen SY, Ho KJ, Hsieh YJ, Wang LT, Mau JL. Contents of lovastatin, y-aminobutyric acid and ergothioneine in mushroom fruiting bodies and mycelia. LWT – Food Science and Technology 2012;47:274-278.

Chen WQ, Luo SH, Li HZ, Yang H. Effects of ganoderma lucidum polysaccharides on serum lipids andlipoperoxidation in ertperimental hyper lipidemic rats. China Journal of Chinese Material Medica 2005.

Chen Y-S, Liu B-L, Chang Y-N. Bioactivities and sensory evaluation of Pu-erh teas made from three tea leaves in an improved pile fermentation process. Journal of Bioscience and Bioengineering 2010;109(6):557-563.

Cheng JT, Lee YY, Hsu FL, Chang W, Niu C-S- Antihypertensive activity of phenolics from the flower of Lonicera japonica. Chin. Pharm. J (Taipei) 1994;46(6):575-82.

Cheng JY, Shih MF. Preventing dyslipidemia by Chlorella pyrenoidosa in rats and hamsters after chronic high fat diet treatment. Life Sci 2005 May 13;76(26):3001-13.

Cheng HH, Huang HY, Chen YY, Huang CL, Chang CJ, Chen HL, Lai MH. Ameliorative effects of stabilized rice bran on type 2 diabetes patients. Ann Nutr Metab 2010;56(1):45-51.

Cheong SH, Kim MY, Sok DE, Hwang SY, Kim JH, Kim HR, Lee JH, Kim YB, Kim MR. Spirulina prevents atherosclerosis by reducing hypercholesterolemia in rabbits fed a high-cholesterol diet. J Nutr Sci Vitaminol (Tokyo) 2010;56(1):34-40.

Cherif S, Rahal N, Haouala M, Hizaoui B, Dargouth F, Gueddiche M, Kallel Z, Balansard G, Boukef K. A clinical trial of a titrated Olea extract in the treatment of essential arterial hypertension. J Pharm. Belg. 1996 Mar – Apr;51(2):69-71.

Cheung PCK. The hypocholesterolemic effect of two edible of mushrooms: *Auricularia auricula* (Tree-ear) and *Tremella fuciformis* (White jelly-leaf) in hypercholesterolemic rats. Nutrition Research 1996;16(10):1721-1725.

Chiang AN, Wu HL, Yeh HI, Chu CS, Lin HC, Lee WC. Antioxidant effects of black rice extract through the induction of superoxide dismutase and catalase activities. Lipids 2006 Aug;41(8):797-803.

Ching LC, Abdullah N, Shuib AS. Characterization of antihypertensive peptides from *Pleurotus cystidiosus* O.K. Miller (Abalone mushroom). Proceedigs of the 7th International Conference on Mushroom Biology and Mushroom Products (ICMBMP7) 2011: 319-328.

Chithra V, Leelamma S. Hypolipidemic effect of coriander seeds (Coriandrum sativum): mechanism of action. Plant Foods Hum Nutr 1997;51(2):167-72.

Chiu YJ, Chi A, Reid IA. Cardiovascular and endocrine effects of acupuncture in hypertensive patients. Clin Exp Hypertens 1997 Oct;19(7):1047-63.

Cho TM, Peng N, Clark JT, Novak L, Roysommuti S, Prasain J, Wyss JM. Genistein Attenutes the Hypertensive Effects of Dietary NaCl in Hypertensive Male Rats. Endocrinology 2007;148(11):5396-5402.

Choi JH, Kim IS, Kim JI, Yoon TH. Studies on anti-aging action of brown algae (Undaria pinnatifida) 2. Dose effedt of alginic acid as a modulator of anti-aging action in liver membranes. Han'guk Susan Hakhoechi 1992;25(3):181-8.

Choi JH, Kim DW, Kim JH, Kim DI, Kim CM. Effect of Brown Algae *(Undaria pinnatifida)*-Noodle on Lipid Metabolism in Serum of SD-Rats. J. Korean Fish. Soc. 1999;32(1):42-45.

Choi YY, Osada K, Ito Y, Nagasawa T, Choi MR, Nishizawa N. Effects of Dietary Protein of Korean Foxtail Millet on Plasma Adiponectin, HDL-Cholesterol, and Insulin Levels in Genetically Type 2 Diabetic Mice. Biosci. Biotechnol. Biochem. 2005;69(1):31-37.

Chong CW, Rokiah MY, Mohd AKR, Norhayati AH. The effect of red pitaya *(Hylocereus sp.)* consumption on the total antioxidant status and malondialdehyde level among diabetes, hypertensive and hypercholesterolemic subjects in Universiti Putra Malaysia. Mal J Nutr 2006;12(2):103.

Chong HZ, Rokiah MY, Norhayati AH, Mohd AKR. Effect of red pitaya *(Hylocereus sp.)* consumpton on blood pressure, blood glucose and lipid profile of hypertensive staff of UPM, Serdang. Mal J Nutr. 2006;12(2):10.

Chou TW, Ma CY, Cheng HH, Chen YY, Lai MH. A rice bran oil diet improves lipid abnormalities and suppress hyperinsulinemic responses in rats with streptozotocin/nicotinamide-induced type 2 diabetes. J Clin Biochem Nutr 2009 Jul;45(1):29-36.

Choudhary R. Benificial effect of allium sativum and allium tuberosum on experimental hyperlipidemia and atherosclerosis. Pak J Physiol 2008;4(2):7-9.

Christiansen B, Muguerza NB, Petersen AM, Kveiborg B, Madsen CR, Thomas H, Ihlemann N, Sørensen JC, Køber L, Sørensen H, Torp-Pedersen C, Dominguez H. Ingestion of Broccoli Sprouts Does Not Improve Endothelial Function in Humans with Hypertension. PloS ONE 2010 Aug;5(8):1-8.

Chu S-L, Fu H, Yang J-X, Liu G-X, Dou P, Zhang L, Tu P-F, Wang X-M. Chinese Journal of Integrative Medicine 2011 Jul;17(7):492-498.

Chu TT, Benzie IF, Lam CW, Fok BS, Lee KK, Tomlinson B. Study of potential cardioprotective effects of Ganoderma lucidum (Lingzhi): results of a controlled human intervention trial. Br J Nutr. 2011 Aug 1:1-11.

Chung IM, Lim JW, Pyun WB, Kim H. Korean Red Ginseng Improves Vascular Stiffness in Patients with Coronary Artery Disease. J. Ginseng Res. 2010;34(3):212-218.

Cicero AF, Vitale G, Savino G, Arletti R. Panax notoginseng (Burk.) effects on fibrinogen and lipid plasma level in rate fed on a high-fat diet. Phytother Res. 2003 Feb;17(2):174-8.

Cignarella A, Nastasi M, Cavalli E, Puglisi L. Novel lipid-lowering properties of *Vaccinium myrtillus* L. Leaves, a traditional antidiabetic treatment, in several models of rat dyslipidaemia: a comparison with ciprofibrate. Thrombosis Research 1996;84(5):311-322.

Circosta C, Pasquale RD, Samperi S, Pino A, Occhiuto F. Biological and analytical characterization of two extracts from *Valeriana officinalis*. Journal of Ethnopharmacology 2007;112:361-367.

Clarke R, Frost C, Collins R, Appleby P, Peto R. Dietary lipids and blood cholesterol: quantitative meta-analysis of metabolic ward studies. BMJ 1997 Jan 11;314(7074):112-7.

Clifton-Bligh PB, Baber RJ, Fulcher GR, Nery ML, Moreton T. Menopause 2001 Jul-Aug;8(4):259-65.

Clifton PM, Bastiaans K, Keogh JB. High protein diets decrease total and abdominal fat and improve CVD risk profile in overweight and obese men and women with elevated triacylglycerol. Nutrition, Metabolism & Cardiovascular Disease 2009;19:548-554.

Coelho CC. Effects of HMB supplementation on LDL-cholesterol, strength and body composition of patiens with hypercholesterolemia. Medicine & science in sports & exercise 2001;33(5):340.

Cohen DL, Bloedon LT, Rothman RL, Farrar JT, Galantino ML, Volger S, Mayor C, Szapary PO, Townsend RR. Iyengar Yoga versus Enhanced Usual Care on Blood Pressure in Patients with Prehypertension to Stage I Hypertension: a Randomized Controlled Trial. Evidence-Based Complementary and Alternative Medicine 2011.

Coimbra S, Santos-Silva A, Rocha-Pereira P, Rocha S, Castro E. Green tea consumption improves plasma lipd profiles in adults. Nutrition Research 2006;26:604-607.

Coimbra SR, Lage SH, Brandizzi L, Yoshida V, da Luz PL. The action of red wine and purple grape juice on vascular reactivity is independent of plasma lipids in hypercholesterolemic patients. Brazilian Journal of Medical and Biological Research 2005;38:1339-1347.

Colquhoun DM, Moores D, Somerset SM, Humphries JA. Comparison of the effects on lipopoteins and apolipoproteins of a diet high in monounsaturated fatty acids, enriched with avocade, and a high-carbohydrate diet. Am J Clin Nutr. 1992 Oct;56(4):671-7.

Corder R, Douthwaite JA, Lees DM, Khan NQ, Viseu Dos Santos AC, Wood EG, Carrier MJ. Endotelin-1 synthesis reduced by red wine. Nature 2001 Dec 20-27;414(6866):863-4.

Cornish SM, Chilibeck PD, Paus-Jennsen L, Biem HJ, Khozani T, Senanayake V, Vatanparast H, Little JP, Whiting SJ, Pahwa P. A randomized controlled trial of the effects of flaxseed lignan complex on metabolic syndrome composite score and bone mineral in older adults. Appl Physiol Nutr Metab, 2009 Apr;34(2):89-98.

Corona G, Boddi V, Balercia G, Rastelli G, De Vita G, Sforza A, Forti G, Mannucci E, Maggi E. The effect of statin therapy on testosterone levels in subjects consulting for erectile dysfunction. J Sex Med. 2010 Apr;7(4 Pt 1):1547-56.

Coronel F, Tornero F, Torrente J, Naranjo P, De Oleo P, Macia M, Barrientos A. Treatment of hyperlipemia in diabetic patients on dialysis with a physiological substace. Am J Nephrol 1991;11(1):32-6.

Coruzzi P, Brambilla L, Brambilla V, Gualerzi M, Rossi M, Parati G, Di Rienzo M, Tadonio J, Novarini A. Potassium depletion and salt sensitivity in essential hypertension. J Clin Endocrinol Meta 2001 Jun;86(6):2857-62.

Costa CA, Bidinotto LT, Takahira RK, Salvadori DM, Barbisan LF, Costa M. Cholesterol reduction and lack of genotoxic or toxic effects i mice after repeated 21-day oral intake of lemongrass (Cymbopogon citratus) essential oil. Food Chem Toxicol 2011 Sep;49(9):2268-72.

Cropley M, Cave Z, Ellis J, Middleton RW. Effect of kava and valerian on human physiological and psychological responses to mental stress assessed under laboratory conditions. Phytother Res. 2002 Feb;16(1):23-7.

Czerwinski J, Bartnikowska E, Leontowicz H, Lange E, Leontowicz M, Katrich E, Trakhtenberg S, Gorinstein S. Oat *(Avena staiva L.)* and amaranth *(Amaranthus hypochondriacus)* meals positively affect plasma lipid profile in rats fed cholesterol-containing diets. Journal of Nutritional Biochemstry 2004;15:622-629.

Daher CF, Baroody KG, Baroody GM. Effect of Urtica dioica extrct intake upon blood lipid profile in the rats. Fitoterapia 2006 Apr;77(3):183-8.

Dai M, Liu Q, Li D, Liu L. Research of material bases on antifebrile and hypotensive effects of flos chrysanthemi. Zhong Yao Cai 2001 Jul;24(7):505-6.

Dai W, Yin J, Hu YM. Clinical Efficacy of Apocynum Tea on Patients with Hypertension. Practical Preventive Medicine 2010.

Daleprane JB, Batisa A, Pacheco JT, da Silva AFE, Costa CA, Resende AC, Boaventura GT. Dietary flaxseed supplementation improves endothelial function in the mesenteric arterial bed. Food Research International 2010;43:2052-2056.

Das M, Sarma BP, Rokeya B, Parial R, Nahar N, Mosihuzzaman M, Khan A, Ali L. Antihyperglycemic and antihyperlipidemic activity of Urtica dioica on type 2 diabetic model rats. Journal of Diabetology 2011 Jun;2:2.

Dattilo AM, Kris-Etherton PM. Effects of weight reduction on blood lipids and lipoproteins: a meta-analysis. Am J Clin Nutr. 1992 Aug;56(2):320-8.

Dehkordi FR, Kamkhah AF. Antihypertensive effect of Nigella sativa seed extract in patients with mild hypertension. Fundam Clin Pharmacol. 2008 Aug;22(4):447-52.

De Morais EC, Stefanuto A, Klein GA, Boaventura BC, de Andrade F, Wazlawik E, Di Pietro PF, Maraschin M, da Silva EL. Comsumption of yerba mate (Ilex paraguariensis) improves serum lipid parameters in healthy dyslipidemic subjects and provides an addtional LDL-cholesterol reduction in individuals on statin therapy. J Agric Food Chem. 2009 Sep 23;57(18):8316-24.

De Moura RS, Miranda DZ, Pinto AC, Sicca RF, Souza MA, Rubenich LM, Carvalho LC, Rangel BM, Tano T, Madeira SV, Resende AC. Mechanism of the endothelium-dependent vasodilation and the antihypertensive effect of Brazilian red wine. J Cardiovasc Pharmacol 2004 Sep;44(3):302-9.

De Tommasi N. Studies on the constituents of *Cyclanthera pedata* (caigua) seeds: isolation and characterizatio of six new Cucurbitacin glycosides. J. Agr. Food Chem. 1996;44(8):2020-2025.

Derosa G, Maffioli P, Ferrari I, D'Angelo A, Fogari E, Palumbo I, Randazzo S, Cicero AF. Comparison between orlistat plus l-carnitine and orlistat alone on inflammation parameters in obese diabetic patients. Fundam Clin Pharmacol. 2011 Oct;25(5):642-51.

Desai F, Vyas O. A Study to determine the effectivenes of yoga, biofeedback & music therapy in management of hypertension. The Indian Journal of Occupational Therapy 2001;33(2):3-7.

Devasankaraiah G, Hanin I, Haranath PS, Ramanamurthy PS. Cholinomimetic effects of aqueous extracts from Carum copticum seeds. Br J Pharmacol 1974 Dec;52(4):613-4.

Devasena I, Narhare P. Effect of yoga on heart rate and blood pressure and its clinical significance. Int J Biol Med Res. 2011;2(3):750-753.

Deyhim F, Lopez E, Gonzalez J, Garcia M, Patil BS. Citrus juice modulates antioxidant enzymes and lipid profiles in orchidectomized rats. J Med Food. 2006;9(3):422-6.

Dhandapani R. Hypolipidemic activity of *Eclipta prostrata* (L.) L. leaft extract in atherogenic diet induced hyperlipidemic rats. Indian Journal of Experimental Biology 2007;45:617-619.

Dhandapani S, Suramanian VR, Rajagopal S, Namasivayam N. Hypolipidemic effect of Cuminum cymimum L. on alloxan-induced diabetic rats. Pharmacol Res. 2002 Sep;46(3):251-5.

Dhanapakiam P, Joseph JM, Ramaswamy VK, Moorthi M, Kumar AS. The cholesterol lowering property of coriander seeds (Coriandrum sativum): mechanism of action. J Environ Biol 2008;29(1):53-6.

Dhar P, Chattopadhya K, Bhattacharyya D, Biswas A, Roy B, Ghosh S. Ameliorative influence of sesame lignans on lipid profile and lipid peroxidation in induced diabetic rats. J Agric Food Chem 2007 Jul 11;55 (14):5875-80.

Dhungel UK, Malhotra V, Sarkar D, Prajapati R. Effect of alternate nostril breathing exercise on cardiorespiratory functions. Nepal Med Coll J. 2008 Mar;10(1):25-7.

Di Donna L, De Luca G, Mazzotti F, Napoli A, Salerno R, Taverna D, Sindona G. Statin-like principles of bergamot fruits (Citrus bergamia): isolation of 3-hydroxymethylglutaryl flavonoid glycosides. J Nat Prod. 2009 Jul;72(7):1352-4.

Diao LH, Yang ZB, Zhou GX, Chen Y, Fan LY, Zhang YY, Liu H, Liu ST. Observation on therapeutic effects of electroacupuncture at Neiguan (PC6) on silent myocardial ischemia. Zhongguo Zhen Jiu 2011 Jul;31(7):591-4.

Diaz-Juárez JA, Tenorio-López FA, Zarco-Olvera G, Valle-Mondragón LD, Torres-Narváez JC. Effect of Citrus paradisi extract and juice on arterial pressure both in vitro and in vivo. Phytother Res. 2009 Jul;23(7):948-54.

Dierberger B, Schach M, Anadere I, Brandle M, Jacob R. Effect of a diet rich in linseed oil on complex viscosity and blood pressure in spontaneously hypertensive rats (SHR). Basic Res Cardiol 1991;86(6):561-6.

Digiesi V, Cantini F, Bisi G, Guarino GC, Oradei A, Littarru GP. Mechanism of action of coenzyme Q_{10} in essential hypertension. Current Therapeutic Research 1992;51(5):668-672.

Digiesi V, Cantini F, Oradei A, Bisi G, Guarino GC, Brocchi A, Bellandi F, Mancini M, Littarru GP. Coenzyme Q10 in essential hypertension. Mol Aspects Med 1994;15:257-63.

Digiesi V, Cantini F, Bisi G, Guarino G, Brodbeck B. L-carnitine adjuvant therapy in essential hypertension. Clin Ter. 1994

211

May;144(5):391-5.

Dineshkumar B, Analava M, Manjunatha M. Antidiabetic and hypolipidaemic effects of few common plants extract in Type 2 diabetic patients at Bengal. Int J Diabetes & Metab 2010;18:59-65.

Diniz YS, Rocha KK, Souza GA, Galhardi CM, Ebaid GM, Rodrigues HG, Novelli Filho JL, Cicogna AC, Novelli EL. Effects of N-acetylcysteine on sucrose-rich diet-induced hyperglycaemia, dyslipidemia and oxidative stress in rats. Eur J Pharmacol 2006 Aug 14;543(1-3):151-7.

Dixit VP, Joshi SC. Antiatherosclerotic effects of alfalfa meal ingestion in chicks; a biochemical evaluation. Indian J Physiol Pharmacol 1985 Jan;29(1):47-50.

Dixit VP, Joshi SC, Prabha Jain. Prevention of aortic lesions and hyperlipidaemia by alfalfa seed extract in cholesterol fed rabbit. J. Biosci. 1986 Jun;10(2):251-256.

Dixit Y, Kar A. Protective role of three vegetable peels in alloxan induced diabetes mellitus in male mice. Plant Foods Hum Nutr. 2010 Sep;65(3):284-9.

Do GM, Kwon EY, Kim HJ, Jeon SM, Ha TY, Park T, Choi MS. Long-term effects of resveratrol supplementation on suppression of atherogenic lesion formation and cholesterol synthesis in apo E-deficient mice. Biochem Biophys Res Commun 2008 Sep 12;374(1):55-9.

Dokusova OK, Krivoruchenko IV. The effect of biotin on the level of cholesterol in the blood of patients with atherosclerosis and essential hyperlipidemia. Kardiologiaa 1972;12(12):113.

Donati C, Barbi G, Cairo G, Prati GF, Degli Esposti E. Pantethine improves the lipid abnormalities of chronic hemodialysis patients: results of a multicenter clinical trial. Clin Nephrol 1986 Feb;25(2):70-4.

Dong JY, Qin LQ, Zhang Z, Zhao Y, Wang J, Arigoni F, Zhang W. Effect of oral l-arginine supplementation on blood pressure: A meta-analysis of randomized, double-blind, placebo-controlled trials. Am Heart J. 2011 Dec;162(6):959-65.

Dong MY, Lumz, Yin QH, Feng WM, Xu JX, Xu WM. Jiangsu J Agricultural Sciences 1995;Vol.1(3):46-55.

Duarte J, Pérez-Palencia R, Vargas F, Ocete MA, Pérez-Vizcaino F, Zarzuelo A, Tamargo J. Antihypertensive effects of the flavonoid quercetin in spontaneously hypertensive rats. British Journal of Pharmacology 2001;133:117-124.

Dubey AK, Devi A, Kutty G, Shankar RP. Hypolipidemic Activity of Ginkgo biloba Extract, Egb 761 in Hypercholesterolemic Wistar Rats. Iranian Journal of Pharmacology & Therapeutics 2005 Jan;4(1):9-12.

Duncan AC, Jäger AK, Staden van J. Screening of Zulu medicinal plants for angiotensin converting enzyme (ACE) inhibitors. Journal of Ethnopharmacology 1999;68:63-70.

Ďuračková Z, Trebatický B, Novotný V, Žitňanová I, Breza J. Lipid metabolism and erectile function improvement by Pycnogenol, extract from the bark of *Pinus pinaster* in patients suffering from erectile dysfuncton-a pilot study. Nutrition Research 2003;23:1189-1198.

Durak I, Kavutcu M, Aytac B, Avci A, Devrim E, Özbek H, Öztürk HS. Effects of garlic extract consumption on blood lipid and oxidant/antioxidan parameters in humans wih high blood cholesterol. Journal of Nutritional Biochemistry 2004;15:373-377.

Duttaroy AK, Jørgensen A. Effects of kiwi fruit consumption on platelet aggregation and plasma lipids in healthy human volunteers. Platelets 2004 Aug;15(5):287-92.

Dwivedi S, Agarwal MP. Antianginal and cardioprotective effects of Terminalia arjuna, an indigenous drug, in coronary artery disease. J Assoc Physicians India 1994 Apr;42(4):287-9.

Dwivedi S, Pachori SB, Amrita. Medicinal plants with hypotensive activity. Indian Pract. 1994;6:117-134.

Dykes L, Rooney LW. Phenolic compounds in cereal grains and their health benefits. Cereal Foods World, May-June 2007;52(3):105-111.

Eady S, Wallace A, Willis J, Scott R, Frampton C. Consumption of plant sterol-based spread derived from rice bran oil is effective at reducing plasma lipid levels in mildly hypercholesterolaemic individuals. Br J Nutr 2011 Feb 15;1-12.

Eddouks M, Lemhadri A, Michel J-B. Hypolipidemic activity of aqueous extract of *Capparis spinosa* L. in normal and diabetic rats. Journal of Ethnopharmacology 2005;98:345-350.

Edwards RL, Lyon T, Litwin SE, Rabovsky A, Symons JD, Jalili T. Quercetin reduces blood pressure in hypertensive subjects. J Nutr. 2007 Nov;137(11):2405-11.

Egert S, Bosy-Westphal A, Seiberl J, Kürbitz C, Settler U, Plachta-Danielzik S, Wagner AE, Frank J, Schrezenmeir J, Rimbach G, Wolffram S, Müller MJ. Quercetin reduces systolic blood pressure and plasma oxidised low-density lipoprotein concentrations in overweight subjects with a high-cardiovascular disease risk phenotype: a double-blinded, placebo-controlled cross-over study. Br J Nutr. 2009 Oct;102(7):1065-74.

Eidi A, Eidi M. Antidiabetic effects of sage *(Salvia officinalis* L.) leaves in normal and streptozotocin-induced diabetic rats. Diabetes & Metabolic Syndrome: Clinical Research & Reviews 2009;3:40-44.

Ejtahed H, Nia JM, Rad AH, Niafar M, Jafarabadi MA, Mofid V. The effects of probiotic yoghurt consumption on blood pressure and serum lipids in type 2 diabetic patiets. Iranian Journal of Nutrition Sciences & Food Technology 2012;6(4).

El Bardai S, Lyoussi B, Wibo M, Morel N. Pharmacological evidence of hypotensive activity of *Marrubium vulgare* and *Foeniculum vulgare* in spontaneously hypertensive rat. Clin. and Exper. Hypertension 2001;23(4):329-343.

El Bardai S, Morel N, Wilbo M, Fabre N, Llabres G, Lyoussl B, Quetin-Leclercq J. The Vasorelaxant Activity of Marrubenol and Marrubiin from *Marrubium vulgare*. Planta Med 2003;69:75-77.

El Bardai S, Lyoussi B, Wibo M, Morel N. Comparative study of the antihypertensive activity of Marrubium vulgare and of the dihydropyridine calcium antagonist amlodipine in spontaneously hypertensive rat. Clin Exp Hypertens. 2004 Aug;26(6):465-74.

El-Bassossy HM, Fahmy A, El-Fawal R. Arginase inhibition alleviates hypertension associated with diabetes. Effect on endothelial dependent relaxation and NO production. Vascular Pharmacology 2012.

El-Dakhakhny M, Mady NI, Halim MA. Nigella sativa L. oil protects against induced hepatotoxicity and improves serum lipid profile in rats. Arzneimittelforschung. 2000 Sep;50(9):832-6.

El-Khayat Z, Ezzat AR, Arbid MS, Rasheed WI, Elias TR. Potential Effects of Bee Honey and Propolis Against the Toxicity of Ochratoxin A in Rats. Macedonian Journal of Medical Sciences 2009 Dec 15;2(4):311-318.

El-Khayat Z, Hussein J, Ramzy T, Ashour M. Antidiabetic antioxidant effect of *Panax ginseng*. Journal of Medicinal Plants Research 2011 Sep;5(18):4616-4620.

El-Mosallamy AEMK, Sleem AA, Abdel-Salam OME, Shaffie N, Kenawy SA. Antihypertensive and Cardioprotective Effects of Pumpkin Seed Oil. Journal of Medicinal Food 2011.

El-Sayed ESM, Abo-Salem OM, Aly HA, Mansour AM. Potential antidiabetic and hypolipidemic effects of propolis extract in streptozotocin-induced diabetic rats. Pak. J. Pharm. Sci. 2009 Apr;22(2):168-174.

El-Tahir KE, Ashour MM, al-Harbi MM. The cardiovascular actions of the volatile oil of the black seed (Nigella sativa) in rats: elucidation of the mechanism of action. Gen Pharmacol. 1993 Sep;24(5):1123-31.

El-Tahir AM, Kamel EH, Abdurahaman A. Effects of volatile oil of *Carum carvi* L. on arterial blood pressure and heart rate. Saudi Pharmacol 1994;2:163-168.

Elberry AA, Harraz FM, Ghareib SA, Gabr SA, Nagy AA, Abdel-Sattar E. Methanolic extract of *Marrubium* vulgare ameliorates hyperglycemia and dyslipidemia in streptozotocin-induced diabetic rts. International Journal of Diabetes Mellitus 2011.

Elgazzar UB, Ghanema IIA, kalaba ZM. Effect of Dietary L-carnitine Supplementation on the Concentration of Circulating Serum Metabolites in Growing New Zealand Rabbits. Australian Journal of Basic and Applied Sciences 2012;6(2):80-84.

Eliasson K, Ryttig KR, Hylander B, Rossner S. A Dietary Fibre Supplement in the Treatment of Mild Hypertension: A Randomized, Double Blind, Placebo-Controlled Trail. J. Hypertens 1992;10:195-199.

Elliot P, Kesteloot H, Appel LJ, Dyer AR, Ueshima H, Chan Q, Brown IJ, Zhao L, Stamler J. Dietary phosphorus and blood pressure: international study of macro- and micro-nutrients and blood pressure. Hypertension 2008 Mar:51 (3);669-75.

Emmanuel UC, James O. Comparative Effects of Aqueous Garlic (*Allium sativum)* and Onion *(Allium cepa)* Extracts on Some Haematological and Lipid Indices of Rats. Annual Review & Research in Biology 2011;1(3):37-44.

Engler MM, Engler MB, Erickson SK, Paul SM. Dietary gamma-linolenic acid lowers blood pressure and alters aortic reactivity and cholesterol metabolism in hypertension. J Hypertens. 1992 Oct;10(10):1197-204.

Engler MM, Schambelan M, Engler MB, Ball DL, Goodfriend TL. Effects of dietary gamma-linolenic acid on blood pressure and adrenal angiotensin receptors in hypertensive rats. Proc Soc Exp Biol Med. 1998 Jul;218(3):234-7.

Eno AE, Owo OI, Itam EH, Konya RS. Blood pressure depression by the fruit juice of Carica papaya (L) in renal and DOCA-induced hypertenson in the rat. Phytother Res. 2000 Jun;14 (4):235-9.

Eno AE, Ibokette UE, Ofem OE, Unoh FB, Nkanu E, Azah N, Ibu JO. The effects of a nigerian specie of *Viscum album* (Mistletoe) leaf extract on the blood pressure of normotensive and doca-induced hypertensive rats. Nigerian Journal of Physiological Sciences 2004;19(1-2):33-38.

Erejuwa OO, Sulaiman SA, Wahab MS, Sirajudeen KN, Salleh MS, Gurtu S. Differential responses to blood pressure and oxidative stress in streptozotocin-induced diabetic wistar-kyoto rats and spontaneously hypertensive rats: effects of antioxidant (honey) treatment. Int J Mol Sci 2011;12(3):1888-907.

Esmaillzadeh A, Tahbaz F, Gaieni I, Alavi-Majd H, Azadbakht L. Cholesterol-lowering effect of concentrated pomegranate juice consumption in type II diabetic patients with hyperlipidemia. Int J Vitam Nutr Res 2006 May;76(3):147-51.

Ester AVH, Soralys C, Rosa L, Inciarte G, Coromoto L. Efecto del consumo de aguacate *(Persea Americana Mill)* sobre el perfil lipidico en adultos con dislipidemia. Anales Venezolanos de Nutricion 2009;22(2):84-89.

Eto M, Watanabe K, Chonan N, Ishii K. Lowering effect of pantethine on plasma beta-thromboglobulin and lipids in diabetes mellitus. Artery 1987;15(1):1-12.

Fallahi F, Roghani M, Bagheri A. Time-Dependent Hypoglycemic and Hypolipidemic Effect of Allium Ascalonicum L. Feeding in Diabetic Rats. J Babol Univ Med Sci 2010 Apr-May;12(1)

Fatehi M, Saleh TM, Fatehi-Hassanabad Z, Farrokhfal K, Jafarzadeh M, Davodi S. A pharmacological study on Berberis vulgaris fruit extract. J Ethnopharmacol 2005 Oct 31;102(1):46-52.

Fatehi-Hassanabad Z, Jafarzadeh M, Tarhini A, Fatehi M. The antihypertensive and vasodilator effects of aqueous extract from Berberis vulgaris fruit on hypertensive rats. Phytother Res. 2005 Mar;19(3):222-5.

Fazila H, Rokiah MY, Norhayati AH, Mohd AKR. Effect of red pitaya *(Hylocereus sp.)* on blood lipid profiles in mild hypercholesterolaemia and hypercholesterolaemia subjects. Mal J Nutr 2006;12(2):104.

Feltkamp H, Meurer KA, Godehardt E. Tryptophan-induced lowering of blood pressure and changes of serotin uptake by platelets in patients with essential hypertension. Klin Wochenschr 1984 Dec 3;62(23):1115-9.

Fenfangetal T. Study on the Reducing the Blood Lipids of the Ganoderma Luidum. Food Science 2003.

Feng JH, Nirmala DM, Rosemary C, Jeffrey B, Graham AM. Effect of Short-Term Supplementation of Potassium Chloride and Potassium Citrate on Blood Pressure in Hypertensives. Hypertension 2005;45:571.

Feringa HH, Laskey DA, Dickson JE, Coleman CI. The effect of grape seed extract on cardiovascular risk markers: a meta-analysis of randomized controlled trials J Am Diet Assoc. 2011 Aug;111(8):1173-81.

Fernandez AAH, Novelli ELB, Okoshi K, Okoshi MP, Di Muzio BP, Guimarães JFC, Jr. Fernandes A. Influence of rutin treatment on biochemical alteratons in experimental diabetes. Biomedicine & Pharmacotherapy 2010;64:214-219.

Fernandez C, Proto C. L-carnitine in the treatment of chronic myocardial ischemia. An analysis of 3 multicenter studies and a bibliographic review. Clin Ter. 1992 Apr;140(4):353-77.

Fidrianny I, Padmawinata K, Soetarno S, Yulinah dan E. Efek Antihipertensi dan Hipotensi beberapa Fraksi dari Ekstrak Etanol Umbi Lapis. Jurnal Matematika dan Sains 2003 Dec;8(4):147-150.

Fields L, Graham D, McBride M, Dominiczak A. N-Acetylcysteine attenuates the development of hypertension in the SHRSP. Proceedings of the British Pharmacological Society.

Figueroa A, Trivino JA, Sanchez-Gonzalez MA, Vicil F. Oral L-citrulline supplementation attenuates blood pressure response to cold pressor test in young men. Am J Hypertens 2010 Jan;23(1):12-6.

Figueroa A, Sanchez-Gonzales MA, Perkins.Veazie PM, Arjmandi BH. Effects of watermelon supplementation on aortic blood pressure and wave reflection in individuals with prehypertension: a pilot study. Am J Hypertens 2011 Jan;24(1):40-4.

Figueroa A, Sanchez-Gonzales MA, Wong A, Arjmandi BH. Watermelon Extract Supplementation Reduces Ankle Blood Pressure and Carotid Augmentation Index in Obese Adults With Prehypertension or Hypertension. Am J Hypertens 2012 Mar 8.

Finley JW, Burrell JB, Reeves PG. Pinto bean consumption changes SCFA profiles in fecal fermentations, bacterial populations of the lower bowel, and lipid profiles in blood of humans. J Nutr. 2007 Nov;137(11):2391-8.

Fintelmann V. Therapeutic profile and mechanisms of action of artichoke leaf extract: hypolipemic, antioxidant, hepatoprotective and choleretic properties. Phytomedicine 1996:1.

Fiorina P, Lanfredini M, Montanari A. Plasma homocysteine and folate are related to arterial blood pressure in type 2 diabetes mellitus. *Am J Hypertens* 1998;11:1100-7.

Fitzpatrick DF, Hirschfield SL, Ricci T, Jantzen P, Coffey RG. Endothelium-Dependent Vasorelaxation Caused by Various Plant Extracts. Journal of Cardiovascular Pharmacology 1995;26:90-95.

Fki I, Bouaziz M, Sahnoun Z, Sayadi S. Hypocholesterolemic effects of phenolic-rich extract of *Chemlali* olive cultivar in rats fed a cholesterol-rich diet. Bioorganic & Medicinal Chemistry 2005;13:5362-5370.

Flachskampf FA, Gallasch J, Gefeller O, Gan J, Mao J, Pfahlberg AB, Wortmann A, Klinghammer L, Pflederer W, Daniel WG. Randomized trial of acupuncture to lower blood pressure. Circulation 2007 Jun 19;115(24):3121-9.

Folkers K, Drzewoski J, Richardson PC, Ellis J, Shizukuishi S, Baker L Bioenergetics in clinical medicine. XVI. Reduction of hypertension in patients by therapy with coenzyme Q10. Res Commun Chem Pathol Pharmacol 1981 Jan;31(1):129-40.

Foppa M, Fuchs FD, Preissler L, Andrighetto A, Rosito GA, Duncan BB. Red wine with the noon meal lowers post-meal blood pressure: a randomized trial in centrally obese, hypertensive patients. J Stud Alcohol 2002 Mar;63(2):247-51.

Fortes RC, Novaes MRCG. The effects of *Agricus sylvaticus* fungi dietary supplementation on the metabolism and blood pressure of patients with colorectal cancer during post surgical phase. Nutr Hosp. 2011;26(1):176-186.

Franceschini G, Werba JP, Safa O, Gikalov I, Sirtori CR. Dose-related increase of HDL-cholesterol levels after N-acetylcysteine in man. Pharmacol Res. 1993 Oct – Nov;28(3):213-8.

Frasetto LA, Schloetter M, Mietus-Syder M, Morris Jr RC, Sebastian A. Metabolic and physiologic improvements from consuming a paleolithic, hunter-gatherer type diet. European Journal of Clinical Nutrition 2009;1-9.

Friedman M, Fitch TE, Levin CE, Yokoyama WH. Feeding Tomatoes to Hamsters Reduces their Plasma Low-density Lipoprotein Cholesterol and Triglycerides. Journal of Food Science 2000;65(5):897-899.

Fritz M, Vecchi B, Rinaldi G, Añón MC. Amaranth seed protein hydrolysates have in vivo and vitro antihypertensive activity. Food Chemistry 2011;126:878-884.

Frühbeck G, Monreal I, Santidrián S. Hormonal implications of the hypocholesterolemic effect of intake of field beans (Vicia faba L.) by young men with hypercholesterolemia. Am J Clin Nutr 1997 Dec;66(6):1452-60.

Fuhrman B, Elis A, Aviram M. Hypocholesterolemic Effect of Lycopene and B-Carotene Is Related to Suppression of Cholesterol Synthesis and Augmentation of LDL Receptor Activity in Macrophages. Biochemical and Biophysical Research Communications 1997;233:658-662.

Fujita H, Yamagami T. Efficacy and Safety of Chinese Black Tea (Pu-Ehr) Extract in Healthy and Hypercholesterolemic Subjets. Ann Nutr Metab. 2008;53:33-42.

Fujita T, Sato Y. Natriuretic and antihypertensive effects of potassium in DOCA-salt hypertensive rats. Kidney Int 1983 Dec;24(6):731-9.

Fujita T, Ando K, Noda H, Ito Y, Sato Y. Effects of increased adrenomedullary activity and taurine in young patients with borderline hypertension. Circulation 1987 Mar;75(3):525-32.

Fukumitsu S, Aida K, Shimizu H, Toyoda K. Flaxseed lignan lowers blood cholesterol and decreases liver disease risk factors in moderately hypercholesterolemic men. Nutr Res 2010 Jul;30(7):441-6.

Fukunaga T, Nishiya K, Kajikawa I, Takeya K, Itokawa H. Studies on the Constituents of Japanese Mistletoes from Different Host Trees and Their Antimicrobial and Hypotensive Properties. Chem. Pharm. Bull. 1989;37(6):1543-1546.

Fukushima M, Nakano M, Morii Y, Ohashi T, Fujiwara Y, Sonoyama K. Hepatic LDL receptor mRNA in rats is increased by dietary mushroom (Agaricus bisporus) fiber and sugar beet fiber. J Nutr. 2000 Sep;130(9):2151-6.

Fukushima M, Ohashi T, Fujiwara Y, Sonoyama K, Nakano M. Cholesterol-lowering effects of maitake (Grifola frondosa) fiber, shiitake (Lentinus edodes) fiber, and enokitake (Flammulina velutipes) fiber in rats. Exp Biol Med (Maywood) 2001 Sep;226(8):758-65.

Fuliang HU, Hepburn HR, Xuan H, Chen M, Daya S, Radloff SE. Effects of propolis on blood glucose, blood lipid and free radicals in rat with diabetes mellitus. Pharmacological Research 2005;51:147-152.

Fumio E, Watanabe Y, Zhang J, Miyamoto K, Yoshimoto H, Fukuhara T, Higaki M. Inhibitory effects of hot water extract from Agaricus blazei fruiting bodies (CJ-01) on hypertension development in Spontaneously Hypertensive Rats. Journal of Traditional Medicines 1999;16(5):201-207.

Gaddi A, Descovich GC, Noseda G, Fragiacomo C, Colombo L, Craveri A, Montanari G, Sirtori CR. Controlled evaluation of pantethine, a natural hypolipidemic compound, in patients with different forms of hyperlipoprotenemia. Atherosclerosis 1984 Jan;50(1):73-83.

Galduróz JCF, Antunes HK, Santos RF. Gender- and age-related variations in blood viscosity in normal volunteers: A study of the effects of *Allium sativum* and *Ginkgo biloba.* Phytomedicine 2007;14:447-451.

Gallaher CM, Gallaher DD. Dried plums (prunes) reduce atherosclerosis lesion area in apolipoprotein E-deficient mice. Br J Nutr 2009 Jan;101(2):233-9.

Gamarallage VKS, Banigesh A, Wu L, Lee P, Juurlink BHJ. The Dietary Phase 2 Protein Inducer Sulforaphane Can Normalize the Kidney Epigenome and Improve Blood Pressure in Hypertensive Rats. *American Journal of Hypertension* 2012 Feb;25:229-235.

Gao F, Zhang K, Song XT, Wu XG, Zhang JY, Cui ZY, Yu F. Study on Assistant Anti-hypertension Effect of Apocynum among Hypertensions Patients. Occupation and Health 2010.

Garg K, Gupta A, Rao HK, Sharma K. Efficacy of hypericum perforatum (St. John's wort) in patients of hypertension with associated anxiety. Journal of Herbal Medicine and Toxicology 2010;4(1):103-108.

Gasparotto Junior A, Aurelio BM, Botelho LEL, Alves SME, Leite KCA, Andrade MMC. Natriuretic and diuretic effects of *Tropaeolum majus* (Tropaeolaceae) in rats. Journal of Ethnopharmacology 2009;122:517-522.

Gasparotto Junior A, Gasparotto FM, Lourenco EL, Crestani S, Stefanello ME, Salvador MJ, da Silva-Santos JE, Marques MC,

Kassuya CA. Antihypertensive effects of isoquercitrin and extracts from Tropaeolum majus L.: evidence for the inhibition of angiotensin converting enzyme. J Ethnopharmacol. 2011 Mar 24;134(2):363-72.

Gasparotto Junior A, Gasparotto FM, Lourenco EL, Crestani S, Stefanello ME, Salvador MJ, da Silva-Santos JE, Marques MC, Kassuya CA. Diuretic and potassium-sparing effect of isoquercitrin – an active flavonoid of Tropaeolum majus L. J Ethnopharmacol 2011 Mar 24;134(2):210-5.

Gavez M, Efectos terapéuticos de *Cyclanthera pedata* ("caigua") deshidratada a dosis bajas y unitomas en pacientes hiperlipidémicos. Segundo Simposium Internacional de Plantas Medicinales y Fitoterapia 2004 Aug:23.

Gebhardt R. Hepatocellular actions of artischoke extracts: stimulation of biliary secretion, inhibition of cholesterol biosynthesis and antioxidant properties. Phytomedicine 1996:1.

Geng F, He Y, Yang L, Wang Z. A rapid assay for angiotensin-converting enzyme activity using ultra-performance liquid chromatography-mass spectrometry. Biomed. Chromatogr. 2010;24:312-317.

Geohas J, Daly A, Juturu V, Finch M, Komorowski JR. Chromium picolinate and biotin combination reduces atherogenic inde of plasma in patients with type 2 diabetes mellitus: a placebo-controlled, double-blinded, randomized clinical trial. Am J Med Sci. 2007 Mar;333(3):145-53.

Georgina EO, Kingsley O, Esosa US, Helen NK, Frank AO, Anthony OC. International Journal of Nutrition and Metabolism 2011 Sep 13;3(8):97-102.

Gerhardt AL, Gallo NB. Full-fat rice bran and oat bran similarly reduce hypercholesterolemia in humans. J Nutr. 1998 May;128(5):865-9.

Ghayur MN, Gilani AH. Radish seed extract mediates its cardiovascular inhibitory effects via muscarinic receptor activation. Fundam Clin Pharmacol 2006 Feb;20(1):57-63.

Ghule BV, Ghante MH, Saoji AN, Yeole PG. Hypolipidemic and antihyperlipidemic effects of Lagenaria siceraria (Mol.) fruit extracts. Indian J Exp Biol. 2006 Nov;44(11):905-9.

Ghule BV, Ghante MH, Yeole PG, Saoji AN. Diuretic activity of *Lagenaria siceraria* fruit extracts in rats. Indian Journal of Pharmaceutical Sciences 2007;69(6):817-819.

Ghule BV, Ghante MH, Saoji AN, Yeole PG. Antihyperlipidemic effect of the methanolic extract from Lagenaria siceraria Stand. Fruit in hyperlipidemic rats. J Ethnopharmacol. 2009 Jul 15;124(2):333-7.

Gilani AH, Shaheen E, Saeed SA, Bibi S, Irfanullah, Sadiq M, Faizi S. Hypotensive action of coumarin glycosides from Daucus carota. Phytomedicine 2000 Oct;7(5):423-6.

Gilani AH, Khan AU, Jabeen Q, Subhan F, Ghafar R. Antispasmodic and blood pressure lowering effects of *Valeriana wallichii* are mediated through K$^+$ channel activation. Journal of Ethnopharmacology 2005;100:347-352.

Gilani AH, Khan AU, Shah AJ, Connor J, Jabeen Q. Blood pressure lowering effect of olive is mediated through calcium channel blockade. International Journal of Food Sciences and Nutrition 2005 Dec;56(8):613-620.

Gilani AH, Jabeen Q, Ghayur MN, Janbaz KH, Akhtar MS. Studies on the antihypertensive, antispasmodic, bronchodilator and hepatoprotective activities of th Carum copticum seed extract. J Ethnopharmacol 2005 Apr 8;98(1-2):127-35.

Gilani AH, Jabeen Q, Khan A-U, Shah AJ. Gut modularity, blood pressure lowering, diuretic and sedatve activities of cardamom. Journal of Ethnopharmacology 2008;115:463-472.

Ginter E, Kubec FJ, Vozár J, Bobek P. Natural hypocholesterolemic agent: pectin plus ascorbic acid.Int J Vitam Nutr Res. 1979;49(4):406-12.

Girija K, Lakshman K, Udaya Chandrika, Sabhya Sachi Ghosh, Divya T. Anti-diabetic and anti-cholesterolemic activity of methanol extracts of three species of *Amaranthus*. Asian Pasific Journal of Tropical Biomedicine 2011;:133-138.

Goldhamer A, Lisle D, Parpia B, Anderson SV, Campbell TC. Medically Supervised Water-only Fasting in the Treatment of Hypertension. Journal of Manipulative and Physiological Therapeutics 2001 Jun;24(5):335-339.

Gonez C. Efectos de la Caigua *(Cyclantera pedata)* sobre el perfil lipidico en adultos. Instituto de Investigación de Altura. UPCH. Rev. Per. Endocr. Meta. 1997;3:30-35.

Gonzales F, Chlimper D, Goñez C, Takara M. Estudio de los efectos la caigua deshidratada (Cycladin) sobre el perfil lipidico de adultos de mediana edad de Lima. Instituto de Investigaciones de la Altura. Universidad Peruana Cayetano Heredia. Laboratorios Farmindutria; Lima Peru, 1994.

Gonzales GF, Góñez C, Villena A. Serum lipid and lipoprotein levels in postmenopausal women: short-course effect of caigua. Menopause 1995;2(4):225-234.

Gonzales GF. Ethnobiology and Ethnopharmacology of *Lepidium meyenii* (Maca), a Plant from the Peruvian Highlands. Evidence-Based Complementary and Alternative Medicine 2012:1-10.

Gordon EA, Guppy LJ, Nelson M. The antihypertensive effects of the Jamaican Cho-Cho (Sechium edule). West Indian Med J. 2000 Mar;49(1):27-31.

Gorguc M, Celik I. Effects of Fresh Butter Consumption on the Lipid Profile in Healthy Human Male. J. Clin. Biochem. Nutr. 2005;36:79-82.

Gorinstein S, Yamamoto K, Katrich E, Leontowicz H, Lojek A, Leontowicz M, Čiž M, Goshev I, Shalev U, Trakhtenberg S. Antioxidative Properties of Jaffa Sweeties and Grapefruit and Their Influence on Lipid Metabolism and Plasma Antioxidative Potential in Rats. Biosci. Biotechnol. Biochem. 2003;67(4):907-910.

Gorinstein S, Bartnikowska E, Kulasek G, Zemser M, Trakhtenberg S. Dietary Persimmon Improves Lipid Metabolism in Rats Fed Diets Containing Cholesterol. J. Nutr. 1998 Nov 1;128(11):2023-2027.

Gorinstein S, Kulasek GW, Bartnikowska E, Leontowicz M, Zemser M, Morawiec M, Trakhtenberg S. The effects of diets, supplemented with either whole persimmon or phenol-free persimmon, on rats fed cholesterol. Food Chemistry 2000;70:303-308.

Gorinstein S, Caspi A, Libman I, Katrich E, Lerner HT, Trakhtenberg S. Fresh Israeli Jaffa Sweetie Juice Consumption Improves Lipid Metabolism and Increases Antioxidant Capacity in Hypercholesterolemic Patients Suffering from Coronary Artery Disease: Studies in Vitro and in Humans and Positive Changes in Albumin and Fibrinogen Fractions. J. Agric. Food Chem 2004;52: 5215-5222.

Gossell-Williams M, Lyttle K, Clarke T, Gardner M, Simon O. Supplementation with pumpkin seed oil improves plasma lipid

215

profile and cardiovascular outcomes of female non-ovariectomized and ovariectomized Sprague-Dawley rats. Phytotherapy Research 2008 Jul;22(7):873-877.

Gossell-Williams M, Hyde C, Hunter T, Simms-Stewart D, Fletcher H, McGrowder D, Walters CA. Improvement in HDL cholesterol in postmenopausal women supplemented with pumpkin seed oil: pilot study. Climacteric 2011 Oct;14(5):558-564.

Graham JDP. Brit. Med. Jour. 1939;4114:951-953.

Graham JDP. Quart. Jour. Pharm. and Pharmacol. 1940;13(1):49-56.

Green CO, Wheatley AO, McGrowder DA, Dilworth LL. Asemota HN. Hypolipidemic effects of ortanique peel polymethoxylated flavones in rats with diet-induced hypercholesterolemia. Journal of Food Biochemistry 2011 Oct;35(5):1555-1560.

Greenway F, Liu Z, Yu Y, Gupta A. A clinical trial testing the safety and efficacy of a standardized Eucommia ulmoides Oliver bark extract to treat hypertension. Altern Med Rev. 2011 Dec;16(4):338-47.

Grigorova S, Kashamov B, Sredkova V, Surdjiiska S, Zlatev H. Effect of tribulus terrestris extract on semen quality and serum total cholesterol content in white plymouth rock-mini cocks. Biotechnology in Animal husbandry 2008;24(3-4):139-146.

Grimsgaard S, Bønaa KH, Jacobsen BK, Bjerve KS. Plasma Saturated and Linoleic Fatty Acids Are Independently Associated with Blood Pressure. Hypertension 1999;34:478-483.

Gropalan R, Gracias D, Madhavan M. Serum lipid and lipoprotein fractions in bengal gram and biochanin A induced alterations in atherosclerosis. Indian Heart J 1991 May – Jun;43(4):185-9.

Grossman E, Grossman A, Schein MH, Zimlichman R, Gavish B. Breathing-control lowers blood pressure. Journal of Human Hypertension 2001 Apr;15(4):263-269.

Grossman E, Laudon M, Zisapel N. Effect of melatonin on noctural blood pressure; meta-analysis of randomized controlled trials. Vasc Health Risk Manag. 2011;7:577-84.

Gu D, He J, Wu X, Duan X, Whelton PK. Effect of potassium supplementation on blood pressure in Chinese: a randomized, placebo-controlled trial. J Hypertens 2001 Jul;19(7):1325-31.

Guo W, Ni G. The effects of acupuncture on blood pressure in different patients. J Tradit Chin Med. 2003 Mar;23(1):49-50.

Gudej J, Tomczyk M. Determination of Flavonoids, Tannins and Ellagic acid in leaves from *Rubus* L. species. Archives of Pharmacal Research 2004;27(11):1114-1119.

Guivernau M, Meza N, Barja P, Roman O. Clinical and Experimental Study on the Long-term Effect of Dietary Gamma-linolenic Acid on Plasma Lipids, Platelet Aggregation, Thromboxane Formation, and Prostacyclin Production. Prostaglandis Leukotrienes and Essential Fatty Acids 1994;51:311-316.

Gulmarães PR, Galvão AMP, Batista CM, Azevedo GS, Oliveira RD, Lamounier RP, Freire N, Barros AMD, Sakurai E, Oliveira JP, Vieira EC, Alvarez-Leite JI. Eggplant *(Solanum melongena)* infusion has a modest and transitory effect on hypercholesterolemic subjects. Brazilian Journal of Medical and Biological Research 2000;33;1027-1036.

Guo H, Saiga A, Sato M, Miyazawa I, Shibata M, Takahata Y, Morimatsu F. Royal Jelly Supplementation Improves Lipoprotein Metabolism in Humans. J Nutr Sci Vitaminol 2007;53:345-348.

Guo W, Ni G. The effects of acupuncture on blood pressure in different patients. J Tradit Chin Med 2003 Mar;23(1):49-50.

Gupta R, Singhal S, Goyle A, Sharma VN. Antioxidant and hypocholesterolaemic effects of Terminalia arjuna tree-bark powder: a randomized placebo-controlled trial. J Assoc Physicians India 2001 Feb;49:231-5.

Gursu MF, Onderci M, Gulcu F, Sahin K. Effects of vitamin C and folic acid supplementation on serum paraoxonase activity and metabolites induced by heat stress in vivo. Nutrition Research 2004;24:157-164.

Gutierrez OG Jr, Ikeda K, Nara Y, Deguan GU, Yamori Y. Fish protein-rich diet attenuates hypertension induced by dietary NG-nitro-L-arginine in normotensive Wistar-Kyoto rats. Clin Exp Pharmacol Physiol. 1994 Nov;21(11):875-9.

Hagander B, Asp NG, Ekman R, Nilsson-Ehle P, Scherstén B. Dietary fibre enrichment, blood pressure, lipoprotein profile and gut hormones in NIDDM patients. Eur J Clin Nutr. 1989 Jan;43(1):35-44.

Haidari F, Seyed-Sadjadi N, Taha-Jalali M, Mohammed-Shahi M. The effect of oral administration of Carum carvi on weight, serum glucose, and lipid profile in streptozotocin-induced diabetic rats. Saudi Med J 2011;32(7):695-700.

Hajhashemi V, Abbasi N. Hypolipidemic activity of Anethum graveolens in rats. Phytother Res. 2008 Mar;22(3):372-5.

Hajjaj H, Macé C, Roberts M, Niederberger P, Fay LB. Effect of 26-Oxygenosterols from *Ganoderma lucidum* and Their Activity as Cholesterol Synthesis Inhibitors. Applied and Environmental Microbiology 2005 Jul;71(7):3653-3658.

Haji-Faraji M, Haji-Tarkhani A. The effect of sourtea *(Hibiscus sabdarriffa)* on essential hypertension. Journal of Ethnopharmacology 1999;65:231-236.

Halbert JA, Silagy CA, Finucane P, Withers RT, Hamdorf PA, Andrews GR. The effectiveness of exercise training in lowering blood pressure: a meta-analysis of randomized controlled trials of 4 weeks or longer. J Hum Hypertens 1997 Oct;11(10):641-9.

Hallebeek JM, Beynen AC. Influence of dietary beetpulp on the plasma level of triacylglycerols in horses. J Anim Physiol Anim Nutr (Berl). 2003 Jun;87(5-6):181-7.

Hallfrisch J, Scholfield DJ. Behall KM. Blood pressure reduced by whole grain diet containing barley or whole wheat and brown rice in moderately hypercholesterolemic men. Nutrition Research 2003;23:1631-1642.

Haloui M, Louedec L, Michel JB, Lyoussi B. Experimental diuretic effects of *Rosmarinus officinalis* and *Centaurium erythraea*. Journal of Ethnopharmacology 2000;71:465-472.

Hamedan WAA. Protective Effect of *Lepidium sativum L.* Seeds Powder and Extract on Hypercholesterolemic Rats. Journal of American Science 2010;6(11):873-879.

Han KH, Choe SC, Kim HS, Sohn DW, Nam KY, Oh BH, Lee MM, Park YB, Choi YS, Seo JD, Lee YW. Effect of red ginseng on blood pressure in patients with essentia hypertension and white coat hypertension. Am J Chin Med. 1998;26(2):199-209.

Han KH, Iijuka M, Shimada K, Sekikawa M, Kuramochi K, Ohba K, Ruvini L, Chiji H, Fukushima M. Adzuki resistant starch lowered serum cholesterol and hepatic 3-hydroxy-3-methylglutaryl-CoA mRNA levels and increased hepatic LDL-receptor and cholesterol 7alpha-hydroxylase mRNA levels in rats fed a cholesterol diet. Br J. Nutr. 2005 Dec;94(6):902-8.

Han LK, Xu BJ, Kimura Y, Zheng Y, Okuda H. Platycodi radix affects lipid metabolism in mice with high fat diet-induced obesity. J Nutr. 2000 Nov;130(11):2760-4.

Han LK, Zheng YN, Xu BJ, Okuda H, Kimura Y. Saponins from platycodi radix ameliorate high fat diet-induced obesity in mice. J

Nutr. 2002 Aug;132(8):2241-5.

Handayani D, Chen J, Meyer BJ, Huang XF. Dietary Shiitake Mushroom *(Lentinus edodes)* Prevents Fat Deposition and Lowers Triglyceride in Rats Fed a High-Fat Diet. Journal of Obesity 2011.

Hansen AS, Marckmann P, Dragsted LO, Finné Nielsen IL, Nielsen SE, Grønbaek M. Effect of red wine and red grape extract on blood lipids, haemostatic factors, and other risk factors for cardiovascular disease. Eur J Clin Nutr. 2005 Mar;59(3):449-55.

Hansen K, Adsersen A, Smitt UW, Nyman U, Christensen SB, Schwartner C, Wagner H. Angiotensin Converting Enzyme (ACE) inhibitory flavonoids from *Erythroxylum laurifolium.* Phytomedicine 1996;2(4):313-317.

Hartley TR, Sung BH, Pincomb GA, Whitsett TL, Wilson MF, Lovallo WR. Hypertension risk status and effect of caffeine on blood pressure. Hypertension 2000 Jul;36(1);137-41.

Hartley TR, Locallo WR, Whitsett TL. Cardiovascular effects of caffeine in men and women. Am J Cardiol 2004 Apr 15;93(8):1022-6.

Hassall CH, Kirtland SJ. Dihomo-y-linolenic acid is more potent than an equivalent amount of linoleic acid in reversing hypertension induced with saturated fat. Prog. Lipid Res. 1986;25:515-517.

Hata Y, Yamamoto M, Ohni M, Nakajima K, Nakamura Y, Takano T. A placebo-controlled study of the effect of sour milk on blood pressure in hypertensive subjects. Am J Clin Nutr 1996 Nov;64(5):767-771.

Hata Y, Nakajima K, Uchida JI, Hidaka H, Nakano T. Clinical Effects of Brown Seaweed, *Undaria pinnatifida* (wakame), on Blood Pressure in Hypertensive Subjects. Journal of Clinical Biochemistry and Nutrition 2001;30:43-53.

Hayakawa K, Kimura M, Kamata K. Mechanism underlying y-aminobutyric acid-induced antihypertensive effect in spontaneously hypertensive rats. European Journal of Pharmacology 2002;438:107-113.

He D, Huang Y, Ayupbek A, Gu D, Yang Y, Aisa HA, Ito Y. Separation and Purification of Flavonoids from Black Currant Leaves by High-Speed Countercurrent Chromatography and Preparative HPLC. J Liq Chromatogr Relat Technol. 2010 March 1;33(5): 615-628.

He FJ, MacGregor GA. Effect of modest salt reduction on blood pressure: a meta-analysis of randomized trials. Implications for public health. Journal of Human Hypertension 2002 Nov;16(11):761-770.

He J, Gu D, Wu X, Chen J, Duan X, Chen J, Whelton PK. Effect of soybean protein on blood pressure: A randomized, controlled trial. Ann Intern Med. 2005 Jul 5;143(1):1-9.

He SY, Qian ZY, Tang FT, Wen N, Xu GL, Sheng L. Effect of crocin on experimental atherosclerosis in quails and its mechanisms. Life Sci. 2005 Jul 8;77(8):907-21.

Hermsdorff HH, Zulet MA, Abete I, Martinez JA. A legume-based hypocaloric diet reduces proinflammatory status and improves metabolic features in overweight/obese subjects. Eur J Nutr. 2011 Feb;50(1):61-9.

Hidaka S, Okamoto Y, Arita M. A hot water extract of Chlorella pyrenoidosa reduces body weight and serum lipids in ovariectomized rats. Phytother Res. 2004 Feb;18(2):164-8.

Higasa S, Fujihara S, Hayashi A, Kimoto K, Aoyagi Y. Distributon of a novel angiotensin I-converting enzyme inhibitory substance (2"-hydroxynicotianamine) in the flour, plant parts, and processed products of buckwheat. Food Chemistry 2011;125:607-613.

Hiramatsu K, Nozaki H, Arimori S. Influence of pantethine on platelet volume, microviscosity, lipid composition and functions in diabetes mellitus with hyperlipidemia. Tokai J Exp Clin Med 1981 Jan;6(1):49-57.

Hodson L, Skeaff CM, Chisholm WA. The effect of replacing dietary saturated fat with polyunsaturated or monounsaturated fat on plasma lipids in free-living young adults. Eur J Clin Nutr. 2001 Oct;55(10):908-15.

Hoe SZ, Kamaruddin MY, Lam SK. Inhibition of Angiotensin-Convertin Enzyme Activity by a Partially Purified Fraction of *Gynura procumbens* in Spontaneously Hypertensive Rats. Med Princ Pract 2007;16:203-208.

Hoe SZ, Lee CN, Mok SL, Kamaruddin MY, Lam SK. *Gynura procumbens* Merr. decreases blood pressure in rats by vasodilatation via inhibition of calcium channels. Clinics 2011;66(1):143-150.

Hopkins PN. Effects of dietary cholesterol on serum cholesterol: a meta-analysis and review. Am J Clin Nutr 1992;55:1060-70.

Hosomi R, Fukunaga K, Arai H, Kanda S, Nishiyama T, Yoshida M. Fish Protein Decreases Serum Cholesterol in Rats by Inhibition of Cholesterol and Bile Acid Absorption. Journal of Food Science 2011 May;76(4):116-121.

Hossain S, Hashimoto M, Choudhury EK, Alam N, Hussain S, Hasan M, Choudhury SK, Mahmud I. Dietary mushroom (Pleurotus ostreatus) ameliorates atherogenic lipid in hypercholesterolaemic rats. Clin Exp Pharmacol Physiol 2003 Jul;30(7):470-5.

Hosseini S, Lee J, Sepulveda RT, Rohdewald P, Watson RR. A randomized, double-blind, placebo-controlled, prospective, 16 week crossover study to determine the role of Pycnogenol in modifying blood pressure in mildly hypertensive patients. Nutrition Research 2001;21:1251-1260.

Hou Y, Shao W, Xiao R, Xu K, Ma Z, Johnstone BH, Du Y. Pu-erh tea aqueous extracts lower atherosclerotic risk factors in a rat hyperlipidemia model. Experimental Gerontology 2009;44:434-439.

Houston M. The role of magnesium in hypertension and cardiovascular disease. J Clin Hypertens (Greenwich) 2011 Nov;13 (11):843-7.

Howes JB, Tran D, Brillante D, Howes LG. Effects of dietary supplementation with isoflavones from red clover on ambulatory blood pressure and endothelial function in postmenopausal type 2 diabetes. Diabetes Obes Metab. 2003 Sep;5(5):325-32.

Hsieh MH, Chan P, Sue YM, Liu JC, Liang TH, Huang TY, Tomlinson B, Chow MS, Kao PF, Chan YJ. Efficacy and tolerability of oral stevioside in patients with mild essential hypertension: a two-year, randomized, placebo-controlled study. Clin Ther. 2003 Nov;25(11):2797-808.

Hsu CH, Tsai TH, Kao YH, Hwang KC, Tseng TY, Chou P. Effect of green tea extract on obese women: A randomized, double-blind, placebo-controlled clinical trial. Clinical Nutrition 2008;27:363-370.

Hsu F-L, Lin Y-H, Lee M-H, Lin C-L, Hou W-C. Both Dioscorin, the Tuber Storage Protein of Yam *(Dioscorea alata* cv. Tainong No. 1), and Its Peptic Hydrolysates Exhibited Angiotensin Converting Enzyme Inhibitory Activities. J Agric. Food Chem. 2002;50:6109-6113.

Hsu G-SW, Lu Y-F, Chang S-H, Hsu S-Y. Antihypertensive effect of mung bean sprout extracts in spontaneously hypertensive rats. Journal of Food Biochemistry 2011;35:278-288.

Hsu Y-M, Lai C-H, Chang C-Y, Fan C-T, Chen C-T, Wu C-H. Characterizing the Lipid-Lowering Effects and Antioxidant Mechanisms of Tomato Paste. Biosci. Biotechnol. Biochem. 2008;72(3):677-685.

Hu C, Wei H, Kong H, Bouwman J, Gonzalez-Covarrubias V, van der Heijden R, Reijmers TH, Bao X, Verheij ER, Hankemeier T, Xu G, van der Greef J, Wang M. Linking biological activity with herbal constituents by systems biology-based approaches: effects of Panax ginseng in type 2 diabetic Goto-Kakizaki rats. Mol Biosyst. 2011 Nov;7(11):3094-103.

Hu L, Zhang Y, Lim PS, Miao Y, Tan C, McKenzie KU, Schyvens CG, Whitworth JA. Apocynin but not L-arginine prevents and reverses dexamethasone-induced hypertension in the rat. Am J Hypertens 2006 Apr;19(4):413-8.

Hu Y, Davies GE. Berberine inhibits adipogenesis in high-fat diet-induced obesity mice. Fitoterapia 2010;81:358-366.

Huang HY, Tso TK, Tsai YC, Chang CK. Antioxidant and angiotensin-converting enzyme inhibition capacities of various parts of *Benincasa hispida* (wax gourd). Nahrung 2004;48:230-233.

Huang L, Wen K, Gao X, Liu Y. Hypolipidemic effect of fucoidan from *Laminaria japonica* in hyperlipidemic rats. Pharmaceutical Biology 2010 Apr;48(4):422-426.

Huang R, Wang Y. Preventive effect of laminaria japonica polysaccharides on experimental atherosclerosis in rat. Journal of Nantong University (Medical Sciences) 2008.

Husain GM, Chatterjee SS, Singh PN, Kumar V. Hypolipidemic and Antiobesity-Like Activity of Standardised Extract of *Hypericum perforatum* L. in Rats. International Scholarly Research Network 2011

Huseini HF, Larijani B, Heshmat R, Fakhrzadeh H, Radjabipour B, Toliat T, Raza M. The Efficacy of *Silybum marianum* (L.) Gaertn. (silymarin) in the treatment of type II diabetes: a randomized, double-blind, placebo-controlled, clinical trial. Phytother Res. 2006 Dec;20(12):1036-9.

Huseini HF, Kianbakht S, Hajiaghaee R, Dabaghian FH. Anti-hyperglycemic and Anti-hypercholesterolemic Effects of Aloe vera Leaf Gel in Hyperlipidemic Type 2 Diabetic Patients: A Randomized Double-Blind Placebo-Controlled Clinical Trial. Planta Med 2011 Dec 23

Hussein A. Purslane Extract Effects on Obesity-Induced Diabetic Rats Fed a High-Fat Diet. Mal J Nutr 2010;16(3):419-429.

Hussein GME, Matsuda H, Nakamura S, Hamao M, Akiyama T, Tamura K, Yoshikawa M. Mate Tea *(Ilex paraguariensis)* Promotes Satiety and Body Weight Lowering in Mice: Involvement of Glucagon-Like Peptide-1. Biol. Pharm. Bull. 2011;34(12):1849-1855.

Hussein GME, Matsuda H, Nakamura S, Akiyama T, Tamura K, Yoshikawa M. Protective and ameliorative effects of maté (*Ilex paraguariensis)* on metabolic syndrome in TSOD mice. Phytomedicine 2011;19:88-97.

Hussein G, Nakamura M, Zhao Q, Iguchi T, Goto H, Sankawa U, Watanabe H. Antihypertensive and neuroprotective effects of astaxanthin in experimental animals. Biol Pharm Bull. 2005 Jan;28(1):47-52.

Hussin M, Hamid AA, Mohamad S, Saari N, Bakar F, Dek SP. Modulation of Lipid Metabolism by *Centella Asiatica* in Oxidative Stress Rats. Journal of Food Science 2009 Mar;74(2):72-78.

Ichimura T, Yamanaka A, Ichiba T, Toyokawa T, Kamada Y, Tamamura T, Maruyama S. Antihypertensive Effect of an Extract of *Passiflora edulis* Rind in Spontaneously Hypertensive Rats. Biosci. Biotechnol. Biochem. 2006;70(3):718-721.

Ifansyah N. Comparative effects of total flavonoids extracted from Ribes nigrum leaves, rutin and isoquercitrin on biosynthesis and release of prosiaglandins in the ex vivo rabbit heart. Thèse de Doct. 3Ème cycle ès Sci. Pharm. Tolouse 1982.

Iftekhar ASMM, Rayhan I, Quadir MA, Akhteruzzaman S, Hasnat A. Effect of *Tamarindus Indica* fruits on blood pressure and lipid-profile in human model: an *in vivo* approach. Pak. J. Pharm. Sci. 2006;19(2):125-129.

Igarashi K, Satoh A, Numazawa S, Takahashi E. Effects of cabbage leaf protein concentrate on the serum and liver lipid concentrations in rats. J Nutr Sci Vitaminol (Tokyo) 1997 Apr;43(2):261-70.

Imafidon EK, Okunrobo OL. Biochemical Evaluation of the Tradomedicinal Uses of the Seeds of *Persea americana* Mill., (Family: Lauraceae). World Journal of Medical Sciences 2009;4(2):143-146.

Imafidon KE. Liver Function Status of Hypertensive and Normotensive Rats Administered *Persea americana* Mill. (Avocado) Seeds. Academic Journal of Plant Sciences 2010;3(3):130-133.

Imenshahidi M, Hosseinzadeh H, Javadpour Y. Hypotensive effect of aqueous saffron extract (Crocus sativus L.) and its constituents, safranal and crocin, in normotensive and hypertensive rats. Phytother Res. 2010 Jul;24(7):990-4.

Inanaga K, Ichiki T, Matsuura H, Miyazaki R, Hashimoto T, Takeda K, Sunagawa K. Resveratrol attenuates angiotensin II-induced interleukin-6 expression and perivascular fibrosis. Hypertens Res. 2009 Jun;32(6):466-71.

Inoue M, Wu CZ, Dou DQ, Chen YJ, Ogihara Y. Lipoprotein lipase activation by red Ginseng saponins in hyperlipidemia model animals. Phytomedicine 1999;6(4):257-265.

Interaminense LF, Leal-Cardoso JH, Magalhães PJ, Duarte GP, Lahlou S. Enhanced hypotensive effects of the essential oil of Ocimum gratissimum leaves and its main constituent, eugenol, in DOCA-salt hypertensive conscious rats. Planta Med. 2005 Apr;71(4):376-8.

Iraz M, Fadillioğlu E, Taşdemir S, Ateş B, Erdoğan S. Dose dependent effects of caffeic acid phenethyl ester on heart rate and blood pressure in rats. Eur J Gen Med 2005;2(2):69-75.

Iritani N, Nogi J. Effect of Spinach and Wakame on Cholesterol Turnover in the Rat. Atherosclerosis 1972;15:87-92.

Ishaq GM, Zia-ul-Arifeen S, Ahmad BD, Moinuddin G, Ahmad A, Devi K. Hypotensive Potential of Aqueous Extract of *Emblica Officinalis* On Anaesthetized Dogs. JK-Practitioner 2005;12(4):213-215.

Israni DA, Patel KV, Gandhi TR. Anti-hyperlipidemic activity of aqueous extract of *Terminalia chebula* & gaumutra in high cholesterol diet fed rats. Pharma science monitor 2010;1(1):48-59.

Iswald I, Arráez-Román D, Rodriguez-Medina I, Beltrán-Debón R, Joven J, Segura-Carretero A, Fernández-Gutiérrez A. Identification of phenolic compounds in aqueous and ethanolic rooibos extracts (Aspalathus linearis) by HPLC-ESI-MS (TOF/IT). Anal Bioanal Chem. 2011 Jul;400(10):3643-54.

Itoh T, Furuichi Y. Lowering serum cholesterol level by feeding a 40% ethanol-eluted fraction from HP-20 resin treated with hot water extract of aduki beans *(Vigna angularis)* to rats fed a high-fat cholesterol diet. Nutrition 2009;25:318-321.

Iyer D, Sharma BK, Patil UK. Effect of ether- and water-soluble fractions of Carica papaya ethanol extract in experimentally induced hyperlipidemia in rats. Pharm Biol. 2011 Dec;49 (12):1306-10.

Jabeen Q, Bashir S, Lyoussi B, Gilani AH. Coriander fruit exhibits gut modulatory, blood pressure lowering and diuretic activities. J

Ethnopharmacol 2009 Feb 25;122(1):123-130.

Jacob A, Pandey M, Kapoor S, Saroja R. Effect of the Indian gooseberry (amla) on serum cholesterol levels in men aged 35-55 years. Eur J Clin Nutr. 1988 Nov;42(11):939-44.

Jadhav GB, Upasani CD. Antihypertensive effect of Silymarin on DOCA salt induced hypertension in unilateral nephrectomized rats. Orient Pharm Exp Med 2011;11:101-106.

Jahodar I, Opletal L, Lukes J, Zdansky P, Solichova D. A study on the anithyper-cholesterolemic and antihyperlipidaemic effects of cabbage extracts and their phytochemical evaluation. Pharmazie 1995;50(12):833-834.

Jain N, Srivastava RD, Singhal A. The effects of right and left nostril breathing on cardiorespiratory and autonomic parameters. Indian J Physiol Pharmacol 2005 Oct-Dec;49(4):469-74.

Jalali-Khanabadi BA, Mozaffari-Khosrav H, Parsaeyan N. Effects of almond dietary supplementation on coronary heart disease lipid risk factors and serum lipid oxidation parameters in men with mild hyperlipidemia. J Altern Complement Med. 2010 Dec;16(12):1279-83.

Jamaatul FH, Rokiah MY, Norhayati AH. Effect of red pitaya *(Hylocereus sp.)* supplementation on blood glucose level and lipid profile of induced hyperglycaemic rats. Malaysian Journal of Nutrition 2005;11(1):585.

Jayanthi S, Varalakshmi P. Tissue lipids in experimental calcium oxalate lithiasis and the effect of DL alpha-lipoic acid. Biocem Int 1992 Apr;26(5):913-21.

Jayasree T, Kishore KK, Vinay M, Vasavi P, Dixit R, Rajanikanth M, Manohar VS. Diuretic effect of chloroform extract of *Benincasa hispidarind* (Pericarp) in Sprague-Dawley rats. International Journal of Applied Biology and Pharmaceutical Technology 2011;Volume 2.Issue 2.:94-99.

Jeon BH, Kim CS, Kim HS, Park JB, Nam KY, Chang SJ. Effect of Korean red ginseng on blood pressure and nitric oxide production. Acta Pharmacol Sin 2000;21:1095-1100.

Jeon BH, Kim CS, Park KS, Lee JW, Park JB, Kim KJ, Kim SH, Chang SJ, Nam KY. Effect of Korean red ginseng on the blood pressure in conscious hypertensive rats. Gen Pharmacol 2000;35:135-141.

Jeong SC, Jeong YT, Yang BK, Islam R, Koyyalamudi SR, Pang G, Cho KY, Song CH. White button mushroom *(Agaricus bisporus)* lowers blood glucose and cholesterol levels in diabetic and hypercholesterolemic rats. Nutrition Research 2010;30:49-56.

Jeng K-C, Chen C-S, Fang Y-P, Hou RC-W, Chen Y-S. Effect of Microbial Fermentation on Content of Statin, GABA, and Polyphenols in Pu-Erh Tea. J. Agric. Food Chem. 2007;55:8787-8792.

Jenkins DJ, Kendall CW, Marchie A, Parker TL, Connelly PW, Qian W, Haight JS, Faulkner D, Vidgen E, Lapsley KG, Spiller GA. Dose response of almonds on coronary heart disease risk factors: blood lipids, oxidized low-density lipoproteins, lipoprotein(a), homocysteine and pulmonary nitric oxide: a randomized, controlled, crossover trial. Circulation 2002 Sep 10;106(11):1327-32.

Jenkins DJA, Popovich DG, Kendall CWC, Vidgen E, Tariq N, Ransom TPP, Wolever TMS, Vuksan V, Mehling CC, Boctor DL, Bolognesi C, Huang J, Patten R. Effect of a Diet High in Vegetables, Fruit and Nuts on Serum Lipids. Metabolism 1997 May;46(5):530-537.

Jensen EN, Buch-Andersen T, Ravn-Haren G, Dragsted LO. The effects of apples on plasma cholesterol levls and cardiovascular risk – a review of the evidence. Journal of Horticultural Science & Biotechnology 2009:34-41.

Jensen T, Retterstøl LJ, Sandset PM, Godal HC, Skjønsberg OH. A daily glass of red wine induces a prolonged reduction in plasma viscosity: a randomized controlled trial. Blood Coagul Fibrinolysis. 2006 Sep;17(6):471-6.

Jemai H, Bouaziz M, Fki I, El Feki A, Sayadi S. Hypolipidimic and antioxidant activities of oleuropein and its hydrolysis derivative-rich extracts from Chemlali olive leaves. Chem Biol Interact. 2008 Nov 25;176(2-3):88-98.

Jemai H, El Feki A, Sayadi S. Antidiabetic and antioxidant effects of hydroxytyrosol and oleuropein from olive leaves in alloxan-diabetic rats. J Agric Food Chem. 2009 Oct 14;57(19):8798-804.

Jezova D, Duncko R, Lassanova M, Kriska M, Moncek F. Reduction of rise in blood pressure and cortisol release during stress by ginkgo biloba extract (EGB 761) in healthy volunteers. Journal of Physiology and Pharmacology 2002;53(3):337-348.

Ji W, Gong BQ. Hypolipidemic effects and mechanisms of Panax notoginseng on lipid profile in hyperlipidemic rats. J Ethnopharmacol 2007 Sep 5;113(2):318-24.

Jiang HD, Cai J, Xu JH, Zhou XM, Xia Q. Endothelium-dependent and direct relaxation induced by ethyl acetate extract from Flos Chrysanthemi in rat thoracic aorta. Journal of Ethnopharmacology 2005;101221-226.

Jiménez R, López-Sepúlveda R, Kadmiri M, Romero M, Vera R, Sánchez M, Vargas F, O'Valle F, Zarzuelo A, Dueñas M, Santos-Buelga C, Duarte J. Polyphenols restore endothelial function in DOCA-salt hypertension: Role of endothelin-1 and NADPH oxidase. Free Radical Biology & Medicine 2007;43:462-473.

Jiménez-Ferrer E, Badillo FH, González-Cortazar M, Tortoriello J, Herrera-Ruiz M. Antihypertensive activity of *Salvia elegans* Vahl. (Lamiaceae): ACE inhibition and angiotensin II antagonism. Journal of Ethnopharmacology 2010;130:340-346.

Jin H, Zhang G, Cao X, Zhang M, Long J, Luo B. Treatment of hypertension by Linzhi combined with hypotensor and its effects on arterial, arteriolar and capillary pressure and microcirculation. Microcirculatory approach to Asian traditional medicine: Strategy for the scientific evaluation: selected proceedings from the 2nd Asian Congress for Microcirculation (ACM'95). Amsterdam; New York: Elsevier 1996:131-8.

Johnkennedy N, Adamma E, Austin A, Chukwunyere NE. Influence of Xylopia Aethiopica Fruits on Some Hematological and Biochemical Profile. Al Ameen J Med Sci 2011;4(2):191-196.

Joo IW, Ryu JH, Oh HJ. The influence of Sam-Chil-Geun (Panax notoginseng) on the serum lipid levels and inflammations of rats with hyperlipidemia induced by poloxamer-407. Yonsei Med J. 2010 Jul;51(4):504-10.

Jovanovski E, Jenkins A, Dias AG, Peeva V, Sievenpiper J, Arnason JT, Rahelic D, Josse RG, Vuksan V. Effects of Korean Red Ginseng (Panax ginsneg C.A. Mayer) and Its Isolated Ginsenosides and Polysaccharides on Arterial Stiffness in Healthy Individuals. American Journal of Hypertension 2010 May;23:469-472.

Juárez-Oropeza MA, Mascher D, Torres-Durán PV, Farias JM, Paredes-Carbajal MC. Effects of dietary Spirulina on vascular reactivity. J Med Food 2009 Feb;12(1):15-20.

Juhasz B, Das DK, Kertesz A, Juhasz A, Gesztelyi R, Varga B. Reduction of blood cholesterol and ischemic injury in the hypercholesteromic rabbits with modified resveratrol, longevinex. Mol Cell Biochem 2011 Feb;348(1-2):199-203.

Jung EH, Kim SR, Hwang IK, Ha TY. Hypoglycemic effects of phenolic acid fraction of rice bran and ferulic acid in C57BL/KsJ-db/db mice. J Agric Food Chem 2007 Nov 28;55(24):9800-4.

Jung F, Mrowietz C, Kiesewetter H, Wenzel E. Effect of Ginkgo biloba on fluidity of blood and peripheral microcirculation in volunteers. Arzneimittelforschung 1990 May;40(5):589-93.

Jung KA, Song TC, Han D, Kim IH, Kim YE, Lee CH. Cardiovascular Protective Properties of Kiwifruit Extract *in Vitro*. Biol. Pharm. Bull. 2005;28(9):1782-1785.

Jurgoński A, Juśkiewicz J, Zduńczyk Z. Ingestion of black chokeberry fruit extract leads to intestinal and systemic changes in a rat model of prediabetes and hyperlipidemia. Plant Foods Hum Nutr 2008 Dec;63(4):176-82.

Jönssön T, Ahrén B, Pacini G, Sundler F, Wierup N, Steen S, Sjöberg T, Ugander M, Frostegård J, Göransson L, Lindeberg S. A Paleolithic diet confers higher insulin sensitivity, lower C-reactive protein and lower blood pressure than a cereal-based diet in domestic pigs. Nutr Metab (Lond) 2006 Nov 2;3:39.

Jönssön T, Granfeldt Y, Ahrén B, Branell UC, Pålsson G, Hansson A, Söderström M. Beneficial effects of a Paleolithic diet on cardiovascular risk factors in type diabetes: a randomized cross-over pilot study. Cardiovasc Diabetol. 2009 Jul 16;8:35.

Kabir Y, Yamaguchi M, Kimura S. Effect of Shiitake (*Lentinus edodes*) and Maitake (*Grifola frondosa*) Mushrooms on Blood Pressure and Plasma Lipids of Spontaneously Hypertensive Rats. J Nutr Sci Vitaminol (Tokyo) 1987 Oct;33(5):341-6.

Kabir Y, Kimura S, Tamura T. Dietary Effects of *Ganoderma lucidum* Mushroom on Blood Pressure and Lipid Levels in Spontaneously Hypertensive Rats (SHR). Journal of Nutritional Science and Vitaminology 1988;34(4):433-438.

Kabir Y, Kimura S. Dietary mushrooms reduce blood pressure in spontaneously hypertensive rats (SHR). J Nutr Sci Vitaminol (Tokyo) 1989 Feb;35(1):91-4.

Kabiri N, Asgary S, Madani H, Mahzouni P. Effects of *Amaranthus caudatus* l. extrat and lovastatin on atherosclerosis in hypercholesterolemic rabbits. Journal of Medicinal Plants Research 2010 Mar;4(5):355-361.

Kabiri N, Asgary S, Setorki M. Lipid lowering by hydroalcoholic extracts of *Amaranthus Caudatus* L. induces regression of rabbits atherosclerotic lesions. Lipids in Health and Disease 2011;10(89)

Kalsait RP, Khedekar PB, Saoji AN, Bhusari KP. Isolation of phytosterols and antihyperlipidemic activity of Lagenaria siceraria. Arch Pharm Res. 2011 Oct;34(10):1599-604.

Kalus U, Pindur G, Jung F, Mayer B, Radtke H, Bachmann K, Mrowietz C, Koscielny J. Influence of the onion as an essential ingredient of the Mediterranean diet on arterial blood pressure and blood fluidity. Arzneimittelforschung 2000 Sep;50(9):795-801.

Kaneda T, Tokuda S. Effect of Various Mushroom Preparations on Cholesterol Levels in Rats. The Journal of Nutrition 1966;90:371-376.

Kanmatsuse K, Kajiwara N, Hayashi K, Shimogaichi S, Fukinbara I, Ishikawa H, Tamura T. Studies on Ganoderma lucidum. I. Efficacy against hypertension and side effects. Yakugaku Zasshi 1985 Oct;105(10):942-7.

Kar P, Laight D, Rooprai HK, Shaw KM, Cummings M. Effects of grape seed extract in Type 2 diabetic subjects at high cardiovascular risk: a double blnd randomized placebo controlled trial examining metabolic markers, vascular tone, inflammation, oxidative stress and insulin sensitivity. Diabet Med. 2009 May;26(5):526-31.

Kareem MA, Krushna GS, Hussain SA, Devi KL. Effect of Aqueous Extract of Nutmeg on Hyperglycaemia, Hyperlipidaemia and Cardiac Histology Associated with Isoproterenol-induced Myocardial Infarction in Rats. Tropical Journal of Pharmaceutical Research 2009 Aug;8(4):337-344.

Karlsen A, Svendsen M, Seljeflot I, Laake P, Duttaroy AK, Drevon CA, Arnesen H, Tonstad S, Blomhoff R. Kiwifruit decreases blood pressure and whole-blood platelet aggregation in male smokers. J Hum Hypertens 2012 Jan 19.

Kas'ianenko VI, Komisarenko IA, Dubtsova EA. Correction of atherogenic dyslipidemia with honey, pollen and bee bread in patients with different body mass. Ter Arkh 2011;83(8):58-62.

Kaškoniene V, Maruška A, Kornyšova O. Quantitative and qualitative determination of phenolic compounds in honey. Chemine Technologija 2009;3:52-74.

Kassaian N, Azadbakht L, Forghani B, Amini M. Effect of fenugreek seeds on blood glucose and lipid profiles in type 2 diabetic patients. Int J Vitam Nutr Res. 2009 Jan;79(1):34-9.

Kawasaki T, Uezono K, Nakazawa Y. Antihypertensive mechanism of food for specified health use: "Eucommia leaf glycoside" and its clinical application. Journal of Health Science 2000;22:29-36.

Kawase M, Hashimoto H, Hosoda M, Morita H, Hosono A. Effect of administration of fermented milk containing whey protein concentrate to rats and healthy men on serum lipids and blood pressure. J Dairy Sci. 2000 Feb;83(2):255-63.

Kechagias S, Zanjani S, Gjellan S, Leinhard OD, Kihlberg J, Smedby O, Johansson L. Effects of moderate red wine consumption on liver fat and blood lipids: a prospective randomized study. Ann Med. 2011 Nov;43(7):545-54.

Keenan JM, Pins JJ, Frazel C, Moran A, Turnquist L. Oat Ingestion Reduces Systolic and Diastolic Blood Pressure in Patients with Mild or Borderline Hypertension: A Pilot Trial. J Fam. Pract. 2002;51:369.

Keiichi H, Toshio N, Mitsuhiro T, Hiroyasu E, Hiroshi O, Hiromichi S, Takao S, Ryuichi K. Effect of systemic L-arginine administration on hemodynamics and nitric oxide release in man. Jpn. Heart J. 1992;33(1):41-8.

Kelley GA, Kelley KS. Aerobic exercice and lipids and lipoproteins in men: a meta-analysis of randomized controlled trials. J Mens Health Gend. 2006;3(1):61-70.

Kermanshahi H, Riasi A. Effect of Dietary Dried Berberis Vulgaris Fruit and Enzyme on Some Blood Parameters of Laying Hens Fed Wheat-Soybean Based Diets. International Journal of Poultry Science 2006;5(1):89-92.

Kesari AN, Kesari S, Singh SK, Gupta RK, Watal G. Studies on the glycemic and lipidemic effect on Murraya koenigii in experimental animals. J Ethnopharmacol 2007 Jun 13;112 (2):305-11.

Kesteloot H, Joossens JV. Relationship of serum sodium, potassium, calcium, and phosphorus with blood pressure. Hypertension 1988;12:589-593.

Khadem-Ansari MH, Rasmi Y, Ramezani F. Effects of Red Grape Juice Consumption on High Density Lipoprotein-Cholesterol, Apolipoprotein AI, Apolipoprotein B and Homocysteine in Healthy Human Volunteers. The Open Biochemistry Journal 2010;4: 96-99.

Khalil R. The Effect of *Crataegus Aronica* Aqueous Extract in Rabbits Fed with High Cholesterol Diet. European Journal of

Scientific Research 2008;22(3):352-360.

Khan A, Safdar M, Khan MMA, Khattak KN, Anderson RA. Cinnamon Improves Glucose and Lipids of People With Type 2 Diabetes. Diabetes Care 2003 Dec;26(12):3215-3218.

Khan AU, Gilani AH. Selective bronchodilatory effect of Rooibos tea (Aspalathus linearis) and its flavonoid, chrysoeriol. Eur J Nutr. 2006 Dec;45(8):463-9.

Khan AU, Gilani AH. Pharmacodynamic Evaluation of *Terminalia bellerica* for Its Antihypertensive Effect. Journal of Food and Drug Analysis 2008;16(3):6-14.

Khan AU, Khan M, Subhan F, Gilani AH. Antispasmodic, bronchodilator and blood pressure lowering properties of *Hypericum oblongifolium* – possible mechanism of action. Phytotherapy Researh 2010 Jul;24(7):1027-1032.

Khan N, Monagas M, Andres-Lacueva C, Casas R, Urpi-Sardà M, Lamuela-Raventós RM, Estruch R. Regular consumption of cocoa powder with milk increases HDL cholesterol and reduces oxidized LDL levels in subjects at high-risk of cardiovascular disease. Nutr Metab Cardiovasc Dis 2011 May 5.

Khan NQ, Lees DM, Douthwaite JA, Carrier MJ, Corder R. Comparison of red wine extract and polyphenol constituents on endothelin-1 synthesis by cultured endothelial cells. Clin Sci (Lond) 2002 Aug;103(48):72-75.

Khan Y, Khan RA, Afroz S, Siddiq A. Evaluation of Hypolipidemic effect of citrus lemon. Journal of Basic and Applied Sciences 2010;6(1):39-43.

Khanam AA, Sachdeva U, Guleria R, Deepak KK. Study of pulmonary and autonomic functions of asthma patients after yoga training. Indian J Physiol Pharmacol 1996 Oct;40(4):318-24.

Khanna N, Arora D, Halder S, Mehta AK, Garg GR, Sharma SB, Mahajan P. Comparative effect of *Ocimum sanctum, Commiphora mukul,* folic acid and ramipril on lipid peroxidation in experimentally-induced hyperlipidemia. Indian J Exp Biol. 2010 Mar;48(3):299-305.

Khattab MM, Nagi MN. Thymoquinone supplementation attenuates hypertension and renal damage in nitric oxide deficient hypertensive rats. Phytother Res. 2007 May;21(5):410-4.

Khatun K, Mahtab H, Khanam PA, Sayeed MA, Khan KA. Oyster mushroom reduced blood glucose and cholesterol in diabetic subjects. Mymensingh Med J 2007 Jan;16(1):94-9.

Khayyal MT, el-Ghazaly MA, Abdallah DM, Nassar NN, Okpanyi SN, Kreuter MH. Blood pressure lowering effect of an olive leaft extract (Olea europaea) in L-NAME induced hypertension in rats. Arzneimittelforschung 2002;52(11):797-802.

Kianbakht S, Abasi B, Perham M, Hashem Dabaghian F. Antihyperlipidemic effects of Salvia officinalis L. leaf extract in patients with hyperlipidemia: a randomized double-blind placeb-controlled clinical trial. Phytother Res. 2011 Dec;25(12):1849-53.

Kieling G, Schneider J, Jahreis G. Long-term consumption of fermented dairy products over 6 months increases HDL cholesterol. Eur. J. Clin. Nutr. 2002;56:843-849.

Kiesewetter H, Jung F, Pindur G, Jung EM, Mrowietz C, Wenzel E. Effect of garlic on thrombocyte aggregation, microcirculation, and other risk factors. Int J Clin Pharmacol Ther Toxicol 1991 Apr;29(4):151-5.

Kiesewetter H, Jung F, Mrowietz C, Wenzel E. Hemorrheological and circulatory effects of Gincosan. Int J Clin Pharmacol Ther Toxicol. 1992 Mar;30(3):97-102.

Kim DI, Lee SH, Choi JH, Lillehoj HS, Yu MH, Lee GS. The butanol fraction of *Eclipta prostrata* (Linn) effectively reduces serum lipid levels and improves antioxidant activities in CD rats. Nutrition Research 2008;28:550-554.

Kim DW, Yokozawa TY, Hattori M, Kadota S, Namba T. Effects of Aqueous Extracts of *Apocynum venetum* Leaves on Hypercholesterolaemic Rats. Phytotherapy Research 1998;12:46-48.

Kim DW, Yokozawa t, Hattori M, Kadota S, Namba T. Effects of aqueous extracts of *Apocynum venetum* leaves on spontaneously hypertensive, renal hypertensive and NaCl-fed-hypertensive rats. Journal of Ethnopharmacology 2000;72:53-59.

Kim DW, Hwang IK, Lim SS, Yoo K-Y, Li H, Kim YS, Kwon DY, Moon WK, Kim D-W, Won M-H. Germinated Buckwheat extract decreases blood pressure and nitrotyrosine immunoreactivity in aortic endothelial cells in spontaneously hypertensive rats. Phytotherapy Research 2009 Jul;23(7):993-998.

Kim EY, Baek IH, Rhyu MR. Cardioprotective effects of aqueous Schizandra chinensis fruit exttract on ovariectomized and balloon-induced carotid artery injury rat models: effects on serum lipid profiles and blood pressure. J Ethnopharmacol 2011 Apr 12;134(3):668-75.

Kim HB, Kim SY, Ryu KS, Lee WC, Moon JY. Effect of Methanol Extract from Mulberry Fruit on the Lipid Metabolism and Liver Function in Cholesterol-Induced Hyperlipidemia Rats. Korean J. Seric. Sci. 2001;43(2):104-108.

Kim HJ, Yokozawa T, Kim HY, Tohda C, Rao TP, Juneja LR. Influence of amla (Emblia officinalis Gaertn.) on hypercholesterolemia and lipid peroxidation in cholesterol-fed rats. J Nutr Sci Vitaminol (Tokyo) 2005 Dec;51(6):413-8.

Kim HK, Kim MJ, Shin DH. Improvement of lipid profile by amaranth (Amaranthus esculantus) supplementation in streptozotocin-induced diabetic rats. Ann Nutr Metab. 2006;50(3):277-81.

Kim HS. Effects of the *Korean Mistletoe* Hot-Water Extract on the Lipid Components and Blood Pressure Level in Spontaneously Hypertensive Rats. Kor. J. Pharmacogn. 2006;37(3):169-176.

Kim HY, Okubo T, Juneja LR, Yokozawa T. The protective role of amla (Emblica officinalis Gaertn.) against fructose-induced metabolic syndrome in a rat model. Br J Nutr. 2010 Feb;103(4):502-12.

Kim JH, Lee DH, Lee SH, Choi SY, Lee JS. Effect of *Ganoderma lucidum* on the Quality and Functionality of Korean Traditional Rice Wine, Yakju. Journal of Bioscience and Bioengineering 2004;97(1):24-28.

Kim JY, Do MH, Lee SS. The effects of a mixture of brown and black rice on lipid profiles and antioxidant status in rats. Ann Nutr Metab 2006;50(4):347-53.

Kim JY, Moon KD, Seo KI, Park KW, Choi MS, Do GM, Jeong YK, Cho YS, Lee MK. Supplementation of SK1 from Platycodi radix ameliorates obesity and glucose intolerance in mice fed a high-fat diet. J Med Food 2009 Jun;12(3):629-36.

Kim KS, Ezaki O, Ikemoto S, Itakura H. Effects of Platycodon grandiflorum feeding on serum and liver lipid concentrations in rats with diet-induced hyperlipidemia. J Nutr Sci Vitaminol (Tokyo) 1995 Aug;41(4):485-91.

Kim KS, Seo EK, Lee YC, Lee TK, Cho YW, Ezaki O, Kim CH. Effect of dietary Platycodon grandiflorum on the improvement of insulin resistance in obese Zucker rats. J Nutr Biochem. 2000 Sep;11(9):420-4.

Kim MJ, Lee HJ, Wiryowidagdo S, Kim HK. Antihypertensive Effects of *Gynura procumbens* Extract in Spontaneously Hypertensive Rats. Journal of Medicinal Food 2006;9(4):587-590.

Kim ND, Kang SY, Schini VB. Ginsenosides evoke endothelium-dependent vascular relaxation in rat aorta. Gen Pharmacol 1994;25:1071-1077.

Kim SH, Park KS. Effects of Panax ginseng extract on lipid metabolism in humans. Pharmacological Research 2003;48:511-513.

Kim SL, Kim S-K, Park C-H. Introduction and nutritional evaluation of buckwheat sprouts as a new vegetable. Food Research International 2004;37:319-327.

Kim SY, Yoon S, Kwon SM, Park KS, Lee-Kim YC. Kale juice improves coronary artery disease risk factors in hypercholesterolemic men. Biomed Environ Sci. 2008 Apr;21(2):91-7.

Klag MJ, Wang NY, Meoni LA, Brancati FL, Cooper LA, Liang KY, Young JH, Ford DE. Coffee intake and risk of hypertension: the Johns Hopkins precursors study. Arch Intern Med. 2002 Mar 25;162(6):657-62.

Klein GA, Stefanuto A, Boaventura BC, de Morais EC, Cavalcante Lda S, de Andrade F, Wazlawik E, Di Pietro PF, Maraschin M, da Silva EL. Mate tea (Ilex paraguariensis) improves glycemic and lipid profles of type 2 diabetes ad pre-diabetes individuals: a pilot study. J Am Coll Nutr. 2011 Oct;30(5):320-32.

Kobayashi Y, Hiroi T, Araki M, Hirokawa T, Miyazawa M, Aoki N, Kojima T, Ohsawa T. Facilitative effects of *Eucommia ulmoides* on fatty acid oxidation in hypertriglyceridaemic rats. Journal of the Science of Food and Agriculture 2012 Jan;92(2):358-365.

Kochhar A, Sharma N, Sachdeva R. Effect of Supplementation of Tulsi *(Ocimum sanctum)* and Neem *(Azadirachta indica)* Leaf Powder on Diabetic Symptoms, Anthropometric Parameters and Blood Pressure of Non Insulin Dependent Male Diabetics. Ethno-Med 2009;3(1):5-9.

Kocyigit Y, Atamer Y, Uysal E. The effect of dietary supplementation of Nigella sativa L. on serum lipid profile in rats. Saudi Med. J. 2009 Jul;30(7):893-6.

Kodama S, Tanaka S, Saito K, Shu M, Sone Y, Onitake F, Suzuki E, Shimano H, Yamamoto S, Kondo K, Ohashi Y, Yamada N, Sone H. Effect of aerobic exercise training on serum levels of high-density lipoprotein cholesterol: a meta-analysis. Arch Intern Med. 2007 May 28;167(10):999-1008.

Koeners MP, van Faassen EE, Wesseling S, de Sain-van der Velden M, Koomans HA, Braam B, Joles JA. Maternal supplementation with citrulline increases renal nitric oxide in young spontaneously hypertensive rats and has long-term antihypertensive effects. Hypertension 2007 Dec;50(6):1077-84.

Kojima M, Nishi S, Yamashita S, Saito Y, Maeda R. Smaller Increase in Serum Cholesterol Level in Rats Fed an Ethanol Extract of Adzuki Bean Seeds. Nippon Shokuhin Kagaku Kogaku Kaishi 2006;53(7):380-385.

Kojuri J, Vosoughi AR, Akrami M. Effects of anethum graveolens and garlic on lipid profile in hyperlipidemic patients. Lipids in Health and Disease 2007;6:1-5.

Kolankaya D, Selmanoğlu G, Sorkun K, Salih B. Protective effects of Turkish propolis on alcohol-induced serum lipid changes and liver injury in male rats. Food Chemistry 2002;78:213-217.

Koltringer P, Langsteger W, Klima G, Reisecker F, Eber O. Hemorheologic effects of ginkgo biloba extract EGb 761. Dose-dependent effect of Egb 761 on microcirculation and viscoelasticity of blood. Fortschr Med 1993 Apr 10;111(10):170-2.

Komatsu W, Miura Y, Yagasaki K. Suppression of hypercholesterolemia in hepatoma-bearing rats by cabbage extract and its components, S-methyl-L-cysteine sulfoxide. Lipids 1998 May;33(5):499-503.

Kondo S, Tayama K, Tsukamoto Y, Ikeda K, Yamori Y. Antihypertensive Effects of Acetic Acid and Vinegar on Spontaneously Hypertensive Rats. Biosci. Biotechnol. Biochem. 2001;65(12):2690-2694.

Korou LM, Agrogiannis G, Pantopoulou A, Vlachos IS, Illiopoulos D, Karatzas T, Perrea DN. Comparative antilipidemic effect of N-acetylcysteine and sesame oil administration in diet-induced hypercholesterolemic mice. Lipids Health Dis. 2010 Mar 6;9:23.

Kothari S, Jain AK, Mehta SC, Tonpay SD. Effect of fresh *Triticum aestivum* grass juice on lipid profile of normal rats. Indian J Pharmacol. 2008 Oct;40(5):235-236.

Kothari S, Jain AK, Mehta SC, Tonpay SD. Hypolipidemic effect of fresh *Triticum aestivum* (Wheat) grass juice in hypercholesterolemic rats. Acta Poloniae Pharmaceutica Mar - Apr;68(2):291-294.

Kouno K, Hirano SI, Kuboki H, Kasai M, Hatae K. Effects of Dried Bonito *(Katsuobushi)* and Captopril, an Angiotensin I-Converting Enzyme Inhibitor, on Rat Isolated Aorta: A Possible Mechanism of Antihypertensive Action. Biosci. Biotechnol. Biochem. 2005;69(5):911-915.

Kow MC, Rokiah MY, Mohd AKR. Effect of red pitaya fruit *(Hylocereussp)* supplementation on lipid profiles of induced hypercholesterolemic rats. Malaysian Journal of Nutrition 2005;11(1):56.

Koya-Miyata S, Arai N, Mizote A, Taniguchi Y, Ushio S, Iwaki K, Fukuda S. Propolis Prevets Diet-Induced Hyperlipidemia and Mitigates Weight Gain in Diet-Induced Obesity in Mice. Biol. Pharm. Bull. 2009;32(12):2022-2028.

Kozakai T, Yamanaka A, Ichiba T, Toyokawa T, Kamada Y, Tamamura T, Ichimura T, Maruyama S. Luteolin Inhibits Endothelin-1 Secretion in Cultured Endothelial Cells. Biosci. Biotechnol. Biochem. 2005;69(8):1613-1615.

Koziróg M, Poliwczak AR, Duchnowicz P, Koter-Michalak M, Sikora J, Broncel M. Melatonin treatment improves blood pressure, lipid profile, and parameters of oxidative stress in patients with metabolic syndrome. J Pineal Res. 2011 Apr;50(3):261-6.

Kozuma K, Tsuchiya S, Kohori J, Hase T, Tokimitsu I. Antihypertensive effect of green coffee bean extract on mildly hypertensive subjects. Hypertens Res. 2005 Sep;28(9):711-8.

Kreydiyyeh SI, Usta J. Diuretic effect and mechanism of action of parsley. Journal of Ethnopharmacology 2002;79:353-357.

Krotkiewski M, Aurell M, Holm G, Grimby G, Szczepanik J. Effects of a sodium-potassium ion-exchanging seaweed preparation in mild hypertension. Am J Hypertens. 1991 Jun;4(6):483-8.

Kuba M, Tanaka K,Sesoko M, Inoue F, Yasuda M. Angiotensin I-converting enzyme inhibitory peptides in red-mold rice made by *Monascus purpureus*. Process Biochemistry 2009;44:1139-1143.

Kubo K, Nanba H. The effect of maitake mushrooms on liver and serum lipids. *Altern Ther Health Med* 1996 Sep;2(5):62-6.

Kubo K, Nanba H. Anti-hyperliposis effect of maitake fruit body (Grifola frondosa). *Biol Pharm Bull* 1997 Jul;20(7):781-5.

Kubota Y, Umegaki K, Kobayashi K, Tanaka N, Kagota S, Nakamura K, Kunitomo M, Shinozuka K. Anti-hypertensive effects of Brazilian Propolis in spontaneously hypertensive rats. Clinical and Experimental Pharmacology and Physiology 2004

Dec;31(2):29-30.

Kubota Y, Tanaka N, Kagota S, Nakamura K, Kunitomo M, Umegaki K, Shinozuka K. Effects of Ginkgo biloba extract feeding on salt-induced hypertensive Dahl rats. Biol. Pharm. Bull. 2006 Feb;29(2):266-9.

Kubota Y, Tanaka N, Kagota S, Kunitomo M, Shinozuka K, Umegaki K. Effects of *Ginkgo biloba* extract on blood pressure and vascular endothelial response by acetylcholine in spontaneously hypertensive rats. Journal of Pharmacy and Pharmacology 2006 Feb;58(2):243-249.

Kudolo GB. The effect of 3-month ingestion of Ginkgo biloba extract on pancreatic beta-cell function in response to glucose loading in normal glucose tolerant individuals. J Clin Pharmacol 2000 Jun;40(6):647-54.

Kumari CS, Govindasamy S, Sukumar E. Lipid lowering activity of *Eclipta prostrata* in experimental hyperlipidemia. Journal of Ethnopharmacology 2006;105:332-335.

Kuo KL, Weng MS, Chiang CT, Tsai YJ, Lin-Shiau SY, Lin JK. Comparative studies on the hypolipidemic and growth suppressive effects if oolong, black, pu-erh, and green tea leaves in rats. J Agric Food Chem. 2005 Jan 26;53(2):480-9.

Kuriyan R, Gopinath N, Vaz M, Kurpad AV. Use of rice bran oil in patients with hyperlipidaemia. Natl Med J India 2005;18(6): 292-6.

Kurowska EM, Spence JD, Jordan J, Wetmore S, Freeman DJ, Piché LA, Serratore P. HDL-cholesterol-raising effect of orange juice in subjects with hypercholesterolemia. Am J Clin Nutr. 2000 Nov;72(5):1095-100.

Kurowska EM, Manthey JA. Hypolipidemic effects and absorption of citrus polymethoxylated flavones in hamsters with diet-induced hypercholesterolemia. J Agric Food Chem 2004 May 19;52(10):2879-86.

Kwak CJ, Kubo E, Fujii K, Nishimura Y, Kobuchi S, Ohkita M, Yoshimura M, Kiso Y, Matsumura Y. Antihypertensive effect of French maritime pine bark extract (Flavangenol): possible involvement of endothelial nitric oxide-dependent vasorelaxation. J Hypertens 2009 Jan;27(1):92-101.

Kwok CY, Wong CNY, Yau MYC, Yu PHF, Au ALS, Poon CCW, Seto SW, Lam TY, Kwan YW, Chan SW. Consumption of dried fruit of *Crataegus pinnatifida* (hawthorn) suppresses high-cholesterol diet-induced hypercholesterolemia in rats. Journal of functional foods 2010;2:179-186.

Kwon SH, Ahn IS, Kim SO, Kong CS, Chung HY, Do MS, Park KY. Anti-obesity and hypolipidemic effects of black soyben anthocyanins. J Med Food 2007 Sep;10(3):552-6.

Kwon Y-I, Vattem DA, Shetty K. Evaluation of clonal herbs of Lamiaceae species for management of diabetes and hypertension. Asia Pac J Clin Nutr 2006;15(1):107-118.

Kwon Y-I, Apostolidis E, Shetty K. In vitro studies of eggplant *(Solanum melongena)* phenolics as inhibitors of key enzymes relevant for type 2 diabetes and hypertension. Bioresource Technology 2008;99;2981-2988.

Lachman J, Hamouz K. Red and purple coloured potatoes as a significant antioxidant source in human nutrition – a review. Plant soil environ. 2005;51(11):477-482.

Lahera V, Khraibi AA, Romero JC. Sulfhydryl group donors potentiate the hypotensive effect of acetylcholine in rats. Hypertension 1993 Aug;22(2):156-60.

Lahlou S, Interaminense Lde F, Leal-Cardoso JH, Morais SM, Duarte GP. Cardiovascular effects of the essential oil of Ocimum gratissimum leaves in rats: role of the autonomic nervous system. Clin Exp Pharmacol Physiol 2004 Apr;31(4):219-25.

Lahlou S, Tahraoui A, Israili Z, Lyoussi B. Diuretic activity of the aqueous extracts of *Carum carvi* and *Tanacetum vulgare* in normal rats. Journal of Ethnopharmacology 2007;110:458-463.

Lal AA, Kumar T, Murthy PB, Pillai KS. Hypolipidemic effect of Coriandrum sativum L. in triton-induced hyperlipidemic rats. Indian J Exp Biol 2004 Sep;42(9):909-12.

Lam SK, Abu Bakar ZA, Chua KS, Ismail R. Acute hypotensive effect of *Gynura procumbens* in the rat: A comparison with synthetic hypotensive agents. *Asia Pacific J Pharmacol*:14(1):19.

Lam SK, Idris A, Abu Bakar ZA, Ismail R. *Gynura procumbens* and blood pressure in the rat: Preliminary study. *Asia Pacific J Pharmacol*:13(1):14.

Lang C, Liu Z, Taylor HW, Baker DG. Effect of Eucommia ulmoides on systolic blood pressure in the spontaneous hypertensive rat. Am J Chin Med. 2005;33(2):215-30.

Langsjoen P, Langsjoen P, Willis R, Folkers K. Treatment of essential hypertension with coenzyme Q10. Mol Aspects Med 1994;15:265-72.

Lans CA. Ethnomedicines used in Trinidad and Tobago for urinary problems and diabetes mellitus. Journal of Ethnobiology and Ethnomedicine 2006;2(45):1-11.

Lansley KE, Winyard PG, Fulford J, Vanhatalo A, Bailey SJ, Blackwell JR, DiMenna FJ, Gilchrist M, Benjamin N, Jones AM. Dietary nitrate supplementation reduces the O2 cost of walking and running: placebo-controlled study. J Appl Physiol 2011 Mar;110(3):591-600.

Lara JJ, Economou M, Wallace AM, Rumley A, Lowe G, Slater C, Caslake M, Sattar N, Lean MEJ. Benefits of salmon eating on traditional and novel vascular risk factors in young, non-obese healthy subjects. Atherosclerosis 2007;193:213-221.

Lata S, Saxena KK, Bhasin V, Saxena RS, Kumar A, Srivastava VK. Beneficial effects of Allium sativum, Allium cepa and Commiphora mukul on experimental hyperlipidemia and atherosclerosis – a comparative evaluation. J Postgrad Med. 1991 Jul;37(3):132-5.

Latha RCR, Daisy P. Influence of *Terminalia bellerica* Roxb. Fruit Extracts on Biochemical Parameters in Streptozotocin Diabetic Rats. International Journal of Pharmacology 2010;6(2):89-96.

Lavy A, Fuhrman B, Markel A, Danker G, Ben-Amotz A, Presser D, Aviram M. Effect of dietary supplementation of red or white wine on human blood chemistry, hematology and coagulation: favorable effect of red wine on plasma high-density lipoprotein. Ann Nutr. Metab. 1994;38(5):287-94.s

Lee EH, Park JE, Choi YJ, Huh KB, Kim WY. A randomized study to establish the effects of spirulina in type 2 diabetes mellitus patients. Nutr Res Pract. 2008;2(4):295-300.

Lee IA, Lee JH, Baek NI, Kim DH. Antihyperlipidemic Effect of Crocin Isolated from the Fructus of *Gardenia jasminoides* and Its Metabolite Crocetin. Biol. Pharm. Bull. 2005;28(11);2106-2110.

Lee JR, Shin JH, Byun SH, Park SJ, Jo MJ, Park SM, Ku SK, Kim SC. Anti-obese and Hypolipemic Effects of the Aqueous Extracts of Raphani Semen in Mice Fed High Fat Diet. J. Korean Soc. Appl. Biol. Chem 2009;52(1):50-57.

Lee HS, Park HJ, Kim MK. Effect of Chlorella vulgaris on lipid metabolism in Wistar rats fed high fat diet. Nutr Res Pract. 2008;2(4):204-10.

Lee KH, Park E, Lee HJ, Kim MO, Cha YJ, Kim JM, Lee H, Shin MJ. Effects of daily quercetin-rich supplementation on cardiometabolic risks in male smokers. Nutr Res Pract. 2011 Fe;5(1):28-33.

Lee NA, Reasner CA. Beneficial effect of chromium supplementation on serum triglyceride levels in NIDDM. Diabetes Care 1994 Dec;17(12):1449-52.

Lee SH, Chung IM, Cha YS, Park Y. Millet consumption decreased serum concentration of triglyceride and C-reactive protein but not oxidative status in hyperlipidemic rats. Nutrition Research 2010;30:290-296.

Lee SJ, Kim CW, Jang HJ, Cho SY, Choi JW. Anti-hyperlipidemia and Anti-arteriosclerosis Effects of *Laminaria japonica* in Sprague-Dawley Rats. Fish Aquat Sci 2011;14(4):235-241.

Lee SY, Rhee HM. Cardiovascular effects of mycelium extract of Ganoderma lucidum: inhibition of sympathetic outflow as a mechanism of its hypotensive action. Chem Pharm Bull (Tokyo) 1990 May;38(5):1359-64.

Lee YA, Cho EJ, Yokozawa T. Effects of proanthocyanidin preparations on hyperlipidemia and other biomarkers in mouse model of type 2 diabetes. J Agric Food Chem. 2008 Sep 10;56(17):7781-9.

Lei XL, Chiou GC. Cardiovascular pharmacology of Panax notoginseng (Burk) F.H. Chen and Salvia miltiorrhiza. Am J Chin Med. 1986;14(3-4):145-52.

Leikert JF, Räthel TR, Wohlfart P, Cheynier V, Vollmar AM, Dirsch VM. Red wine polyphenols enhance endothelial nitric oxide synthase expression and subsequent nitric oxide release from endothelial cells. Circulation 2002 Sep 24;106(13):1614-7.

Lemhadri A, Hajji L, Michel J-B, Eddouks M. Cholesterol and triglycerides lowering activities of caraway fruits in normal and streptozotocin diabetic rats. Journal of Ethnopharmacology 2006 Jul 19;106:321-326.

Leng GC, Lee AJ, Frowkes FGR, Jepson RG, Lowe GDO, Skinner ER, Mowat BF. Randomized controlled trial of gamma-linolenic acid and eicosapentaenoic acid in peripheral arterial disease. Clinical Nutrition 1998;17(6):265-271.

Lerman-Garber I, Ichazo-Cerro S, Zamora-González J, Cardoso-Saldaña G, Posadas-Romero C. Effect of a high-monounsaturated fat diet enriched with avocado in NIDDM patients. Diabetes Care. 1994 Apr;17(4):311-5.

Leuchtengs H. Crataegus Special Extract WS 1442 in NYHA II heart failure. A placebo controlled randomized double-blind study. Fortschr. Med 1993;111:352-354.

Li C, Gao Y, Li M, Shi W, Liu Z. Effect of Laminaria japonica polysaccharides on lowing serum lipid and anti-atherosclerosis in hyperlipemia quails. Zhong Yao Cai 2005 Aug;28(8):676-9.

Li CH, Matsui T, Matsumoto K, Yamasaki R, Kawasaki T. Latent production of angiotensin I-converting enzyme inhibitors from buckwheat protein. Journal of Peptide Science 2002 Jun;Volume 8, Issue 6:267-274.

Li F, Zhang Y, Zhong Z. Antihyperglycemic effect of ganoderma lucidum polysaccharides on streptozotocin-induced diabetic mice. Int J Mol Sci 2011;12(9):6135-45.

Li H, Xia N, Brausch I, Yao Y Förstermann U. Flavonoids from Artichoke *(Cynara scolymus L.)* Up-Regulate Endothelal-Type Nitric-Oxide Synthase Gene Expression in Human Endothelial Cells. The Journal of Pharmacology and Experimental Therapeutics 2004;310(3):926-932.

Li P, Anyannusi O, Reid C, Longhurst JC. Inhibitory effect of electroacupuncture (EA) on the pressor response induced by exercise stress. Clin Auton Res. 2004 Jun;14(3):182-8.

Li P, Longhurst JC. Neural mechanism of electroacupuncture's hypotensive effects. Autonomic Neuroscience: Basic and Clinical 2010;157:24-30.

Li RW, Theriault AG, Au K, Douglas TD, Casaschi A, Kurowska EM, Mukherjee R. Citrus polymethoxylated flavones improve lipid and glucose homeostasis and modulate adipocytokines in fructose-induced insulin resistant hamsters. Life Sci. 2006 Jun 20;79(4):365-73.

Li SC, Liu YH, Liu JF, Chang WH, Chen CM, Chen CY. Almond consumption improved glycemic control and lipid profiles in patients with type 2 diabetes mellitus. Metabolism 2011 Apr;60(4):474-9.

Li TY, Li TG, Zhang GX, Guo HY, Liu J, Li BG, Piao ZY, Gai GG. Experimental Study of Hypotensive Effect of Soluble Semen Raphani Alkaloids in Spontaneous Hypertensive Rats. World J. Integrated Traditional and Western Med. 2007;2(1):25.

Li Y, Bai Q, Jin X, Wen H, Gu Z. Effects of cultivar and culture conditions on – aminobutyric acid accumulation in germinated fava beans (*Vicia faba* L.). Journal of the Science of Food and Agriculture 2010 Jan 15;90(1):52-57.

Lin LZ, Harnly JM. Identification of the phenolic components of chrysanthemum flower *(Chrysanthemum morifolium* Ramat). Food Chemistry 2010;120:319-326.

Lin Y, Vermeer MA, A Trautwein E. Triterpenic Acids Present in Hawthorn Lower Plasma Cholesterol by Inhibiting Intestinal ACAT Activity in Hamsters. Evid Based Complement Alternat Med. 2009 Feb 19.

Liang MT, Podolka TD, Chuang WJ. Panax notoginseng supplementation enhances physical performance during endurance exercise. J Strength Cond Res. 2005 Feb;19(1):108-14.

Liang YR, Xu JY, Luo XY, Zheng XQ, Sun QL, Ma SC, Lu JL. Effect of green tea on angiotensin II level and myocardial microstructure in spontaneous hypertensive rats. Journal of Medicinal Plants Research 2010 Sep;4(18):1843-1846.

Liang YR, Ma SC, Luo XY, Xu JY, Wu MY, Luo YW, Zheng XQ, Lu JL. Effects of Green Tea on Blood Pressure and Hypertensive-induced Cardiovascular Damage in Spontaneously Hypertensive Rat. Food Sci. Biotechnol. 2011;20(1):93-98.

Lin C-C, Li T-C, Lai M-M. Efficacy and safety of *Monascus purpureus* Went rice in subjects with hyperlipidemia. European Journal of Endocrinology 2005;153:679-686.

Lin C-L, Lin S-Y, Lin Y-H, Hou W-C. Effects of tuber storage protein of yam *(Dioscorea alata* cv. Tainong No. 1) and its peptic hydrolyzates on spontaneously hypertensive rats. Journal of the Science of Food and Agriculture 2006 Aug 15;86(10):1489-1494.

Lin T-L, Lin H-H, Chen C-C, Lin M-C, Chou M-C, Wang C-J. *Hibiscus sabdariffa* extract reduces serum cholesterol in men and women. Nutrition Research 2007;27:140-145.

Ling WH, Cheng QX, Ma J, Wang T. Red and black rice decrease atherosclerotic plaque formation and increase antioxidant status in rabbits. J Nutr. 2001 May;131(5):1421-6.

Liu D-Z, Liang H-J, Han C-H, Lin S-Y, Chen C-T, Fan M, Hou W-C. Feeding trial of instant food containing lyophilised yam powder in hypertensive subjects. J Sci Food Agric 2009;89:138-143.

Liu JC, Hsu FL, Tsai JC, Chan P, Liu JYH, Thomas GN, Tomlinson B, Lo MY, Lin JY. Antihypertensive effects of tannins isolated from traditional Chinese herbs as non-specific inhibitors of angiontensin converting enzyme. Life Sciences 2003;73:1543-1555.

Liu HG, Liu K, Zhou YN, Xu YJ. Effect of NADPH oxidase activity inhibitor apocynin on blood pressure in rats exposed to chronic intermittent hypoxia and the possible mechanisms. Zhonghua Jie He He Xi Za Zhi 2008 Dec;31(12):921-5.

Liu X, Wei J, Tan F, Zhou S, Würthwein G, Rohdewald P. Pycnogenol, French maritime pine bark extract, improves endothelial function of hypertensive patients. Life Sciences 2004;74:855-862.

Liu Y, Fukuwatari Y, Okumura K,Takeda K, Ishibashi KI, Furukawa M, Ohno N, Mori K, Gao M, Motoi M. Immunomodulating Activity of *Agaricus brasiliensis* KA21 in Mice and in Human Volunteers. ECAM 2008,5(2):205-219.

Liu Y, Xu X, Bi D, Wang X, Zhang X, Dai H, Chen S, Zhang W. Influence of squalene feeding on plasma leptin, testosterone & blood pressure in rats. Indian J Med Res 2009 Feb;129:150-153.

Liu Z-F, Li C-M, Gao Y-L, Li M, Han B. Effect of polysaccharides from Laminaria japonica on hemorheology and microcirculation. Chinese Journal of New Drugs 2006.

Liya W. Pharmacological Study of Semi-Sythetic Luteolin in Reducing Blood Pressure. Chinese Pharmacological Bulletin 1986.

Loizzo MR, Said A, Tundis R, Rashed K, Statti GA, Hufner A, Menichini F. Inhibition of Angiotensin Converting Enzyme (ACE) by Flavonoids isolated from *Ailanthus excelsa* (Roxb) (Simaroubaceae). Phytother. Res. 2007;21:32-36.

Longhurst JC, Li P. Neural mechanism of electroacupuncure's hypotensive effects. Autonomic Neuroscience: Basic and Clinical 010;157:24-30.

López Ledesma R, Frati Munari AC, Hernández Dominguez BC, Cervantes Montalvo S, Hernández Luna MH, Juárez C, Morán Lira S. Monounsaturated fatty acid (avocado) rich diet for mild hypercholesterolemia. Arch Med Res. 1996;27(4):519-23.

Lucas EA, Mahajan SS, Soung DY, Lightfoot SA, Smith BJ, Arjmandi BH. Flaxseed bu Not Flaxseed Oil Prevented the Rise in Serum Cholesterol Due to Ovariectomy in the Golden Syrian Hamsters. Journal of Medicinal Food 2011;14(3)

Luo LF, Wu WH, Zhou YJ, Yan J, Yang GP, Ouyang DS. Antihypertensive effect of *Eucommia ulmoides* Oliv. extracts in spontaneously hypertensive rats. Journal of Ethnopharmacology 2010;129:238-243.

Lupattelli G, Marchesi S, Lombardini R, Roscini AR, Trinca F, Gemelli F, Vaudo G, Mannarino E. Artichoke juice improves endothelial function in hyperlipemia. Life Sciences 2004;76:775-782.

Lupton JR, Robinson MC, Morin JL. Cholesterol-lowering effect of barley bran flour and oil. J Am Diet Assoc. 1994 Jan;94(1): 65-70.

Ma Q, Ma J. Effect of Semen Raphani on anti-hypertension. Tradit Chin Med 1998;39:454.

Ma YX, Chen SY. Observations on the anti-aging, antihypertensive and antihyperlipemic effect of Apocynum venetum leaf extract. Zhong Xi Yi Jie He Za Zhi 1989 Jun;9(6):335-7.

Maas JL, Wang SY, Galletta GJ. Evaluation of Strawberry Cultivars for Ellagic Acid Content. HortScience 1991;26(1):6668.

Macarulla MT, Medina C, De Diego MA, Chávarri M, Zulet MA, Martine JA, Nöel-Suberville C, Higueret P, Portillo MP. Effets of the whole seed and a protein isolate of faba bean (Vicia faba) on the cholesterol metabolism of hypercholesterolaemic rats. Br J Nutr. 2001 May;85(5):607-14.

Mackraj I, Ramesar S, Singh M, Govender T, Baijnath H, Singh R, Gathiram P. The *in vivo* effects of *Tulbhagia violacea* on blood pressure in a salt-sensitive rat model. Journal of Ethnopharmacology 2008;117:263-269.

Madanmohan, Udupa K, Bhavanani AB, Vijayalakshmi P, Surendiran A. Effect of slow and fast pranayams on reaction time and cardiorespiratory variables. Indian J Physiol Pharmacol 2005;49(3):313-318.

Magda RA, Awad AM, Selim KA. Evaluation of Mandarin and Navel Orange Peels as Natural Sources of Antioxidant in Biscuits. Alex. J. Fd. Sci. & Technol. Special Volume Conference 2008 Mar:75-82.

Maghrani M, Zeggwagh N-A, Michel J-B, Eddouks M. Antihypertensive effect of *Lepidium sativum* L. in spontaneously hypertensive rats. Journal of Ethnopharmacology 2005;100:193-197.

Maisont S, Narkrugsa W. The Effect of Germination on GABA Content, Chemical Composition, Total Phenolics Content and Antioxidant Capacity of Thai Waxy Paddy Rice. Kasetsart J. (Nat. Sci.) 2010;44:912-923.

Makihara H, Shimada T, Machida E, Oota M, Nagamine R, Tsubata M, Kinoshita K. Preventive effect of Terminalia bellirica on obesity and metabolic disorders in spontaneously obese type diabetic model mice. J Nat Med. 2011 Nov 22.

Malaguarnera M, Vacante M, Avitabile T, Malaguarnera M, Cammalleri L, Motta M. L-Carnitine supplementation reduces oxidized LDL cholesterol in patients with diabetes[1-3]. Am J Clin Nutr 2009;89:1-6.

Malaguarnera M, Gargante MP, Russo C, Antic T, Vacante M, Malaguarnera M, Avitabile T, Li Volti G, Galvano F. L-carnitine supplementation to diet: a new tool in treatment of nonalcoholic steatohepatitis – a randomized and controlled clinical trial. Am J Gastroenterol 2010 Jun;105(6):1338-45.

Malhotra V, Dhungel KU, Ganga J. Does The Effect of Pranayama Differ in Yoga Practitioner And Naive? Journal of Clinical and Diagnostic Research 2010 Dec;4:3503-3506.

Mali VR, Bodhankar SL. Effect of *Lagenaria siceraria* (LS) powder on dexamethasone induced hypertension in rats. International Journal of Advances in Pharmaceutical Sciences 2010;1:50-53.

Malinow MR, McLaughlin P, Stafford C, Livingston AL, Kohler GO. Alfalfa saponins and alfalfa seeds. Dietary effects in cholesterol-fed rabbits. Atherosclerosis 1980 Nov;37(3):433-8.

Malve H, Kerkar P, Mishra N, Loke S, Rege NN, Marwaha-Jaspal A, Jainani KJ. LDL-cholesterol lowering activity of a blend of rice bran oil and safflower oil (8:2) in patients with hyperlipidaemia: a proof of concept, double blind, controlled, randomised parallel group study. J Indian Med Assoc 2010 Nov;108(11):785-8.

Mamaghani-E, Arefhosseini, Golzarand, Aliasgarzadeh, Jabbary-V. Long-term Effects of Processed Berberis Vulgaris on Some Metabolic Syndrome Components. Iranian Journal of Endocrinology and Metabolism 2009; 11(1);41-47.

Mancilha-Carvalho JJ, Silva NAS. The Yanomami Indians in the INTERSALT Study. Arq Bras Cardiol 2003;80(3):295-300.

Mangoni AA, Sherwood RA, Swift CG, Jackson SHD. Folic acid enhances endothelial function and reduces blood pressure in smokers: a randomized controlled trial. Journal of Internal Medicine 2002;252;497-503.

Mansour SM, Bahgat AK, El-Khatib AS, Khayyal MT. *Ginkgo biloba* extract (Egb 761) normalizes hypertension in 2K, 1C hypertensive rats: Role of antioxidant mechanisms, ACE inhibiting activity and improvement of endothelial dysfunction. Phytomedicine 2011;18:641-647.

Mark DA, Maki K. Concord grape juice reduces blood pressure in men with high systolic blood pressure. Abstract No. 693. Presented at Experimental Biology 2003, April 11-15, San Diego, CA, USA.

Margetts BM, Beilin LJ, Vandongen R, Armstrong BK. Vegetarian diet in mild hypertension: a randomized controlled trial. Br Med J (Clin Res Ed). 1986 Dec 6;293(6560):1468-71.

Marhazlina M, Rokiah MY, Norhayati AH, Mohd AKR. Effects of red pitaya *(Hylocereus sp.)* consumption on blood pressure, blood glucose level in type 2 diabetes subjects. Mal J Nutr 2006;12(2):105.

Marlene MM, Tulley R, Morales S, Lefevre M. Rice bran oil, not fiber, lowers cholesterol in humans. Am J Clin Nutr 2005;81:64-8.

Marnewick JL, Rautenbach F, Venter I, Neethling H, Blackhurst DM, Wolmarans P, Macharia M. Effects of rooibos *(Aspalathus linearis)* on oxidative stress and biochemical parameters in adults at risk for cardiovascular disease. Journal of Ethnopharmacology 2011;133:46-52.

Maron DJ, Lu GP, Cai NS, Wu ZG, Li YH, Chen H, Zhu JQ, Jin XJ, Wouters BC, Zhao J. Cholesterol-lowering effect of a theaflavin-enriched green tea extract: a randomized controlled trial. Arch Intern Med. 2003 Jun 23;163(12):1448-53.

Marshall MW, Kliman PG, Washington VA. Effects of biotin on lipids and other constituents of plasma of healthy men and women. Artery 1980;7:330-351.

Marthur R, Sharma A, Dixit VP, Varma M. Hypolipidaemic effect of fruit juice on Emblica officinalis in cholesterol-fed rabbits. J Ethnopharmacol 1996 Feb;50(2):61-8.

Martin DS, Breitkopf NP, Eyster KM, Williams JL. Dietary soy exerts an antihypertensive effect in spontaneously hypertensive female rats. Am J Physiol Regul Integr Comp Physiol. 2001 Aug;281(2):553-60.

Martin N, Pantoja C, Chiang L, Bardisa L, Araya C, Roman R. Hemodynamic effects of a boiling water dialysate of maize silk in normotensive anaesthetized dogs. Journal of Ethnopharmacology 1991;31:259-262.

Martina V, Masha A, Gigliardi VR, Brocato L, Manzato E, Berchio A, Massarenti P, Settanni F, Casa LD, Bergamini S, Iannone A. Long-Term N-Acetylcysteine and L-Arginine Administration Reduces Endothelial Activation and Systolic Blood Pressure in Hypertensive Patients With Type 2 Diabetes. Diabetes Care 2008 May;31(5):940-944.

Martinello F, Soares SM, Franco JJ, Santos AC, Sugohara A, Garcia SB, Curti C, Uyemura SA. Hypolipemic and antioxidant activities from Tamarindus indica L. pulp fruit extract in hypercholesterolemic hamsters. Food Chem Toxicol. 2006 Jun;44(6): 810-8.

Martirosyan DM, Miroshnichenko LA, Kulakova SN, Pogojeva AV, Zoloedov VI. Amaranth oil application for coronary heart disease and hypertension. Lipids in Health and Disease 2007;6(1):1-12.

Maruthappan V, Shree KS. Hypolipidemic activity of haritaki *(Terminalia chebula)* in atherogenic diet induced hyperlipidemic rats. J Adv Pharm Technol Res. 2010 Apr-Jun;1(2):229-235.

Maruyama C, Araki R, Kawamura M, Kondo N, Kigawa M, Kawai Y, Takanami Y, Miyashita K, Shimomitsu T. Azuki bean juice lowers serum triglycerde concentrations in healthy young women. J Clin Biochem Nutr. 2008 Jul;43(1):19-25.

Maruyama H, Sumitou Y, Sakamoto T, Araki Y, Hara H. Antihypertensive Effects of Flavonoids Isolated from Brazilian Green Propolis in Spontaneously Hypertensive Rats. Biol. Pharm. Bull. 2009;32(7):1244-1250.

Mate A, Miguel-Carrasco JL, Monserrant MT, Vázquez CM. Systemic antioxidant properties of L-carnitine in two differen models of arterial hypertension. J Physiol. Biochem 2010 Jun;66(2):127-36.

Matsubara F, Ueno H, Muneyuki S, Suzuki T, Magata K, Kikuchi N, Nakamichi N, Kumagai H, Saruta T. Effects of GABA Supplementation on Blood Pressure and Safety in Adults with Mild Hypertension. Japanese Pharmacology & Therapeutics 2002;30(11):963-972.

Matsui T, Li CH, Tanaka T, Maki T, Osajima Y, Matsumoto K. Depressor effect of wheat germ hydrolysate and its novel angiotensin I-converting enzyme inhibitory peptide, Ile-Val-Tyr, and the metabolism in rat and human plasma. Biol Pharm Bull 2000 Apr;23(4):427-31.

Matsumoto K, Yokoyama S, Gato N. Bile acid-binding activity of young persimmon (Diospyros kaki) fruit and its hypolipidemic effect in mice. Phytother Res. 2010 Feb;24(2):205-10.

Matsumura Y, Kita S, Ono H, Kiso Y, Tanaka T. Preventive Effect of a Chicken Extract on the Development of Hypertension in Stroke-prone Spontaneously Hypertensive Rats. Biosci. Biotechnol. Biochem. 2002;66(5):1108-1110.

Matsuura M, Kimura Y, Nakata K, Baba K, Okuda H. Artery relaxation by chalcones isolated from the roots of Angelica keiskei. Planta Med. 2001 Apr;67(3):230-5.

Mcackin CJ, Widlansky ME, Hamburg NM, Huang AL, Weller S, Holbrook M, Gokce N, Hagen TM, Keaney Jr. JF, Vita JA. Effect of Combined Treatment with Alpha Lipoic Acid and Acetyl-L-Carnitine on Vascular Function and Blood Pressure in Coronary Artery Disease Patients. J Clin Hypertens (Greenwich) 2007 Apr;9(4):249-255.

McKiernan F, Lokko P, Kuevi A, Sales RL, Costa NM, Bressa J, Alfenas RC, Mattes RD. Effects of peanut processing on body weight and fasting plasma lipids. Br J Nutr. 2010 Aug;104(3):418-26.

McMahon FG, Vargas R. Can garlic lower blood pressure? A pilot study. Pharmacotherapy 1993 Jul – Aug;13(4):406-7.

McPherson L. Effects of the consumption of fully cooked red kidney beans (*Phaseolus vulgaris*) on the growth rate of rats and the morphology of the gut wall. Journal of the Science of Food and Agriculture 1991;57(4):611-621.

McRae MP. Treatment of hyperlipoproteinemia with pantethine: A review and analysis of efficacy and tolerability. Nutrition Research 2005;25:319-333.

Meckling KA, Sherfey R. A randomized trial of a hypocaloric high-protein diet, with and without exercise, on weight loss, fitness, and without exercise, on weight loss, fitness, and markers of the Metabolic Syndrome in overweight and obese women. Appl Physiol Nutr Metab 2007 Aug;32(4):743-52.

Medhin DG, Hadházy, Bakos P, Verzár-Petri G. Hypertensive effects of Lupinus termis and Coriandrum sativum in Anaesthetized Rats. A preliminary study. Acta Pharm Hung 1986 Mar;56(2):59-63.

Meissner HO, Reich-Bilinska H, Mscisz A, Kedzia B. Therapeutic Effects of *Lepidium peruvianum* Chacon (Pre-Gelatinized Maca) used as a non-hormonal alternative to HRT in perimenopausal women – Clinical Pilot Study. IJBS 2006 May;2(2).

Meliani N, Dib MA, Allali H, Tabti B. Hypoglycaemic effect of *Berbers vulgaris* L. in normal and streptozotocin-induced diabetic rats. Asian Pacific Journal of Tropical Biomedicine 2011;468-471.

Melis MS. Chronic administration of aqueous extract of *Stevia rebaudiana* in rats: renal effects. Journal of Ethnopharmacology 1995;47:129-134.

Melita Rodriguez S, Acosta H, Barroso C. Diuretic effect of chayote juice (Sechium edule) in rats. Rev Med Panama 1984 Jan;9(1):68-74.

Mendonca S, Saldiva PH, Cruz RJ, Arêas JAG. Amaranth protein presents cholesterol-lowering effet. Food Chemistry 2009;116:738-742.

Mengheri E, Scarino ML, Vignolini F, Spadoni MA. Modifications in plasma cholesterol and apolipoproteins of hypercholesterolaemic rats induced by ethanol-soluble factors of Vicia faba. Br J Nutr. 1985 Mar;53(2):223-32.

Merchant RE, Andre CA. A revie of recent clinical trials of the nutritional supplement Chlorella pyrenoidosa in the treatment of fibromyalgia, hypertension, and ulcerative colitis. Altern Ther Health Med 2001;7(3):79-91.

Merchant RE, Andre CA, Sica DA. Nutritional supplementation with Chlorella pyrenoidosa for mild to moderate hypertension. J Med Food 2002;5(3):141-52.

Messripour M, Mesripour A. Effects of vitamin B6 on age associated changes of rat brain glutamate decarboxylase activity. African Journal of Pharmacy and Pharmacology 2011 Mar;5(3):454-456.

Metwalli OM, Al-Okbi SY, Abbas AE. Effect of some sources of dietary fibers on rat plasma lipids. Egypt. J. Pharm. Sci. 1994; 35(1-6):31-8.

Metwally MAA, El-Gellal AM, El-Sawaisi SM. Effects of Silymarin on Lipid Metabolism in Rats. World Applied Sciences Journal 2009;6(12):1634-1637.

Miceli N, Mondello MR, Monforte MT, Sdrafkakis V, Dugo P, Crupi ML, Taviano MF, De Pasquale R Trovato A. Hypolipidemic effects of Citrus bergamia Risso et Poiteau juice in rats fed a hypercholesterolemic diet. J Agric Food Chem. 2007 Dec 26;55(26):10671-7.

Miguel-Carrasco JL, Monserrat MT, Mate A, Vázquez CM. Comparative effects of captopril and L-carnitine on blood pressure and antioxidant enzyme gene expression in the heart of spontaneously hypertensive rats. European Journal of Pharmacology 2010;63:65-72.

Milkowska-Leyck K, Filipek B, Strzelecka H. Pharmacological effects of lavandulifolioside from *Leonurus cardiaca*. Journal of Ethnopharmacology 2002;80:85-90.

Miloradovic Z, Bugarski B, Komes D, Grujic Milanovic J, Ivanov M, Jovovic DJ, Mihailovic-Stanojevic N. Thyme extract improves blood pressure and oxidative stress in spontaneously hypertensive rats. Journal of Hypertension 2010 Jun;28.

Mirmiran P, Fazeli MR, Asghari G, Shafiee A, Azizi F. Effect of pomegranate seed oil on hyperlipidaemic subjects: a double-blind placebo-controlled clinical trial. Br J Nutr. 2010 Aug;104(3):402-6.

Mishima S, Yoshida C, Akino S, Sakamoto T. Antihypertensive Effects of Brazilian Propolis: Identification of Caffeoylquinic Acids as Constituents Involved in Hypotension in Spontaneously Hypertensive Rats. Biol. Pharm. Bull. 2005;28(10):1909-1914.

Mishra RC, Tripathy S, Quest D, Desai KM, Akhtar J, Dattani ID, Gopalakrishnan V. L-Serine lowers while glycine increases blood pressure in chronic L-NAME-treated and spontaneously hypertensive rats. J Hypertens 2008 Dec;26(12):2339-48.

Mishra RC, Tripathy S, Desai KM, Quest D, Lu Y, Akhtar J, Gopalakrishnan V. Nitric oxide synthase inhibition promotes endothelium-dependent vasodilatation and the antihypertensive effect of L-serine. Hypertension 2008 Mar;51(3):791-6.

Mishra RC, Tripathy S, Gandhi JD, Balsevich J, Akhtar J, Desai KM, Gopalakrishnan V. Decreases in splanchnic vascular resistance contribute to hypotensive effects of L-serine in hypertensive rats. Am J Physiol Heart Circ Physiol 2010;298:1789-1796.

Mitra A, Bhattacharya D. Dose-dependent effects of Fenugreek composite in Diabetes with dislipidaemia. Internet Journal of Food Safety 2006;8:49-55.

Miwa Y, Yamada M, Sunayama T, Mitsuzumi H, Tsuzaki Y, Chaen H, Mishima Y, Kibata M. Effects of glucosyl hesperidin on serum lipids in hyperlipidemic subjects: preferential reduction in elevated serum triglyceride level. J Nutr Sci Vitaminol (Tokyo) 2004 Jun;50(3):211-8.

Miwa Y, Mitsuzumi H, Sunayama T, Yamada M, Okada K, Kubota M, Chaen H, Mishima Y, Kibata M. Glucosyl hesperidin lowers serum triglyceride level in hypertriglyceridemic subjects through the improvement of very low-density lipoprotein metabolic abnormality. J Nutr Sci Vitaminol (Tokyo) 2005 Dec;51(6):460-70.

Mitwalli AH, Al-Wakeel JS, Alam A, Tarif N, Abu-Aisha H, Rashed M, Nahed NA. L-Carnitine Supplementation in Hemodialysis Patients. Saudi J Kidney Dis Transplant 2005;16(1):17-22.

Miyake Y, Kuzuya K, Ueno C, Katayama N, Hayakawa T, Tsuge H, Osawa T. Suppressive Effect of Components in Lemon Juice on Blood Pressure in Spontaneously Hypertensive Rats. Food Sci. Technol. Int. Tokyo 1998;4(1):29-32.

Miyake Y, Kono S, Nishiwaki M, Hamada H, Nishikawa H, Koga H, Ogawa S. Relationship of coffee consumption with serum lipids and lipoproteins in Japanese men. Ann Epidemiol. 1999 Feb;9(2):121-6.

Miyake Y, Suzuki E, Ohya S, Fukumoto S, Hiramitsu M, Sakaida K, Osawa T, Furuichi Y. Lipid-Lowering Effect of Eriocitrin, the Main Flavonoid in Lemon Fruit, in Rats on a High-Fat and High-Cholesterol Diet. Journal of Food Science 2006 Dec;71(9): 633-637.

Miyawaki T, Aono H, Toyoda-Ono Y, Maeda H, Kiso Y, Moriyama K. Antihypertensive effects of sesamin in humans. J Nutr Sci Vitaminol (Tokyo) 2009 Feb;55 (1):87-91.

Miyazawa N, Okazaki M, Ohga S. Antihypertensive effect of Pleurotus nebrodensis in spontaneously hypertensive rats. J Oleo Sci. 2008;57(12):675-81.

Mizoguchi T, Takehara I, Masuzawa T, Saito T, Naoki Y. Nutrigenomic studies of effects of Chlorella on subjects with high-risk factors for lifestyle-related disease. J Med Food 2008 Sep;11(3):395-404.

Mizushima S, Ohshige K, Watanabe J, Kimura M, Kadowaki T, Nakamura Y, Tochikubo O, Ueshima H. Randomized controlled trial of sour milk on blood pressure in borderline hypertensive men. Am. J Hypertens 2004;17:701-706.

Mizutani K, Ikeda K, Kawai Y, Yamori Y. Resveratrol attenuates ovariectomy-induced hypertension and bone loss in stroke-prone spontaneously hypertensive rats. J Nutr Sci Vitaminol (Tokyo) 2000 Apr;46(2):78-83.

Modaghegh MH, Shahabian M, Esmaeili HA, Rajbai O, Hosseinzadeh H. Safety evaluation of saffron (Crocus sativus) tablets in healthy volunteers. Phytomedicine 2008 Dec;15(12):1032-7.

Mohamed MS, Afifi AA. Influence of Mackerel Fish and Potato Starch in Lipid Profile and Glucose Level in Normal Rats. Journal of Applied Sciences Research 2011;7(3):369-375.

Mohan M, Waghulde H, Kasture S. Effect of pomegranate juice on Angiotensin II-induced hypertension in diabetic Wistar rats. Phytother Res 2010 Jun;24(2):196-203.

Mollac V, Sacco I, Janda E, Malara C, Ventrice D, Colica C, Visalli V, Muscoli S, Ragusa S, Muscoli C, Rotiroti D, Romeo F. Hypolipemic and hypoglycaemic activity of bergamot polyphenols: From animal models to human studies. Fitoterapia 2011;82:309-316.

Monroy-Ruiz J, Sevilla MA, Carrón R, Montero MJ. Astaxanthin-enriched-diet reduces blood pressure and improves cardiovascular parameters in spontaneously hypertensive rats. Pharmacol Res. 2011 Jan;63(1):44-50.

Montenegro MF, Pessa LR, Tanus-Santos JE. Isoflavone genistein inhibits the angiotensin-converting enzyme and alters the vascular responses to angotensin I and bradykinin. European Journal of Pharmacology 2009;607:173-177.

Moore CS, Bryant SP, Mishra GD, Krebs JD, Browning LM, Miller GJ, Jebb SA. Oily fish reduces plasma triacylglycerols: a primary prevention study in overweight men and women. Nutrition 2006;22:1012-1024.

Morand C, Dubray C, Milenkovic D, Lioger D, Martin JF, Scalbert A, Mazur A. Hesperidin contributes to the vascular protective effects of orange juice: a randomized crossover study in healthy volunteers. Am J Clin Nutr. 2011 Jan;93(1):73-80.

Moreira FV, Bastos JFA, Blan AF, Alves PB, Santos MRV. Chemical composition and cardiovascular effects induces by the essential oil of *Cymbopogon citratus* DC. Stapf. Poacea, in rats. Revista Brasileira de Farmacognosia 2010 Marc.

Morello S, Vellecco V, Alfieri A, Mascolo N, Cicala C. Vasorelaxant effect of the flavonoid galangin on isolated rat thoracic aorta. Life Sciences 2006;78:825-830.

Moreno-Loaiza O, Paz-Aliaga A. Vasodilator effect mediated by nitric oxide of the Zea mays L *(Andean Purple Corn)* hydroalcoholic extract in aortic rings of rat. Rev Peru Med Exp Salud Publica 2010 Oct-Dec;27(4):527-31.

Morigiwa A, Kitabatake K, Fujimoto Y, Ikekawa N. Angiotensin converting enzyme-inhibitory triterpenes from *Ganoderma lucidum.* Chemical and Pharmaceutical Bulletin (Tokyo) 1986;34:3025-3028.

Morris MC, Sacks F, Rosner B. Does fish oil lower blood pressure? A meta-analysis of controlled trials. Circulation 1993 Aug;88(2):523-33.

Motoyama T, Sano H, Fukuzaki H. Oral magnesium supplementation in patients with essential hypertension. Hypertension 1989;13:227-232.

Mourad AM, de Carvalho Pincinato E, Mazzola PG, Sabha M, Moriel P. Influence of soy lecithin administration on hypercholesterolemia. Cholesterol 2010;2010:824813.

Movahedian A, Ghannadi A, Vashirnia M. Hypocholesterolemic Effects of Purslane Extract on Serum Lipids in Rabbits Fed with High Cholesterol Levels. International Journal of Pharmacology 2007;3(3):285-289.

Mozaffari-Khosravi H, Jalali-Khanabadi B-A, Afkhami-Ardekani M, Fatehi F, Noori-Shadkam M. The effects of sour tea (Hibiscus sabdariffa) on hypertenson in patients with type II dibetes Sour tea for hypertension in diabetic patients. Journal of Human Hypertension 2009 Jan;23:48-54.

Münstedt K, Hoffmann S, Hauenschild A, Bülte M, von Georg R, Hackethal A. Effect of honey on serum cholesterol and lipid values. J Med Food 2009 Jun;12(3):624-8.

Mukai Y, Sato S. Polyphenol-containing azuki bean (Vigna angularis) extract attenuates blood pressure elevation and modulates nitric oxide synthase and caveolin-1 expressions in rats with hypertension. Nutr Metab Cardiovasc Dis 2009 Sep;19(7):491-7.

Murai A, Miyahara T, Tanaka T, Sako Y, Nishimura N, Kameyama M. The effects of pantethine on lipid and lipoprotein abnormalities in survivors of cerebral infarction. Artery 1985;12(4):234-43.

Muraki E, Chiba H, Tsunoda N, Kasono K. Fenugreek Improves Diet-induced Metabolic Disorders in Rats. Horm Metab Res. 2011 Dec;43(13):950-5.

Murali YK, Anand P, Tandon V, Singh R, Chandra R, Murthy PS. Long-term effects of Terminalia chebula Retz, on hyperglycemia and associated hyperlipidemia, tissue glycogen content and in vitro release of insulin in streptozotocin induced diabetic rats. Exp Clin Endocrinol Diabetes 2007 Nov;115(10):641-6.

Murata M, Ishihara K, Saito H. Hepatic fatty acid oxidation enzyme activities are stimulated in rats fed the brown seaweed, Undaria pinnatifida (wakame). J Nutr 1999 Jan;129(1):146-151.

Mushtaq R, Mushtaq R, Khan ZT. Effect of Walnut on Lipid Profile in Obese Female in Different Ethnic Groups of Quetta, Pakistan. Pakistan Journal of Nutrition 2009;8(10):1617-1622.

Mute V, Awari D, Vawhal P. Kulkarni A, Bartakke U, Shetty R. Evaluation of Diuretic Activity of Aqueous Extract of *Raphanus sativus*. European Journal of Biological Sciences 2011;3(1):13-15.

Mölgaard J, von Schenck H, Olsson AG. Alfalfa seeds lower low density lipoprotein cholesterol and apolipoprotein B concentrations in patients with type II hyperlipoproteinemia. Atherosclerosis 1987 May;65(1-2):173-9.

Nader MA, el-Agamy DS, Suddek GM. Protective effects of propolis and thymoquinone on develpment of atherosclerosis in cholesterol-fed rabbits. Arch Pharm Res. 2010 Apr;33(4):637-43.

Nagai T, Nagashima T. Functional properties of dioscorin, a soluble viscous protein from Japanese yam (Dioscorea opposita thunb.) tuber mucilage Tororo. Z Naturforsch C 2006 Nov-Dec;61(11-12):792-8.

Nagai T, Tanoue Y, Kai N, Suzuki N, Nagashima T. The liquor made from silver vine [Actinidia polygama (Sieb. Et Zucc.) Planch. Ex Maxim.] berries possess strongly antioxidative activity and antihypertensive activity. African Journal of Food Science 2011 Mar;5(3):125-130.

Nagao T, Hase T, Tokimitsu I. A green tea extract high in catechins reduces body fat and cardiovascular risks in humans. Obesity (Silver Spring) 2007 Jun;15(6):1473-83.

Nagaoka S, Kanamaru Y, Kuzuya Y, Kojima T, Kuwata T. Comparative Studies on the Serum Cholesterol Lowering Action on Whey

Protein and Soybean Protein in Rats. Biosci. Biotech. Biochem. 1992;56(9):1484-1485.

Nainwal P, Dhamija K, Tripathi S. Study of antihyperlipidemic effect on the juice of the fresh fruits of *Lagenaria siceraria.* International Journal of Pharmacy and Pharmceutical Sciences 2011;3:88-90.

Naissides M, Mamo JCL, James AP, Pal S. The effect of chronic consumption of red wine on cardiovascular disease risk factors in postmenopausal women. Atherosclerosis 2006;185:438-445.

Nakagawa K, Ueno A, Nishikawa Y. Intractions between Carnosine and Captopril on Free Radical Scavenging Activity and Angiotensin-converting Enzyme Activity *in vtro.* Yakugaku Zasshi 2006;126(1):37-42.

Nakajima K, Hata Y, Osono Y, Hamura M, Kobayashi S, Watanuki M. Antihypertensive Effect of Extracts of *Lactobacillus casei* in Patients with Hypertension. Journal of Clinical Biochemistry and Nutrition 1995;18(3):181-187.

Nakamura Y, Kanazawa M, Liyanage R, Iijima S, Han KH, Shimada K, Sekikawa M, Yamauchi A, Hashimoto N, Ohba K, Fukushima M. Effect of white wheat bread containing sugar beet fiber on serum lipids and hepatic mRNA in rats fed on a cholesterol-free diet. Biosci Biotechnol Biochem 2009 Jun;73(6):1280-5.

Nakashima M, Shigekuni Y, Obi T, Shiraishi M, Miyamoto A, Yamasaki H, Etoh T, Iwai S. Nitric oxide-dependent hypotensive effects of wax gourd juice. Journal of Ethnopharmacology 2011;138:404-407.

Namazi N, Esfanjani AT, Asghari M, Bahrami A. Effect of Hydroalcholic Nettle *(Urtica dioica)* Extract on Some Cardiovascular Risk Factors in Patients With Type 2 Diabetes. J. Med. Sci. 2011 Apr 1;11(3):138-144.

Nammi S, Gudavalli R, Babu BS, Lodagala DS, Boini KM. Possible mechanisms of hypotension produced 70% alcoholic extract of Terminalia arjuna (L.) in anaesthetized dogs. BMC Complement Altern Med. 2003 Oct 16;3(5):1-4.

Nantz MP, Rowe CA, Bukowski JF, Percival SS. Standardized capsule of *Camellia sinensis* lowers cardiovascular risk factors in a randomized, double-blind, placebo-controlled study. Nutrition 2009;25:147-154.

Naoufel AZ, Abderahman M, Jean BM, Mohamed E. Hypotensive Effect of *Chamaemelum Nobile* Aqueous Extract in Spontaneously Hypertensive Rats. Clinical and Experimental Hypertension 2009;31:440-450.

Naseri MKG, Yahyavi H, Arabian M. Antispasmodic Activity of Onion *(Allium cepa* L.) Peel Extract on Rat Ileum. Iranian Journal of Pharmaceutical Research 2008;7(2):155-159.

Naseri MKG, Arabian M, Badavi M, Ahangarpour A. Vasorelaxant and Hypotensive Effects of *Allium cepa* Peel Hydroalcoholic Extract in Rats. Pakistan Journal of Biological Sciences 2008;11(12):1569-1575.

Nassiri-Asl M, Zamansoltani F, Abbasi E, Daneshi MM, Zangivand AA. Effects of Urtica dioica extract on lipid profile in hypercholesterolemic rats. Zhong Xi Yi Jie He Xue Bao 2009 May;7(5):428-33.

Nazni P, Vijayakumar TP, Alagianambi P, Amirthaveni M. Hypoglycemic and Hypolipidemic Effect of Cynara Scolymus among Selected Type 2 Diabetic Individuals. Pakistan Journal of Nutrition 2006;5(2):147-151.

Nemoseck TM, Carmody EG, Furchner-Evanson A, Gleason M, Li A, Potter H, Rezende LM, Lane KJ, Kern M. Honey promotes lower weight gain, adiposity, and triglycerides than sucrose in rats. Nutrition Research 2011;31:55-60.

Nestel PJ, Chronopulos A, Cehu M. Dairy fat in cheese raises LDL cholesterol less than that in butter in mildly hypercholesterolaemic subjects. Eur J Clin Nutr. 2005 Sep;59(9):1059-63.

Newaz MA, Yousefipour Z, Nawal N, Adeeb N. Nitric oxide synthase activity in blood vessels of spontaneously hypertensive rats: antioxidant protection by gamma-tocotrienol. J Physiol Pharmacol. 2003 Sep;54(3):319-27.

Ngondi JL, Oben JE, Minka SR. The effect of *Irvingia gabonensis* seeds on body weight and blood lipids of obese subjects in Cameroon. Lipids in Health and Disease 2005;4(12):1-4.

Ngondi JL, Etoundi BC, Nyangono CB, Mbofung CMF, Oben JE. IGOB131, a novel seed extract of the West African plant *Irvingia gabonensis,* significantly reduces body weight and improves metabolic parameters in overweight humans in a randomized double-blind placebo controlled investigation. Lipids in Health and Disease 2009;8(7):1-7.

Nicolle C, Gueux E, Lab C, Jaffrelo L, Rock E, Mazur A, Amouroux P, Rémésy C. Lyophilized carrot ingestion lowers lipemia and beneficially affects cholesterol metabolism in cholesterol-fed C57BL/6J mice. Eur J Nutr. 2004 Aug;43(4):237-45.

Niijima A, Okui T, Matsumura Y, Yamano T, Tsuruoka N, Kiso Y, Nagai K. Effects of L-carnosine on renal sympathetic nerve activity and DOCA-salt hypertension in rats. Autonomic Neuroscience: Basic and Clinical 2002;97:99-102.

Nishikawa Y, Takata Y, Nagai Y, Mori T, Kawada T, Ishihara N. Antihypertensive Effect of Kurosu Extract, a Traditional Vinegar Produced from Unpolished Rice, in the SHR rats. Nippon Shokuhin Kagaku Kogaku Kaishi 2001;48(1):73-75.

Nishizawa N, Fudamoto Y. The elevation of plasma concentration of high-density lipoprotein cholesterol in mice fed with protein from proso millet. Biosci Biotechnol Biochem 1995 Feb;59(2):333-5.

Nishizawa N, Shimanuki S, Fujihashi H, Watanabe H, Fudamoto Y, Nagasawa T. Proso millet protein elevates plasma level of high-density lipoprotein: a new food function of proso millet. Biomed Environ Sci. 1996 Sep;9(2-3):209-12.

Nissen S, Sharp RI, Panton L, Vukovich M, Trappe S, Fuller JC Jr. Beta-hydroxy-beta-methylbutyrate (HMB) supplementation in humans is safe and may decrease cardiovascular risk factors. J Nutr 2000 Aug;130(8):1937-45.

Niwano Y, Beppu F, Shimada T, Kyan R, Yasura K, Tamaki M, Nishino M, Midorikawa Y, Hamada H. Extensive Screening for Plant Foodstuffs in Okinawa, Japan with Anti-Obese Activity on Adipocytes *In Vitro.* Plant Foods Hum Nutr 2009;64:6-10.

Nkanu EE, Eno AE, Ofem OE, Imoru JO, Unoh FB. Effect of crude extract of *Viscum album* (mistletoe) on plasma lipids: an insight into its possible antihyperglycaemic and antihypertensive properties. Port Harcourt Medical Journal 2007;1:171-177.

Noakes M, Keogh JB, Foster PR, Clifton PM. Effect of an energy-restricted, high-protein, low-fat diet relative to a conventional high-carbohydrate, low-fat diet on weight loss, body composition, nutritional status, and markers of cardiovascular health in obese women. Am J Clin Nutr. 2005;81:1298-306.

Norazmir MN, Ayub MY. Beneficial Lipid-Lowering Effects of Pink Guava Puree in High Fat Diet Induced-Obese Rats. Mal J Nutr 2010;16(1):171-185.

Nouran G, Kimiagar M, Abadi A, Mirzazadeh M, Harrison G. Peanut consumption and cardiovascular risk. Public Health Nutr. 2010 Oct;13(10):1581-6.

Novoa BE, Céspedes AC, de Gracia LA, Olarte C, Jorge E. Quercitrina: Un flavoide con actividad hipotensora, Obtenido del *Croton glabellus.* Rev. Colomb. Cienc. Quim. - Farm. 1985;4(2):7-13.

229

Nurminen ML, Niittynen L, Korpela R, Vapaatalo H. Coffee, caffeine and blood pressure: a critical review. Eur J Clin Nutr. 1999 Nov;53(11):831-9.

Nwaoguikpe RN, Braide W. The effect of aqueous seed extract of *persea americana* (avocado pear) on serum lipid and cholesterol levels in rabbits. African Journal of Pharmacy ad Pharmacology Research 2011 Apr;1(2):23-29.

Nwozo SO, Orojobi BF, Adaramoye OA. Hypolipidemic and antioxidant potentials of Xylopia aethiopica seed extract in hypercholesterolemic rats. J Med. Food. 2011 Jan – Feb;14(1-2):114-9.

Obaidy S. Degree of doctor of medicine: The effect of twice-a-day intake of chayote extract among hypertensive individuals in barangay sto. Niño, liloy Zamboanga del norte. The Faculty Ateneo de Zamboanga University School of Medicine 2007.

Oben J, Kuate D, Agbor G, Momo C, Talla X. The use of a *Cissus quadrangularis* formulation in the management of weight loss and metabolic syndrome. Lipids in Health and Disease 2006;5(24):1-7.

Oben J, Enonchong E, Kothari S, Chambliss W, Garrison R, Dolnick D. *Phellodendron* and *Citrus* extracts benefit cardiovascular health in osteoarthritis patients: a double-blind, placebo-controlled pilot study. Nutrition Journal 2008;7(16):1-8.

Oben JE, Ngondi JL, Momo CN, Agbor GA, Sobgui CSM. The use of *Cissus quadrangularis/Irvingia gabonensis* combination in the management of weight loss: a double-blind placebo-controlled study. Lipids in Health and Disease 2008;7(12):1-7.

Ochani PC, D´Mello P. Antioxidant and antihyperlipidemic activity of *Hibiscus sabdariffa* Linn. Leaves and calyces extracts in rats. Indian Journal of Experimental Biology 2009 Apr;47:276-282.

Ochiai M, Hayashi T, Morita M, Ina K, Maeda M, Watanabe F, Morishita K. Short-term effects of L-citrulline supplementation on arterial stiffness in middle-aged men. International Journal of Cardiology 2012;155:257-261.

O'Dea K. Marked improvement in carbohydrate and lipid metabolism in diabetic Australian aborigines after temporary reversion to traditional lifestyle. Diabetes 1984 Jun;33(6):596-603.

Odetola AA, Iranloye YO, Akinloye O. Hypolipidaemic Potentials of *Solanum melongena* and *Solanum gilo* on Hypercholesterolemic Rabbits. Pakistan Journal of Nutrition 2004; 3(3):180-187.

Ofem OE, Eno AE, Imoru J, Nkanu E, Unoh F, Ibu JO. Effect of crude aqueous leaf extract of *Viscum album* (mistletoe) in hypertensive rats. Indian J Pharmacol 2007 Feb;39(1):15-19.

Ogawa A, Suzuki Y, AoyamaT, Takeuchi H. Dietary alpha-linolenic acid inhibits angiotensin-converting enzyme activity and mRNA expression levels in the aorta of spontaneously hypertensive rats. J Oleo Sci. 2009;58(7):355-60.

Ogawa A, Suzuki Y, Aoyama T, Takeuchi H. Effect of dietary alpha-linolenic acid on vascular reactivity in aorta of spontenously hypertensive rats. J Oleo Sci. 2009;58(5):221-5.

Ogawa H, Watanabe K, Mitsunaga T, Meguro T. Effect of Quinoa on Blood Pressure and Lipid Metabolism in Diet-induced Hyperlipidemic Spontaneously Hypertensive Rats (SHR). Nippon Eiyo Shokuryo Gakkaishi 2001;54(4):221-227.

Ogawa H, Nakashima S, Baba K. Effects of dietary *Angelica keiskei* on lipid metabolism in stroke-prone spontaneously hypertensive rats. Clinical and Experimental Pharmacology and Physiology 2003 Apr;30(4):284-288.

Ogawa H, Nakamura R, Baba K. Beneficial effect of laserpitin, a coumarin compound from *Angelica keiskei,* on lipid metabolism in stroke-prone spontaneously hypertensive rats. Clinical and Experimental Pharmacology and Physiology 2005 Dec;32(12): 1104-1109.

Ogawa H, Ohno M, Baba K. Hypotensive and lipid regulatory actions of 4-hydroxyderricin, a chalcone from *Angelica keiskei,* in stroke-prone spontaneously hypertensive rats. Clinical and Experimental Pharmacology and Physiology 2005 Jan;32(1-2):19-23.

Ogawa H, Okada Y, Kamisako T, Baba K. Beneficial effect of xanthoangelol, a chalcone compound from Angelica keiskei, on lipid metabolism in stroke-prone spontaneously hypertensive rats. Clin Exp Pharmacol Physiol. 2007 Mar;34(3):238-43.

Ogawa M, Takahara A, Ishijima M, Tazaki S. Decrease of plasma sulfur amino acids in essential hypertension. Japanese Circulation Journal 1985 Dec;49:1217-1224.

Ogawa N, Satsu H, Watanabe H, Fukaya M, Tsukamoto Y, Miyamoto Y, Shimizu M. Acetic Acid Suppresses the Increase in Disaccharidase Activity That Occurs during Culture of Caco-2 Cells. J Nutr 2000 Mar;130(3):507-513.

Ohtsuki K, Abe A, Mitsuzuwi H, Kondo M, Uemura K, Iwasaki Y, Kondo Y. Effects of long-term administration of hesperidin and glucosyl hesperidin to spontaneously hypertensive rats. J Nutr Sci Vitaminol (Tokyo) 2002 Oct;48(5):420-2.

Okamoto K, Iizuka Y, Murakami T, Miyake H, Suzuki T. Effects of chlorella alkali extract on blood pressure in SHR. Jpn Heart J 1978 Jul;19(4):622-3.

Olivieri O, Negri M, De Gironcoli M, Bassi A, Guarini P, Stanzial AM, Grigolini L, Ferrari S, Corrocher R. Effects of dietary fish oil on malondialdehyde production and glutathione peroxidase activity in hyperlipidaemic patients. Scand J Cli Lab Invest 1998;48:659-665.

Olszewski AJ, Szostak WB, Bialkowska M, Rudnicki S, McCully KS. Reduction of plasma lipid and homocysteine levels of pyridoxine, folate, cobalamin, choline, riboflavin, and troxerutin in atherosclerosis. Atherosclerosis 1989;75:1-6.

Omujal F, Nnambwayo J, Agwaya MS, Tumusiime RH, Ogwang PE, Katuura E, Nalika N, Nambatya GK. Bioactive components in indigenous African vegetables. Presented in the International Symposium on Biodiversity and Sustainable Diets: United Against Hunger: FAO Headquarters, Rome Italy 2010 November.

Onuegbu AJ, Olisekodiaka JM, Onibon MO, Adesiyan AA, Igbeneghu CA. Consumption of soymilk lowers atherogenic lipid fraction in healthy individuals. J Med Food 2011 Mar;14(3):257-60.

Orozco-Gutiérrez JJ, Castillo-Martinez L, Orea-Tejeda A, Vázquez-Diaz O, Valdespino-Trejo A, Narváez-David R, Keirns-Davis C, Carrasco-Ortiz O, Navarro-Navarro A, Sánchez-Santillan R. Effect of L-arginine or L-citrulline oral supplementation on blood pressure and right ventricular function in heart failure patients with preserved ejection fraction. Cardiology Journal 2010;17(6): 612-618.

Overton PD, Furlonger N, Beety JM, Chakraborty J, Tredger JA, Morgan LM. The effects of dietary sugar-beet fibre and guar gum on lipid metabolism in Wistar rats. Br J Nutr. 1994 Sep;72(3):385-95.

Owoyele BV, Alabi OT, Adebayo JO, Soladoye AO, Abioye AIR, Jimoh SA. Haematological evaluation of ethanolic extract of *Alliu ascalonicum* in male albino rats. Fitoterapia 2004;75:322-326.

Owoyele BV, Yakubu MT, Alonge F, Olatunji LA, Soladoye AO. Effects of Folic Acid Intake on Serum Lipid Profiles of Apparently Healthy Young Adult Male Nigerians. African Journal of Biomedical Research 2005;8:139-142.

Pakdeechote P, Kukongviriyapan U, Berkban W, Prachaney P, Kukongviriyapan V, Nakmareong S. Mentha cordifolia extract inhibits the development of hypertension in L-NAME-induced hypertensive rats. Journal of Medicinal Plant Research 2011 Apr;5(7):1175-1183.

Pal RK, Manoj J. Hepatoprotective activity of alcoholic and aqueous extracts of fruits of *Luffa cylindrica* Linn in rats. Annals of Biological Research 2011;2(1):132-141.

Pal S, Ellis V, Dhaliwal S. Effects of whey protein isolate on body composition, lipids, insulin and glucose in overweight and obese individuals. Br J Nutr. 2010 Sep;104(5);716-23.

Pal S, Ellis V. The chronic effects of whey proteins on blood pressure, vascular function, and inflammatory markers in overweight individuals. Obesity (Silver Spring) 2010 Jul;18(7):1354-9.

Pan A, Yu D, Demark-Wahnefried W, Franco OH, Lin X. Meta-analysis of the effecs of flaxseed interventions on blood lipids. Am J Clin Nutr. 2009 Aug;90(2):288-97.

Pan Z, Zhao L, Guo D, Yang R, Xu C Wu X. Effects of oral calcium supplementation on blood pressure in population. Zhonghua Yu Fang Yi Xue Za Zhi 2000 Mar;34(2):109-12.

Panossian A, Wikman G. Pharmacology of *Schisandra chinensis* Bail: An overview of Russian research and uses in medicine. Journal of Ethnopharmacology 2008;118:183-212.

Paoli A, Cenci L, Grimaldi KA. Effect of ketogenic Mediterranean diet with phytoextracts and low carbohydrates/high-protein meals on weight, cardiovascular risk factors, body composition and diet compliance in Italian council employees. Nutr J. 2011 Oct 12;10:112.

Papandreou D, Malindretos P, Arvanitidou M, Makedou A, Rousso I. Homocysteine lowering with folic acid supplements in children: Effects on blood pressure. International Journal of Food Sciences and Nutrition 2010 Feb;61(1):11-17.

Paradisi G, Cucinelli F, Mele MC, Barini A, Lanzone A, Caruso A. Endothelial function in post-menopausal women: effect of folic acid supplementation. Human Reproduction 2004;19(4):1031-1035.

Paran E, Novack V, Engelhard YN, Hazan-Halevy I. The effects of natural antioxidants from tomato extract in treated but uncontrolled hypertensive patients. Cardiovasc Drugs Ther. 2009 Apr;23(2):145-51.

Park HJ, Lee YJ, Ryu HK, Kim MH, Chung HW, Kim WY. A randomized double-blind, placebo-controlled study to establish the effects of spirulina in elderly Koreans. Ann Nutr Meta 2008;52(4):322-8.

Park JH, Kim HW, Kim YC, Choi EC, Kim BK. Studies on antihypertensive components of *G. lucidum* in Korea. Korean J. Food Hyg. 1987;2:57-65.

Park KO, Ito Y, Nagasawa T, Choi MR, Nishizawa N. Effects of Dietary Korean Proso-Millet Protein on Plasma Adiponectin, HDL Cholesterol, Insulin Levels, and Gene Expression in Obese Type 2 Diabetic Mice. Biosci. Biotechnol. Biochem. 2008;72(11): 2918-2925.

Park SA, Choi MS, Kim MJ, Jung UJ, Kim HJ, Park KK, Noh HJ, Park HM, Park YB, Lee JS, Lee MK. Hypoglycemic ad hypolipidemic action of Du-zhong *(Eucommia ulmoides* Oliver) leaves water extract in C57BL/KsJ-*db/db* mice. Journal of Ethnopharmacology 2006;107:412-417.

Park T, Lee K. Dietary taurine supplementation reduces plasma and liver cholesterol and triglyceride levels in rats fed a high-cholesterol or a cholesterol-free diet. Adv Exp Med Biol. 1998;442:319-25.

Park T, Oh J, Lee K. Dietary Taurine or Glycine supplementation reduces plasma and liver cholesterol and triglyceride concentrations in rats fed a cholesterol-free diet. Nutrition Research 1999;19(2):1777-1789.

Park Y, Kwon HY, Shimi MK, Rhyu MR, Lee Y. Improved lipid profile in ovariectomized rats by red ginseng extract. Pharmazie 2011 Jun;66(6):450-3.

Park YK, Kim J-S, Kang M-H. Concord grape juice supplementation reduces blood pressure in Korean hypertensive men: Double-blind, placebo controlled intervention trial. BioFactors 2004;22(1-4):145-147.

Park YS, Cha MH, Yoon YS, Ahn HS. Effect of Low Calorie Diet and *Platycodon Grandiflorum* Extract on Fatty Acid Biding Protein Expression in Rats with Diet-induced Obesity. Nutritional Sciences 2005 Feb;8(1):3-9.

Park YS, Yoon Y, Ahn HS. *Platycodon grandiflorum* extract represses up-regulated adipocyte fatty acid binding protein triggered by a high fat feeding in obese rats. World J Gastroenterol 2007 Jul;13(25):3493-3499.

Park YS, Leontowicz H, Leontowicz M, Namiesnik J, Libman ACI, Tashma Z, Katrich E, Gorinstein S. Characteristics of Blond and Red Star Ruby Jaffa Grapefruits *(Citrus paradisi)*: Results of the Studies in Vitro, in Vivo and on Patients Suffering from Atherosclerosis. Proc. II IS on Human Health Effects of F&V 2009:137-143.

Parmar HS, Kar A. Antiperoxidative, antithyroidal, antihyperglycemic and cardioprotective role of Citrus sinensis peel extract in male mice. Phytother Res. 2008 Jun;22(6):791-5.

Parmar HS, Kar A. Protective role of Mangifera indica, Cucumis melo and Citrullus vulgaris peel extracts in chemically induced hypothyroidism. Chem Biol Interact. 2009 Feb 12;177(3):254-8.

Paschos GK, Magkos F, Panagiotakos DB, Votteas V, Zampelas A. Dietary supplementation with flaxseed oil lowers blood pressure in dyslipidaemic patients. European Journal of Clinical Nutrition 2007:1-6.

Paśko P, Zagrodzki P, Bartoń H, Chlopicka J, Gorinstein S. Effect of Quinoa Seeds *(Chenopodium quinoa)* in Diet on some Biochemical Parameters and Essential Elements in Blood of High Fructose-Fed Rats. Plant Foods Hum Nutr 2010;65:333-338.

Patade A, Devareddy L, Lucas EA, Korlagunta K, Daggy BP, Arjmandi BH. Flaxseed reduces total and LDL cholesterol concentrations in Native American postmenopausal women. J Womens Health (Larchmt) 2008 Apr;17(3):355-66.

Patel J, Goyal R, Bhatt P. Beneficial effecs of levo-carnitine on lipid metabolism and cardiac function in neonatal streptozotocin rat model of diabetes. Int J Diabetes & Metabolism 2008;16:29-34.

Patel SS, Verma NK, Shrestha B, Gauthaman K. Antihypertensive effect of methanolic extract of *Passiflora nepalensis*. Rev. bras. farmacogn. 2011;21(1)

Patel U, Kulkarni M, Undale V, Bhosale A. Evaluation of Diuretic Activity of Aqueous and Methanol Extracts of *Lepidium sativum* Garden Cress (Cruciferae) in Rats. Tropical Journal of Pharmaceutical Research 2009 Jun;8(3):215-219.

Patil RH, Prakash K, Maheshwari VL. Hypolipidemic effect of Terminalia arjuna (L.) in experimentally induced hypercholesteremic rats. Acta Biologica Szegediensis 2011;552(2):289-293.

Pecháňová O, Zicha J, Kojšová S, Dobešová Z, Jendeková L, Kuneš J. Effect of chronic N-acetylcysteine treatment on the development of spontaneous hypertension. Clinical Science 2006;110:235-242.

Pecháňová O, Jendeková L, Vranková S. Effect of chronic apocynin treatment on nitric oxide and reactive oxygen species production in borderline and spontaneous hypertension. Pharmacol Rep. 2009 Jan – Feb;61(1):116-22.

Pérez Méndez O, Garcia Hernández L. High-density lipoproteins (HDL) size and composition are modified in the rat by a diet supplemented with "Hass" avocade (Persea americana Miller). Arch Cardiol Mex. 2007 Jan – Mar;77(1):17-24.

Perez SC, Vianna LM. Favorable effects of pyridoxine and folic acid supplementation of shr-sp. Arch Neurocien (Mex) 2005;10(3):146-149.

Pérez-Guisado J, Muñoz-Serrano A, Alonso-Moraga A. Spanish Ketogenic Mediterranean Diet: a healthy cardiovascular diet for weight loss. Nutr J. 2008 Oct 26;7:30.

Perez YY. Jimenez-Ferrer E. Alonso D, Botello-Amaro CA, Zamilpa A. *Citrus limetta* leaves extract antagonizes the hypertensive effect of angiotensin II. Journal of Ethnopharmacology 2010;128:611-614.

Perez-Vizcaino F, Duarte J, Jimenez R, Santos-Buelga C, Osuna A. Antihypertensive effects of the flavonoid quercetin. Pharmacological Reports 2009;61:67-75.

Perona JS, Cañizares J, Montero E, Sánchez-Dominguez JM, Catalá A, Ruiz-Gutiérrez V. Virgin olive oil reduces blood pressure in hypertensive elderly subjects. Clinical Nutrition 2004;23:1113-1121.

Perrinjaquet-Moccetti T, Busjahn A, Schmidlin C, Schmidt A, Bradl B, Aydogan C. Food supplementation with an olive (Olea europaea L.) leaf extract reduces blood pressure in borderline hypertensive monozygotic twins. Phytother Res. 2008 Sep;22(9):1239-42.

Persson IA, Josefsson M, Persson K, Andersson RG. Tea flavonoids inhibit angiotensin-converting enzyme activity and increase nitric oxide production in human endothelial cells. J Pharm Pharmacol. 2006 Aug;58(8):1139-44.

Persson IA, Persson K, Hägg S, Andersson RG. Effects of cocoa extract and dark chocolate on angiotensin-converting enzyme and nitric oxide in human endothelial cells and healthy volunteers – a nutrigenomics perspective. J Cardiovasc Pharmacol 2011 Jan;57(1):44-50.

Persson IAL, Dong L, Persson K. Effect of *Panax ginseng* extract (G115) on angiotensin-converting enzyme (ACE) activity and nitric oxide (NO) production. Journal of Ethnopharmacology 2006;105:321-325.

Persson IAL, Persson K, Andersson RGG. Effect of *Vaccinium myrtillus* and its Polyphenols on Angiotensin-Converting Enzyme Activity in Human Endothelial Cells. J. Agric. Food Chem. 2009;57(11):4626-4629.

Persson IAL, Persson K, Hägg S, Andersson RGG. Effects of green tea, black tea and Rooibos tea on angiotensin-converting enzyme and nitric oxide in healthy volunteers. Public Health Nutrition 2010;13(5):730-737.

Peterson JJ, Beecher GR, Bhagwat SA, Dwyer JT, Gebhardt SE, Haytowitz DB, Holden JM. Flavanones in grapefruit, lemons, and limes: A compilation and review of the data from the analytical literature. Journal of Food Composition and Analysis 2006;19: 74-80.

Petit PR, Sauvaire YD, Hillaire-Buys DM, Leconte OM, Baissac YG, Ponsin GR, Ribes GR. Steroid saponins from fenugreek seeds: extraction, purification, and pharmacological investigation on feeding behavior and plasma cholesterol. Steroids 1995 Oct;60(10):674-80.

Pfeifer M, Begerow B, Minne HW, Nachtigall D, Hansen C. Effects of short-term vitamin D(3) and calcium supplementation on blood pressure and parathyroid hormone levels in elderly women. J Clin Endocrinol Metab 2001 Apr;86(4):1633-7.

Pfeuffer M, Auinger A, Bley U, Kraus-Stojanowic I, Laue C, Winkler P, Rüfer CE, Frank J, Bösch-Saadatmandi C, Rimbach G, Schrezenmeir J. Effect of quercetin on traits of the metabolic syndrome, endothelial function and inflammatory parameters in men with different APOE isoforms. Nutr Metab Cardiovasc Dis 2011 Nov 23.

Phillips OA, Mathew KT, Oriowo MA. Antihypertensive and vasodilator effects of methanolic and aqueous extracts of *Tribulus terrestris* in rats. Journal of Ethnopharmacology 2006;104:351-355.

Phillipson BE, Rothrock DW, Connor WE, Harris WS, Illingworth DR. Reduction of plasma lipids, lipoproteins, and apoproteins by dietary fish oils in patients with hypertriglyceridemia. N Engl J Med 1985 May 9;312(19):1210-6.

Pihlanto A, Akkanen S, Korhonen HJ. ACE-inhibitory and antioxidant properties of potato *(Solanum tuberosum).* Food Chemistry 2008;109:104-112.

Pinto MS, de Carvalho JE, Lajolo FM, Genovese MI, Shetty K. Evaluation of antiproliferative, anti-type 2 diabetes, and antihypertension potentials of ellagitannins from strawberries (Fragaria x ananassa Duch.) using in vitro models. J Med Food 2010 Oct;13(5):1027-35.

Pittaway JK, Ahuja KD, Cehun M, Chronopoulos A, Robertson IK, Nestel PJ, Ball MJ. Dietary supplementation with chickpeas for at least 5 weeks results in small but significant reductions in serum total and low-density lipoprotein cholesterols in adult women and men. Ann Nutr Metab 2006;50(6):512-8.

Pittaway JK, Ahuja KD, Robertson IK, Ball MJ. Effects of a controlled diet supplemented with chickpeas on serum lipids, glucose tolerance, satiety and bowel function. J Am Coll Nutr 2007 Aug;26(4):334-40.

Porteri E, Rizzoni D, De Ciuceis C, Boari GEM, Platto C, Pilu A, Miclini M, Rosei CA, Bulgari G, Rosei EA. Vasodilator Effects of Red Wines in Subcutaneous Small Resistance Artery of Patients With Essential Hypertension. American Journal of Hypertension 2010 Apr;23(4):373-378.

Potter AS, Foroudi S, Stamatikos A, Patil BS, Deyhim F. Drinking carrot juice increases total antioxidant status and decreases lipid peroxidation in adults. Nutr J 2011 Sep 24;10:96.

Poudyal H, Panchal S, Brown L. Comparison of purple carrot juice and B-carotene in a high-carbohydrate, high-fat diet-fed rat model of the metabolic syndrome. Br J Nutr. 2010 Nov;104(9):1322-32.

Prakash P, Glupta N. Therapeutic uses of *Ocimum sanctum linn* (Tulsi) with a note on eugenol and its pharmacological actions: a short review. Indian J Physiol Pharmacol 2005;49(2):125-131.

Pramanik T, Sharma HO, Mishra S, Mishra A, Prajapati R, Singh S. Immediate effect of slow pace bhastrika pranayama on blood pressure and heart rate. J Altern Complement Med. 2009 Mar;15(3):293-5.

Pramanik T, Pudasaini B, Prajapati R. Immediate effect of a slow pace breathing exercise *Bhramari pranayama* on blood pressure and heart rate. Nepal Med Coll J 2010;12(3):154-157.

Prasad K, Mantha SV, Muir AD, Westcott ND. Reduction of hypercholesterolemic atherosclerosis by CDC-flaxseed with very low alpha-linolenic acid. Atherosclerosis 1998 Feb;136(29.367-75.

Prasad K. Reduction of serum cholesterol and hypercholesterolemic atherosclerosis in rabbits by secoisolariciresinol diglucoside isolated from flaxseed. Circulation 1999 Mar 16;99(10):1355-62.

Prasad K. Antihypertensive Activity of Secoisolariciresinol Diglucoside (SDG) Isolated from Flaxseed: Role of Guanylate Cyclase. International Journal of Angiology 2004;13(1):7-14.

Prasad K. Hypocholesterolemic and antiatherosclerotic effect of flax lignan complex isolated from flaxseed. Atherosclerosis 2005 Apr;179(2):269-75.

Preuss HG, Wallerstedt D, Talpur N, Tutuncuoglu SO, Echard B, Myers A, Bui M, Bagchi D. Effects of niacin-bound chromium and grape seed proanthocyanidin extract on the lipid profile of hypercholesterolemic subjects: a pilot study. J Med 2000;31(5-6): 227-46.

Preuss HG, Clouatre D, Mohamadi A, Jarrell ST. Wild garlic has a greater effect than regular garlic on blood pressure and blood chemistries of rats. Int Urol Nephrol 2001;32(4):525-30.

Preuss HG, Echard B, Polansky MM, Anderson R. Whole Cinnamon and Aqueous Extracts Ameliorate Sucrose-Induced Blood Pressure Elevations in Spontaneously Hypertensive Rats. Journal of the American College of Nutrition 2006;25(2):144-150.

Preuss HG, Echard B, Bagchi D, Perricone NV. Maitake Mushroom Extracts Ameliorate Progressive Hypertension and Other Chronic Metabolic Perturbations in Aging Female Rats. International Journal of Medical Sciences 2010;7(4):169-180.

Press RI, Geller J, Evans GW. The effect of chromium picolinate on serum cholesterol and apolipoprotein fractions in human subjects. West J Med. 1990 Jan;152(1):41-5.

Przygodda F, Martins ZN, Castaldelli APA, Minella TV, Vieira LP, Cantelli K, Fronza J, Padoin MJ. Effect of erva-mate (*Ilex paraguariensis* A. St.-Hil., Aquifoliaceae) on serum cholesterol, triacylglycerides and glucose in Wistar rats fed a diet supplemented with fat and sugar. Brazilian Journal of Pharmacognosy 2010;20(6):956-961.

Puddley IB, Beilin LJ. Alcohol is bad for blood pressure. Clin Exp Pharmacol Physiol 2006 Sep;33(9):847-52.

Puglisi MJ, Vaishnav U, Shrestha S, Torres-Gonzalez M, Wood RJ, Volek JS, Fernandez ML. Raisins and additional walking have distinct effects on plasma lipids and inflammatory cytokines. Lipids in Health and Disease 2008;7(14):1-9.

Purvis JR, Cummings DM, Landsman P, Carroll R, Barakat H, Bray J, Whitley C, Horner RD. Effect of Oral Magnesium Supplementation on Selected Cardiovascular Risk Factors in Non-Insulin-Dependent Diabetics. Archives of Family Medicine 1994 Jun; Vol. 3 (6):503-508.

Puska P. Fat and heart disease: yes we can make a change – the case of North Karelia (Finland). Ann Nutr Metab 2009;54(1):33-8.

Qin W, Zhiping T, Haidan L, Lei G, Sijie W, Jinwen L, Weizhi Z, Tianli Z, Jiefeng Y, Xinhua X. Chemical characterization of *Auricularia auricula* polysaccharides and its pharmcological effect on heart antioxidant enzyme activities and left ventricular function in aged mice. International Journal of Biological Macromolecules 2010;46:284-288.

Quiñones M, Miguel M, Muguerza B, Aleixandre A. Effect of a cocoa polyphenol extract in spontaneously hypertensive rats. Food Funct. 2011 Nov 3;11:649-53.

Qureshi AA, Sami SA, Salser WA, Khan FA. Dose-dependent suppression of serum cholesterol by tocotrienol-rich fraction (TRF25) of rice bran in hypercholesterolemic humans. Atherosclerosis 2002 Mar;161(1):199-207.

Raghuraj P, Telles S. Immediate effect of specific nostril manipulatig yoga breathing practices on autonomic and respiratory variables. Appl Psychophysiol Biofeedback 2008 Jun;33(2):65-75.

Rajasekaran S, Kasiappan R, Sivagnanam K, Subramanian S. Benefical Effects of Aloevera leaf gel extract on lipid profile status in rats with streptozotocin diabetes. Clinical and Experimental Pharmacology and Physiology 2006;33:232-237.

Raji IA, Mugabo P, Obikeze K. Effect of *Tulbaghia violacea* on the blood pressure and heart rate in male spontaneously hypertensive Wistar rats. Journal of Ethnopharmacology 2012.

Ram A, Lauria P, Gupta R, Sharma VN. Hypolipidaemic effect of *Myristica fragrans* fruit extract in rabbits. J Ethnopharmacol 1996 Dec;55(1):49-53.

Ram B, Singh, Shanti S, Rastogi, Reema Singh, Saraswati Ghosh, Mohammad A. Niaz. Effects of guava intake on serum total and high-density lipoprotein cholesterol levels and on systemic blood pressure. The American Journal of Cardiology 1992 Nov;70(15):1287-1291.

Ramel A, Martinez JA, Kiely M, Bandarra NM, Thorsdottir I. Moderate consumption of fatty fish reduces diastolic blood pressure in overweight and obese European young adults during energy restriction. Nutrition 2010;26:168-174.

Ramesa S, Baijnath H, Govender T, Mackraj I. Angotensin I-converting enzyme inhibitor activity of nutritive plants in KwaZulu-Natal. Journal of Medicinal Food. 2008 Jun;11(2):331-336.

Rangineni V, Sharada D, Saxena S. Diuretic, Hypotensive, and Hypocholesterolemic Effects of *Eclipta alba* in Mild Hypertensive Subjects: A Pilot Study. Journal of Medicina Food 2007 Mar; 10(1):143-148.

Ranilla LG, Kwon YI, Apostolidis E, Shetty K. Phenolic compounds, antioxidant activity and *in vitro* inhibitory potential against key enzymes relevant for hyperglycemia and hypertenson of commonly used medicinal plants, herbs and spices in Latin America. Bioresource Technology 2010;101:4676-4689.

Rao NM. Angiotensin converting enzyme inhibitors from ripened and unripened bananas. Current Science 1999;76:86-88.

Rasool AH, Yuen KH, Yusoff K, Wong AR, Rahman AR. Dose dependent elevaton of plasma tocotrienol levels and its effect on arterial compliance, plasma total antioxidant status, and lipid profile in healthy humans supplemented with tocotrienol rich vitamin E. J Nutr. Sci. Vitaminol (Tokyo) 2006 Dec;52(6):473-8.

Rastopchin IP. Effect of calcium pangamate on the cholesterol index of atherogenicity in cerebral arteriosclerosis patients. Zh Nevropatol Psikhiatr Im S S Korsakova 1984;84(7):1020-3.

Rauchová H, Dobešová Z, Drahota Z, Zicha J, Kuneš J. The effect of chronic L-carnitine treatment on blood pressure and plasma lipids in spontaneously hypertensive rats. European Journal of Pharmacology 1998;342:235-239.

Reddy DBS, Kumar R, Bharavi K, Venkateswarlu U. Hypolipidemic Activity of Methanolic Extract of *Terminalia arjuna* Leaves in Hyperlipidemic Rat Models. Research Journal of Medical Sciences 2011;5(3):172-175.

Ren LK, Vasil'ev AV, Orekhov AN, Tertov VV, Tutel'ian VA. Anti-atherosclerotic properties of higher mushrooms (a clinico-experimental investigation). Vopr Pitan 1989 Jan-Feb;1:16-9.

Ren Y, Li Y, Zhao Y, Yu F, Zhan Z, Yuan Y, Yang J. Effects of resveratrol on lipid metabolism in C57BL/6J mice. Wei Sheng Yan Jiu. 2011 Jul;40(4):495-7.

Reshef N, Hayari Y, Goren C, Boaz M, Madar Z, Knobler H. Antihypertensive Effect of Sweetie Fruit in Patients With Stage I Hypertension Antihypertensive Effect of Sweetie Fruit in Patients With Stage I Hypertension. American Journal of Hypertension 2005 Oct;18:1360-1363.

Rhyu MR, Kim EY, Yoon BK, Lee YJ, Chen SN. Aqueous extract of *Schizandra chinensis* fruit causes endothelium-dependent and -independent relaxation of isolated rat thoracic aorta. Phytotmedicine 2006;13:651-657.

Ried K, Frank OR, Stocks NP, Fakler P, Sullivan T. Effect of garlic on blood pressure: a sysematic review and meta-analysis. BMC Cardiovasc Discord 2008 Jun 16;8:13.

Ried K, Frank OR, Stocks NP. Aged garlic extract lowers blood pressure in patients with treated but uncontrolled hypertension: A randomized conrolled trial. Maturias 2010;67:144-150.

Ried K, Fakler P. Protective effect of lycopene on serum cholesterol and blood pressure: Meta-analyses of intervention trials. Maturitas 2011 Apr;68(4):299-310.

Rietz B, Isensee H, Strobach H, Makdessi S, Jacob R. Cardioprotective actions of wild garlic (allium ursinum) in ischema and reperfusion. Mol Cell Biochem. 1993 Feb 17;119(1-2):143-50.

Rimando AM, Perkins-Veazie PM. Determination of citrulline in watermelon rind. J Chromatogr A. 2005 Jun 17;1078(1-2):196-200.

Rimm EB, Williams P, Fosher K, Criqui M, Stampfer MJ. Moderate alcohol intake and lower risk of coronary heart disease: meta-analysis of effects on lipids and haemostatic factors. BMJ 1999 Dec 11;319(7224):1523-8.

Rivas M, Garay RP, Escanero JF, Cia P Jr, Cia P, Alda JO. Soy milk lowers blood pressure in men and women with mild to moderate essential hypertension. J Nutr. 2002 Jul;132(7):1900-2.

Rivera L, Morón R, Zarzuelo A, Galisteo M. Long-term resveratrol administration reduces metabolic disturbances and blood pressure in obese Zucker rats. Biochem Pharmacol 2009 Mar 15;77(6):1053-63.

Rizvi K, Hampson JP, Harvey JN. Do lipid-lowering drugs cause erectile dysfunction? A systematic review. Fam Pract. 2002 Feb;19(1):95-8.

Roberts KT. The Potential of Fenugreek (Trigonella foenum-graecum) as a Functional Food and Nutraceutical and Its Effects on Glycemia and Lipidemia. J Med Food 2011 Dec;14(12):1485-9.

Robich MP, Chu LM, Chaudray M, Nezafat R, Han Y, Clements RT, Laham RJ, Manning WJ, Coady MA, Sellke FW. Anti-angiogenic effect of high-dose resveratrol in swine model of metabolic syndrome. Surgery 2010 Aug;148(2):453-62.

Robinson M, Lu B, Kappagoda T. Effect of Grape Seed Extract in Subjects with Pre-Hypertension. 13th World congress on heart disease, Vancouver, B.C. Canada, July 28-31,2007:239-242.

Rodriguez L, Muñoz del Rio P, Vela AC. Acción hipocolesterolémia de la caigua (Cyclantera pedata). Hemero Médica 1987;1:4-5.

Roghani M, Khalili M, Baluchnejadmojarad, Aghaie M, Ansari F, Sharayeli M. Effect of oral feeding of *Allium schoenoprasum L.* on blood glucose and lipid level in diabetic Rats. Journal of Gorgan University of Medical Sciences 2010;12(1):9-14.

Roghani-Dehkordi F, Kamkhah AF. Artichoke Leaf Juice Contains Antihypertensive Effect in Patients With Mild Hypertension. Journal of Dietary Supplements 2009 Dec;6(4):328-341.

Rojas J, Ronceros S, Palomino R. Efecto antihipertensivo y dosis letal 50 del jugo del fruto y del etracto etanólico de las hojas de *Passiflora edulis* (maracuyá), en ratas. An. Fac. Med. 2006 jul – sep;67(3):206-213.

Rojas J, Ronceros S, Palomino R, Salas M, Azañero R, Cruz H, Rojas A, Asmat J, Tam J. Efecto coadyuvante del extracto liofilizado de *Passiflora edulis* (maracuyá) en la reducción de la presión arterial en pacientes tratados con enalapril. An Fac med. 2009;70(2):103-8.

Romano M, Vacante M, Cristaldi E, Colonna V, Gargante MP, Cammalleri L, Malaguarnera M. L-carnitine treatment reduces steatosis in patients with chronic hepatitis C treated with alpha-interferon and ribavirin. Dig Dis Sci 2008 Apr;53(4):1114-21.

Roopesh C, Salomi KR, Nagarjuna S, Reddy YP. Diuretic activity of methanolic and ethanolic extracts of *Centella asiatica* leaves in rats. International Research Journal of Pharmacy 2011;2(11):163-165.

Ros E, Núñez I, Pérez-Heras A, Serra M, Gilabert R, Casals E, Deulofeu R. A walnut diet improves endothelial function n hypercholesterolemic subjects: a randomized crossover trial. Circulation. 2004 Apr 6;109(13):1609-14.

Rosa CO, Costa NM, Nunes RM, Leal PF. The cholesterol-lowering effect of black, carioquinha and red beans (Phaseolus vulgaris, L.) in hypercholesterolemic rats. Arch Latinoam Nutr. 1998 Dec;48(4):306-10.

Rosario LSM, Alvarado-Ortiz UCE. Efecto de la Caigua (Cyclantera pedata) Liofilizada y Encapsulada sobre lo niveles de Colesterolemia en sujetos varones entre 40 y 65 años. Horizonte medico 1997:1(2)

Rouse IL, Beilin LJ, Armstrong BK, Vandongen R. Blood-pressure-lowering effect of a vegetarian diet: controlled trial in normotensive subjects. Lancet 1983 Jan 1;1(8314-5):5-10.

Roza JM, Xian-Liu Z, Guthrie N. Effect of citrus flavonoids and tocotrienols on serum cholesterol levels in hypercholesterolemic subjects. Alternative therapies 2007;13(6):44-48.

Rui Y-C. Advances in pharmacological studies of silymarin. Mem. Inst. Oswaldo Cruz 1991;86(2):79-85.

Ruiz-Gutiérrez V, Muriana FJ, Guerrero A, Cert AM, Villar J. Plasma lipids, erythrocyte membrane lipids and blood pressure of hypertensive women after ingestion of dietary oleic acid from two different sources. J Hypertens. 1996 Dec;14(12):1483-90.

Ruiz-Roso B, Quintela JC, de la Fuente E, Haya J, Pérez-Olleros L. Insoluble carob fiber rich in polyphenols lowers total and LDL cholesterol in hypercholesterolemic subjects. Plant Foods Hum Nutr 2010 Mar;65 (1):50-6.

Ruggenenti P, Cattaneo D, Loriga G, Ledda F, Motterlini N, Gherardi G, Orisio S, Remuzzi G. Ameliorating hypertension and insulin resistance in subjects at increased cardiovascular risk: effects of acetyl-L-carnitine therapy. Hypertension 2009 Sep;54(3).567-74.

Rumberger JA, Napolitano J, Azumano I, Kamiya T, Evans M. Pantethine, a derivate of vitamin B_5 used as a nutritional supplement, favorably alters low-density lipoprotein cholesterol metabolism in low- to moderate-cardiovascular risk North American subjects; a triple-blinded placebo and diet-controlled investigation. Nutrition Research 2011;31:608-615.

Ruzaidi A, Amin I, Nawalyah AG, Hamid M, Faizul HA. The effect of Malaysian cocoa extract on glucose levels and lipid profles in diabetic rats. Journal of Ethnopharmacology 2005;98:55-60.

Sá CM, Ramos AA, Azevedo MF, Lime CF, Fernandes-Ferreira M, Pereira-Wilson C. Sage Tea Drinking Improves Lipid Profile and Antioxidant Defences in Humans. Int. J. Mol. Sci. 2009;10:3937-3950.

Sabitha V, Ramachandran S, Naveen KR, Panneerselvam K. Antidiabetic and antihyperlipidemic potential of *Abelmoschus esculentus* (L.) Moench. in streptozotocin-induced diabetc rats. J Pharm Bioallied Sci 2011 Jul;3(3):397-402.

Sadeek EA, El-Razek FHA. The Chemo-Protective Effect of Turmeric, Chili, Cloves and Cardamom on Correcting Iron Overoad-Induced Liver Injury, Oxidative Stress and Serum Lipid Profile in Rat Models. Journal of American Science 2010;6(10):702-712.

Sagesaka-Mitane Y, Sugiura T, Miwa Y, Yamaguchi K, Kyuki K. Effect of tea-leaf saponin on blood pressure of spontaneously hypertensive rats. Yakugaku Zasshi 1996 May;116(5):388-95.

Saito I, Kawabe H, Hasegawa C, Iwaida Y, Yamakawa H, Saruta T, Takeshita E, Nagano S, Sekihara T. Effect of L-dopa in young patients with hypertension. Angiology 1991 Sep;42(9):691-5.

Saito K, Sano H, Furuta Y, Fukuzaki H. Effect of oral calcium on blood pressure response in salt-loaded borderline hypertensive patients. Hypertension 1989 Mar;13(3):219-26.

Sakai Y, Murakami T, Yamamoto Y. Antihypertensive Effects of Onion on NO Synthase Inhibitor-induced Hypertensive Rats and Spontaneously Hypertensive Rats. Biosci. Biotechnol. Biochem. 2003;67(6):1305-1311.

Saleem R, Faizi S, Siddiqui BS, Ahmed M, Hussain SA, Qazi A, Dar A, Ahmad SI, Qazi MH, Akhtar S, Hasnain SN. Hypotensive effect of chemical constituents from Aloe barbadensis. Planta Med 2001 Nov;67(8):757-60.

Saleem R, Ahmad M, Naz A, Siddiqui H, Ahmad SI, Faizi S. Hypotensive and toxicological study of citric acid and other constituents from Tagetes patula roots. Arch Pharm Res. 2004 Oct;27(10):1037-42.

Sales RL, Coelho SB, Costa NMB, Bressan J, Iyer S, Boateng LA, Lokko P, Mattes RD. The Effects of Peanut Oil and Lipid Profile of Normolipidemic Adults: A Three-country Collaborative Study. The Journal of Applied Research 2008;8(2):216-225.

Sallinen K, Arvola P, Wuorela H, Ruskoaho H, Vapaatalo H, Pörsti I. High calcium diet reduces blood pressure in exercised and nonexercised hypertensive rats. Am J Hypertens. 1996 Feb;9(2):144-56.

Samuels R, Mani UV, Iyer UM, Nayak US. Hypocholesterolemic effect of spirulina in patients with hyperlipidemic nephrotic syndrome. J Med Food 2002;5(2):91-6.

Sandhu JS, Shah B, Shenoy S, Chauhan S, Lavekar GS, Padhi MM. Effects of *Withania somnifera* (Ashwagandha) and *Terminalia arjuna* (Arjuna) on physical performance and cardiorespiratory endurance in healthy young adults. Int J Ayurveda Res. 2010 Jul – Sep;1(3):144-149.

Sankar D, Rao MR, Sambandam G, Pugalendi KV. Effect of Sesame Oil on Diuretcs or B-blockers in the Modulation of Blood Pressure, Anthropometry, Lipid Profile, and Redox Status. Yale Journal of Biology and Medicine 2006;79:19-26.

Sankar D, Ali A, Sambandam G, Rao R. Sesame oil exhibits synergistic effect with anti-diabetic medication in patients with type 2 diabetes mellitus. Clin Nutr. 2011 Jun;30(3):351-8.

Sano S, Sugiyama K, Ito T, Katano Y, Ishihata A. Identification of the strong vasorelaing substance scirpusin B, a dimer of piceatannol, from passion fruit (Passiflora edulis) seeds. J Agric Food Chem 2011 Jun 8;59(11):6209-13.

Sano T, Kumamoto Y, Kamiya N, Okuda M, Tanaka Y. Effect of lipophilic extract of Chlorella vulgaris on alimentary hyperlipidemia in cholesterol-fed rats. Artery 1988;15(4):217-24.

Sansawa H, Takahashi M, Tsuchikura S, Endo H. Effect of chlorella and its fractions on blood pressure, cerebral stroke lesions, and life-span in stroke-prone spontaneously hypertensive rats. J Nutr Sci Vitaminol (Tokyo) 2006 Dec;52(6):457-66.

Sarkar C, Bairy KL, Rao NM, Udupa EG. Effect of banana on cold stress test & peak expiratory flow rate in healthy volunteers. Indian J Med Res. 1999 Jul;110:27-9.

Sarr M, Chataigneau M, Martins S, Schott C, Bedoui JE, Oak MH, Muller B, Chataigneau T, Schini-Kerth VB. Red wine polyphenols prevent angiotensin II-induced hypertension and endothelial dysfunction in rats: Role of NADPH oxidase. Cardiovascular Research 2006;71:794-802.

Sato S, Mukai Y, Yamate J, Kato J, Kurasaki M, Hatai A, Sagai M. Effect of polyphenol-containing azuki bean (Vigna angularis) extract on blood pressure elevation and macrophage infiltration in the heart and kidney of spontaneously hypertensive rats. Clin Exp Pharmacol Physiol 2008 Jan;35(1):43-9.

Satoshi I, Kenji O, Yoshihito A, Hitoshi K. Effect of extracts squeezed from Agaricus blazei for high-normal blood pressure or mild hypertension on human blood pressure. Yakuri to chiryo 2006;34(12):1295-1309.

Sattanathan K, Dhanapal CK, Manavalan R. LDL lowering properties of rutin in diabetic patients. International Journal of Pharma and Bio Sciences 2010 Oct – Dec;1(4):467-473.

Sattanathan K, Dhanapal CK, Manavalan R. Antihypertensive and other Beneficial Health Effects of Rutin Supplementation in Diabetic Patients. Research Journal of Pharmaceutical, Biological and Chemical Science 2011 Jan – Mar;2(1):843-849.

Sattanathan K, Dhanapal CK, Umarani R, Manavalan R. Beneficial health effects of rutin supplementation in patients with diabetes mellitus. Journal of Applied Pharmaceutical Science 2011;1(8):227-231.

Schneider I, Kressel G, Meyer A, Krings U, Berger RG, Hahn A. Lipid lowering effects of oyster mushroom *(Pleurotus ostreatus)* in humans. Journal of Functional Foods 2011:3;17-24.

Schussler M, Holzl J, Fricke U. Myocardial effects of flavonoids from Crataegus species. Arzneirninelforschung 1995;45:842-845.

Seals DR, Silverman HG, Reiling MJ, Davy KP. Effect of regular aerobic exercise on elevated blood pressure in postmenopausal women. Am J Cardiol 1997 Jul 1;80(1):49-55.

Sedigheh A, Jamal MS, Mahbubeh S, Somayeh K, Mahmoud RK, Azadeh A, Fatemeh S. Hypoglycaemic and hypolipidemic effects of pumpkin *(Cucurbita pepo* L.) on alloxan-induced diabetic rats. African Journal of Pharmacy and Pharmacology 2011 Dec 22;5(23):2620-2626.

Segermann J, Hotze A, Ulrich H, Rao GS. Effect of alpha-lipoic acid on the peripheral conversion of thyroxine to triiodothyronine and on serum lipid-, protein- and glucose levels. Arzneimittelforschung 1991 Dec;41(12):1294-8.

Sendl A, Schliak M, Löser R, Stanislaus F, Wagner H. Inhibition of cholesterol synthesis in vitro by extracts and isolated compounds prepared from garlic and wild garlic. Atherosclerosis 1992;94:79-95.

Seppo L, Jauhiainen T, Poussa T, Korpela R. A fermented milk high in bioactive peptides has a blood pressure-lowering effect in hypertensive subjects. Am J. Clin. Nutr. 2003;77:326-330.

Sesso HD, Cook NR, Buring JE, Manson JE, Gaziano JM. Alcohol consumptio and the risk of hypertension in women and men. Hypertension 2008 Apr;51(4):1080-7.

Sethi J, Yadav M, Dahiya K, Sood S, Singh V, Bhattacharya SB. Antioxidant effect of Triticum aestivium (wheat grass) in high-fat diet-induced oxidative stress in rabbits. Methods Find Exp Clin Pharmacol 2010 May;32(4):233-5.

Shaila HP, Udupa AL, Udupa SL. Preventive actions of *Terminalia bellerica* in experimentally induced atherosclerosis. Int. J. Cardiol. 1995;49:101-106.

Shaila HP, Udupa SL, Udupa AL. Hypolipidemic activity of three indigenous drugs in experimentally induced atherosclerosis. International Journal of Cardiology 1998;67:119-124.

Shakeri A, Tabibi H, Ossareh SH. Effects of L-Carnitine Supplementation on Serum Lipids and Apoproteins in Hemodialysis Patients with Lp(a) Hyperlipoproteinemia. Iranian Journal of Nutrition Sciences & Food Technology 2007;2(2):1-14.

Sharifi AM, Darabi R, Akbarloo N. Study of antihypertensive mechanism of *Tribulus terrestris* in 2K1C hypertensive rats: Role of tissue ACE activity. Life Sciences 2003;73:2963-2971.

Sharma A, Mathur R, Dixit VP. Preventon of hypercholesterolemia and atherosclerosis in rabbits after supplementation of *Myristica fragrans* seed extract. Indian J Physiol Pharmacol 1995;39(4):407-410.

Sharma RD, Raghuram TC, Rao NS. Effect of fenugreek seeds on blood glucose and serum lipids in type I diabetes. Eur J Clin Nutr. 1990 Apr;44(4):301-6.

Shaughnessy KS, Boswall IA, Scanlan AP, Gottschall-Pass KT, Sweeney MI. Diets containing blueberry extract lower blood pressure in spontaneously hypertensive stroke-prone rats. Nutrition Research 2009;29:130-138.

Shchepotin BM, Shchulipenko IM. Treatment of patients with hypertension with an extract of the leaves of Eucommia ulmoides. Vrach Delo 1983 Jan;1:30-3.

Shen X, Lu R, He G. Effects of lyophilized royal jelly on experimental hyperlipidemia and thrombosis. Chung Hua Yu Fang I Hsueh Tsa Chih 1995 Jan;29(1):27-9.

Sheng L, Qian Z, Zheng S, Xi L. Mechanism of hypolipidemic effect of crocin in rats: crocin inhibits pancreatic lipase. Eur J Pharmacol 2006 Aug 14;543(1-3):116-22.

Sher H, Alyemeni MN. Ethnobotanical and pharmaceutical evaluation of Capparis spinosa L, validity of local folk and Unani system of medicine. Journal of Medicinal Plants Research 2010 Sep 4;4(17):1751-1756.

Sheriff M, Tukur MA, Bilkisu MM, Sera S, Falmata AS. The effet of oral administration of honey and glucophage alone or their combination on the serum biochemical parameters of induced diabetic rats. Research in Pharmaceutical Biotechnology 2011 Oct;3(9):118-122.

Shibata S, Oda K, Onodera-Masuoka N, Matsubara S, Kikuchi-Hayakawa H, Ishikawa F, Iwabuchi A, Sansawa H. Hypocholesterolemic effect of indigestible fraction of Chlorella regularis in cholesterol-fed rats. J Nutr Sci Vitaminol (Tokyo) 2001 Dec;47(6):373-7.

Shibata S, Hayakawa K, Egashira Y, Sanada H. Hypocholesterolemic mechanism of Chlorella: Chlorella and its indigestible fraction enhance hepatic cholesterol catabolism through up-regulation of cholesterol 7alpha-hydroxylase in rats. Biosci Biotechnol Biochem. 2007 Apr;71(4):916-25.

Shidfar F, Homayounfar R, Fereshtehnejad S-M, Kalani A. Effect of Folate Supplementation on Serum Homocysteine and Plasma Total Antioxidant Capacity in Hypercholesterolemic Adults under Lovastatin Treatment: A Double-blind Randomized Controlled Clinical Trial. Archives of Medical Research 2009;40:380-386.

Shidfar F, Froghifar N, Vafa M, Rajab A, Hosseini S, Shidfar S, Gohari M. The effects of tomato consumption on serm glucose, apolipoprotein B, apoliprotein A-I, homocysteine and blood pressure in type 2 diabetic patients. Int J Food Sci Nutr. 2011 May;62(3):289-94.

Shikov AN, Pozharitskaya ON, Makarov VG, Demchenko DV, Shikh EV. Effect of Leonurus cardiaca oil extract in patients with arterial hypertension accompanied by anxiety and sleep disorders. Phytother Res. 2011 Apr;25(4):540-3.

Shimada M, Hasegawa T, Nishimura C, Kan H, Kanno T, Nakamura T, Matsubayashi T. Anti-hypertensive effect of gamma-aminobutyric acid (GABA)-rich Chlorella on high-normal blood pressure and borderline hypertension in placebo-controlled double blind study. Clin Exp Hypertens 2009 Jun;31(4):342-54.

Shimanuki S, Nagasawa T, Nishizawa N. Plasma HDL subfraction levels increase in rats fed proso-millet protein concentrate. Med Sci. Monit. 2006 Jul;12(7):221-6.

Shimizu E, Hayashi A, Takahashi R, Aoyagi Y, Murakami T, Kimoto K. Effects of angiotensin I-converting enzyme inhibitor from Ashitaba (Angelica keiskei) on blood pressure of spontaneously hypertensive rats. J Nutr Sci Vitaminol (Tokyo) 1999 Jun;45(3):375-83.

Shimizu-Ibuka A, Udagawa H, Kobayashi-Hattori K, Mura K, Tokue C, Takita T, Arai S. Hypocholesterolemic Effect of Peanut Skin and Its Fractions: A Case Record of Rats Fed on a High-Cholesterol Diet. Biosci. Biotechnol. Biochem. 2009;73(1):205-208.

Shindo M, Kasai T, Abe A, Kondo Y. Effects of dietary administration of plant-derived anthocyanin-rich colors to spontaneously hypertensive rats. J Nutr Sci Vitaminol (Tokyo) 2007 Feb;53 (1):90-3.

Shirke SS, Jagtap AG. Effects of methanolic extract of *Cuminum cyminum* on total serum cholesterol in ovariectomized rats. Indian Journal of Pharmacology 2009;41(2):92-93.

Shrime MG, Bauer SR, McDonald AC, Chowdhury NH, Coltart CE, Ding EL. Flavonoid-rich cocoa consumption affects multiple cardiovascular risk factors in a meta-analysis of short-term studies. J Nutr. 2011 Nov;141(11):1982-8.

Shukla A, Bettzieche A, Hirche F, Brandsch C, Stangi GI, Eder K. Dietary fish protein alters blood lipid concentrations and hepatic genes involved in cholesterol homeostasis in the rat model. Br J Nutr. 2006 Oct;96(4):574-82.

Shum OL, Chiu KW. Hypotensive action of *Solanum melongena* on normotensive rats. Phytotherapy Research 1991;5(2):76-81.

Si H, Liu D. Genistein, a soy phytoestrogen, upregulates the expression of human endothelial nitri oxide synthase and lowers blood pressure in spontaneously hypertensive rats. J Nutr. 2008 Feb;138(2):297-304.

Si XY, Jia RH, Huang CX, Ding GH, Liu HY. Effects of Valeriana officinalis var. Latifolia on expression of transforming growth

236

factor beta 1 in hypercholesterolemic rats. Zhongguo Zhong Yao Za Zhi 2003 Sep;28(9):845-8.

Siegel G, Walter A, Engel S, Walper A, Michel F. Pleiotropic effects of garlic. Wien Med Wochenschr 1994;149(8-10):217-24.

Siddiqi HS, Mehmood MH, Rehman NU, Gilani AH. Studies on the antihypertensive and antidyslipidemic activities of *Viola odorata* leaves extract. Lipids in Health and Disease 2012;11(6).

Siddiqui MT, Siddiqi M. Hypolipidemic principles of Cicer arietinum: biochanin-A and formononetin. Lipids 1976 Mar;11(3): 243-6.

Silagy CA, Neil HA. A meta-analysis of the effect of garlic on blood pressure. J Hypertens 1994 Apr;12(4):463-8.

Sim MK. Cardiovascular actions of chicken-meat extract in normo- and hypertensive rats. Br J Nutr. 2001 Jul;86(1):97-103.

Simeonov SB, Botushanov NP, Karahanian EB, Pavlova MB, Husianitis HK, Troev DM. Effects of Aronia melanocarpa juice as part of the dietary regimen in patients with diabetes mellitus. Folia Med (Plovdiv) 2002;44(3):20-3.

Singh RB, Rastogi SS, Singh NK, Ghosh S, Gupta S, Niaz MA. Can guava fruit intake decrease blood pressure and blood lipids? J Human Hypertens 1993 Feb;7(1):33-8.

Singh AB, Tamarkar AK, Narender T, Srivastava AK. Antihyperglycaemic effect of an unusual amino acid (4-hydroxyisoleucine) in C57BL/KsJ-db/db mice. Nat Prod Res. 2010 Feb;24(3):258-65.

Singh RB, Niaz MA, Rastogi SS, Shukla PK, Thakur AS. Effect of hydrosoluble coenzyme Q10 on blood pressures and insulin resistance in hypertensive patients with coronary artery disease. J Hum Hypertens 1999 Mar;13(3):203-8.

Singh S, Rehan HM, Majumdar DK. Effect of Ocimum sanctum fixed oil on blood pressure, blood clotting time and pentobarbitone-induced sleeping time. J Ethnopharmacol 2001 Dec;78(2-3):139-43.

Singh S, Gaurav V, Parkash V. Effects of 6-week nadi-shodhana pranayama training on cardio-pulmonary parameters. Journal of Physical Education and Sports Management 2011 Aug;2(4):44-47.

Singi G, Damasceno DD, D'andrea ED, Silva GA. Acute effects of *Allium sativum* L. and *Cympobongon citratus* (DC) Stapf hydroalcoholic extracts on arterial blood pressure of anesthetized rats. Rev. Bras. Farmacogn. 2005;15(2):94-97.

Sireesha Y, Kasetti RB, Nabi SA, Swapna S, Apparao C. Antihyperglycemic and hypolipidemic activities of *Setaria italica* seeds in STZ diabetic rats. Pathophysiology 2011;18:159-164.

Sirtori CR, Zucchi-Dentone C, Sirtori M, Gatti E, Descovich GC, Gaddi A, Cattin L, Da Col PG, Senin U, Mannarino E. Cholesterol-lowering and HDL-raising properties of lecithinated soy proteins in type II hyperlipidemic patients. Ann Nutr Metab 1985;29(6):348-57.

Sivaprakasapillai B, Edirisinghe I, Randolph J, Steinberg F, Kappagoda T Effect of grape seed extract on blood pressure in subjects with the metabolic syndrome. Metabolism 2009 Dec;58(12):1743-6.

Skarpanska-Stejnborn A, Pilaczynska-Szczesniak L, Basta P, Deskur-Smielcka E. The influence of supplementation with artichoke (Cynara scolymus L.) extract on selected redox parameters in rowers. Int J Sport Nutr Exerc Metab. 2008 Jun;18(3):313-27.

Sobenin IA, Andrianova IV, Fomchenkov IV, Gorchakova TV, Orekhov AN. Time-released garlic powder tablets lower systolic and diastolic blood pressure in men with mild and moderate arterial hypertension. Hypertens Res 2009 Jun;32(6):433-7.

Sobolová L, Škottová N, Večeřa R, Urbánek K. Effect of silymarin and its polyphenolic fraction on cholesterol absorption in rats. Pharmacological Research 2006;53:104-112.

Solà R, Godàs G, Ribalta J, Vallvé JC, Girona J, Anguera A, Ostos M, Recalde D, Salazar J, Caslake M, Martin-Luján F, Salas-Salvadó J, Masana L. Effects of soluble fiber (Plantago ovata husk) on plasma lipids, lipoproteins in men with ischemc heart disease. Am J Cln Nutr. 2007 Apr;85(4):1157-63.

Somanadhan B, Varughese G, Palpu P, Sreedharan R, Gudiksen L, Smitt UW, Nyman U. An ethnopharmacological survey for potential angiotensin converting enzye inhibitors from Indian medicinal plants. Journal of Ethnopharmacology 1999;65:103-112.

Song YB, An YR, Kim SJ, Park HW, Jung JW, Kyung JS, Hwang SY, Kim YS. Lipid metabolic effect of Korean red ginseng extract in mice fed on a high-fat diet. J Sci Food Agric 2012 Jan 30;92(2):388-96.

Souza P, Gasparotto A, Crestani S, Stefanello MEA, Marques MCA, Silva-Santos JE, Kassuya CAL. Hypotensive mechanism of the extracts and artemetin isolated from Achillea millefolium L. (Asteraceae) in rats. Phytomedicine 2011;18:819-825.

Spiller GA, Miller A, Olivera K, Reynolds J, Miller B, Morse SJ, Dewell A, Farquhar JW. Effects of plant-based diets high in raw or roasted almonds, or roasted almond butter on serum lipoproteins in humans. J Am Coll Nutr. 2003 Jun;22(3):195-200.

Srivastava RD, Dwivedi S, Sreenivasan KK, Chandrashekhar CN. Cardiovascular effects of *Terminalia* species of plants. Indian Drugs 1992;29:144-149.

Srividya AR, Dhanabal SP, Satish kumar MN, Parth kumar HB. Antioxidant and Antidiabetic Activity of Alpinia Galanga. International Journal of Pharmacognosy and Phytochemical Research 2010;3(1):6-12.

Stacewicz-Sapuntzakis M, Bowen PE, Hussain EA, Damayanti-Wood Bl, Farnsworth NR. Chemical composition and potential health effects of prunes: a functional food ? Crit Rev Food Sci Nutr. 2001 May;41(4):251-86.

Staessen J, Fagard R, Lijinene P, Amery A. Body weight, sodium intake and blood pressure. J Hypertens 1989;7(1):19-23.

Stehouwer CD, van Guldener C. Does homocysteine cause hypertension? Clin Chem Lab Med 2003;41(11):1408-11.

Steiner M, Khan AH, Holbert D, Lin RIS. A double-blind crossover study in moderately hypercholesterolemic men that compared the effect of aged garlic extract and placebo administration on blood lipids. Am J Clin Nutr 1996;64:866-70.

Stensvold I, Tverdal A, Foss OP. The effect of coffee on blood lipids and blood pressure. Results frm a Norwegian cross-sectional study, men and women, 40-42 years. J Clin Epidemiol. 1989;42(9):877-84.

Stephens AM, Dean LL, Davis JP, Osborne JA, Sanders TH. Peanuts, Peanut Oil, and Fat Free Peanut Flour Reduced Cardiovascular Disease Risk Factors and the Development of Atherosclerosis in Syrian Golden Hamsters. Journal of Food Science 2010;75(4):116-122.

Strandhagen E, Thelle DS. Filtered coffee raises serum cholesterol: results from a controlled study. European Journal of Clinical Nutrition 2003;57:1164-1168.

Stravro PM, Hana AK, Vuksan V. P-3: The effect of Korean red ginseng extracts with escalating levels of ginsenoside Rg3 on blood pressure in individuals with high norma blood pressure or hypertension. Am J Hypertens 2002;15:34.

Streppel MT, Arends LR, van't Veer P, Grobbee DE, Gelejinse jM. Dietary fiber and blood pressure: a meta-analysis of randomized placebo-controlled trials. Arch Intern Med. 2005 Jan 24;165(2):150-6.

Suanarunsawat T, Boonnak T, Na Ayutthaya WD, Thirawarapan S. Anti-hyperlipidemic and cardioprotective effects of *Ocimum sanctum L.* fixed oil in rats fed a high fat diet. J Basic Clin Physiol Pharmacol 2010;21(4):387-400.

Subbalakshmi NK, Saxena SK, Urmimala, D'Souza UJA. Immediate effect of 'Nadi-Shodhana Pranayama' on some selected parameters of cardiovascular, pulmonary, and higher functions of brain. Thai Journal of Physiological Sciences 2005 Aug;18(2): 10-16.

Subramaniam S, Subramaniam R, Rajapandian S, Uthrapathi S, Gnanamanickam VR, Dubey GP. Anti-Atherogenic Activity of Ethanolic Fraction of *Terminaia arjuna* Bark on Hypercholesterolemic Rabbits. Evidence-Based Complementary and Alternative Medicine 2011:1-8.

Suda I, Oki T, Masuda M, Kobayashi M, Nishiba Y, Furuta S. Physiological Functionality of Purple-Fleshed Sweet Potatoes Containing Anthocyanins and Their Utilization in Foods. Jarq 2003;37(3):167-173.

Sudheesh S, Presannakumar G, Vijayakumar S, Vijayalakshmi NR. Hypolipidemic effect of flavonoids from *Solanum melongena.* Plant Foods for Human Nutrition 1997;51:321-330.

Suetsuna K, Maekawa K, Chen JR. Antihypertensive effects of *Undaria pinnatifida* (wakame) peptide on blood pressure in spontaneously hypertensive rats. J Nutr Biochem 2004 May;15(5):267-72.

Sugii M, Ohkita M, Taniguchi M, Baba K, Kawai Y, Tahara C, Takaoka M, Matsumura Y. Xanthoangelol D isolated from the roots of Angelica keiskei inhibits endothelin-1 production through the suppression of nuclear factor-kappaB. Biol Pharm Bull. 2005 Apr;28(4):607-10.

Suhong C, Guiyuan L, Xiaodong Z, Xiaoyu L, Han Z, Yunwei Z, Yin W, Saiyue L, Zhunan N. Anti-hypertensive effects of laiju extract in two different rat models. Asia Pac J Clin Nutr 2007;16(1):309-312.

Sui H, Yan W, Geng G. Effect of Apigenin on SBP of Spontaneous Hypertenson Rats and Its Mechanism. Journal of Environment and Health 2009 Feb

Sui H, Yu Q, Zhi Y, Geng G, Liu H, Xu H. Effects of apigenin on the expression of anglotensin-converting enzyme 2 in kidney in spontaneously hypertensive rats. Wei Sheng Yan Jiu 2010 Nov;39(6):693-6.

Sui H, Zhi Y, Liu H, Gao P, Xu H, Yan W. Endothelium-dependent vasorelaxation effects induced by apigenin on the thoracic aorta of rats and its possible mechanism. Wei Sheng Yan Jiu 2011 Jul;40(4):416-9.

Sun T, Simon PW, Tanumihardjo SA. Antioxidant phytochemicals and antioxidant capacity of biofortified carrots (Daucus carota L.) of various colors. J Agric Food Chem. 2009 May 27;57(10):4142-7.

Sung J, Han KH, Zo JH, Park HJ, Kim CH, Oh BH. Effects of red ginseng upon vascular endothelial function in patients with essentia hypertension. Am J Chin Med. 2000;28(2):205-16.

Sung YY, Yoon T, Kim SJ, Yang WK, Kim HK. Anti-obesity activity of Allium fistulosum L. extract by down-regulation of the expression of lipogenic genes in high-fat diet-induced obese mice. Mol Med Report 2011;4(3):431-5.

Susalit E, Agus N, Effendi I, Tjandrawinata RR, Nofiarny D, Perrinjaquet-Moccetti T. Olive (Olea europaea) leaf etract effective in patients with stage-1 hypertension: comparison with Captopril. Phytomedicine 2011 Feb 15;18(4):251-8.

Sutton-Tyrrell K, Boston A, Selhub J, Zeigler-Johnson C. High homocysteine levels are independently related to isolated systolic hypertension in older adults. *Circulation* 1997;96:1745-9.

Suzuki, Atsushi. Chlorogenic acid attenuates hypertension and improves entohelial function in spontaneously hypertensve rats. Journal of Hypertension 2006 Jun;24(6):1075-1082.

Suzuki A, Kagawa D, Fuiji A, Ochiai R, Tokimitsu I, Saito I. Short- and long-term effects of ferulic acid on blood pressure in spontaneously hypertensive rats. Am J Hypertens 2002 Apr;15(4 Pt 1):351-7.

Sved AF, Van Itallie CM, Fernstrom JD. Studies on the antihypertensive action of L-tryptophan. J Pharmacol Exp Ther 1982 May;221(2):329-33.

Tahri A, Yamani S, Legssyer A, Aziz M, Mekhfi H, Bnouham M, Ziyyat A. Acute diuretic, natriuretic and hypotensive effects of a continuous perfusion of aqueous extract of *Urtica dioica* in the rat. Journl of Ethnopharmacology 2000;73:95-100.

Tain YL, Huang LT, Lin IC, Lau YT, Lin CY. Melatonin prevents hypertension and increased asymmetric dimethylarginine in young spontaneous hypertensive rats. J Pineal Res. 2010 Nov;49(4):390-8.

Tain YL, Hsu CN, Huang LT, Lau YT. Apocynin attenuates oxidative stress and hypertension in young spontaneously hypertensive rats independent of ADMA/NO pathway. Free Radic Res. 2012 Jan;46(1):68-76.

Takahashi S, Tanaka H, Hano Y, Ito K, Nomura T, Shigenobu K. Hypotensive effect in rats of hydrophilic extract from *Terminalia arjuna* containing tannin-related compounds. Phytotherapy Research 1997 Sep;11(6):424-427.

Takai M, Suido H, Tanaka T, Kotani M, Fujita A, Takeuchi A, Makino T, Sumikawa K, Origasa H, Tsuji K, Nakashima M. LDL-cholesterol-lowering effect of a mixed green vegetable and fruit beverage containing broccoli and cabbage in hypercholesterolemic subjects. Rinsho Byori 2003 Nov;51(11):1073-83.

Takamitsu C, Hiroyuki A, Osami K, Takashi B. Dose Dependency of Sodium Alginate Oligosaccharides in a Randomized Double-blind Placebo-controlled Clinical Study in Subjects with High Normal Blood Pressure and Mild Hypertension. Japanese Pharmacology & Therapeutics 2006;34(11):1267-1277.

Takao T, Watanabe N, Yuhara K, Itoh S, Suda S, Tsuruoka Y, Nakatsugawa K, Konishi Y. Hypocholesterolemic Effect of Protein Isolated from Quinoa *(Chenopodium quinoa* Willd.) Seeds. Food Sci. Technol. Res. 2005;11(2):161-167.

Takeuchi H, Sakurai C, Noda R, Sekine S, Murano Y, Wanaka K, Kasai M, Watanabe S, Aoyama T, Kondo K. Antihypertensive effect and safety of dietary alpha-linolenic acid in subjects with high-normal blood pressure and mild hypertension. J Oleo Sci. 2007;56(7):347-60.

Talpur N, Echard B, Dadgar A, Aggarwal S, Zhuang C, Bagchi D, Preuss HG. Effects of Maitake mushroom fractions on blood pressure of Zucker fatty rats. Res Commun Mol Pathol Pharmacol 2002;112(1-4):68-82.

Talpur N, Echard B, Ingram C, Bagchi D, Preuss H. Effects of a novel formulation of essential oils on glucose-insulin metabolism in diabetic and hypertensive rats: a pilot study. Diabetes Obes Metab. 2005 Mar;7(2):193-9.

Talpur NA, Echard BW, Fan AY, Jaffari O, Bagchi D, Preuss HG. Antihypertensive and metabolic effects of whole Maitake mushroom powder and its fractions in two rat strains. Mol Cell Biochem 2002 Aug;237(1-2):129-36.

Tam SC, Yip KP, Fung KP, Chang ST. Hypotensive and renal effects of an extract of the edible mushroom Pleurotus sajor-caju. Life

Sci. 1986 Mar 31;38(13):1155-61.

Tamizifar B, Rismankarzadeh M, Vosoughi A-A, Rafieeyan M, Tamizifar B, Aminzade A. A Low-dose almond-based diet decreases LDL-C while preserving HDL-C. Arch Iranian Med 2005;8(1):45-51.

Tanaka H, Watanabe K, Ma M, Hirayama M, Kobayashi T, Oyama H, Sakaguchi Y, Kanda M, Kodama M, Aizawa Y. The effects of γ-Aminobutyric Acid, Vinegar, and Dried Bonito on Blood Pressure in Normotensive and Mildly or Moderately Hypertensive Volunteers. J Clin. Biochem. Nutr. 2009 Jul;45:93-100.

Tanaka Y, Sasaki R, Fukui F, Waki H, Kawabata T, Okazaki M, Hasegawa K, Ando S. Acetyl-L-carnitine supplementation restores decreased tissue carnitine levels and impared lipid metabolism in aged rats. J Lipid Res. 2004 Apr;45(4):729-35.

Tanida M, Niijima A, Fukuda Y, Sawai H, Tsuruoka N, Shen J, Yamada S, Kiso Y, Nagai K. Dose-dependent effects of L-carnosine on the renal sympathetic nerve and blood pressure in urethane-anesthetized rats. American Journal of Physiology – Regulatory, Integrative and Comparative Physiology 2005 Feb;288(2):447-455.

Tanida M, Shen J, Kubomura D, Nagai K. Effects of Anserine on the Renal Sympathetic Nerve Activity and Blood Pressure in Urethane-Anesthetized Rats. Physiol. Res. 2010;59:177-185.

Tang ZL, Shen SF. A study of Laminaria digitata powder on experimental hyperlipoproteinemia and its hemorrheology. Zhong Xi Yi Jie He Za Zhi 1989 Apr;9(4):223-5.

Tapsell LC, Gillen LJ, Patch CS, Batterham M, Owen A, Baré M, Kennedy M. Including walnuts in a low-fat/modified-fat diet improves HDL cholesterol-to-total cholesterol ratios in patients with type 2 diabetes. Diabetes Care 2004 Dec;27(12):2777-83.

Taubert D, Roesen R, Schömig E. Effect of cocoa and tea intake on blood pressure: a meta-analysis. Arch Intern Med. 2007 Apr 9;167(7):626-34.

Taubert D, Roesen R, Lehmann C, Jung N, Schömig E. Effects of low habitual cocoa intake on blood pressure and bioactive nitric oxide: a randomized controlled trial. JAMA 2007 Jul 4;298(1):49-60.

Tazakori Z, Zare M, M Iranparvar, Mehrabi Y. Effect of rice bran on blood glucose and serum lipid parameters in type II diabetic patient. Iranian Journal of Endocrinology and metabolism 2006;8(2):169-174.

Teas J, Baldeón ME, Chiriboga DE, Davis JR, Sarriés AJ, Braverman LE. Could dietary seaweed reverse the metabolic syndrome? Asia Pac J Clin Nutr 2009;18(2):145-157.

Telles S, Nagarathna R, Nagemdra HR, Desiraju T. Physiological changes in sports teachers following 3 months of training in yoga. Indian Journal of Medical Sciences 1993 Oct;47(10)

Teow SS. Effective dosage of the extract of Ganoderma lucidum in the treatment of various ailments. In Royse DJ editor(s). *Mushroom biology and mushroom products.* Pennsylvania: Pennsylvanian State University 1996.

Teres S, Barceló-Coblijn G, Benet M, Álvarez R, Bressani R, Halver JE, Escribá PV. Oleic acid content is responsible for the reduction in blood pressure induced by olive oil. PNAS 2008 Sep 16;105(37):13811-13816.

Terpstra AH, Lapré JA, de Vries HT, Beynen AC. The hypocholesterolemic effect of lemon peels, lemon pectin, and the waste stream material of lemon peels in hybrid F1B hamsters. Eur J Nutr. 2002 Feb;41(1):19-26.

Terzic MM, Dotlic J, Maricic S, Mihailovic T, Tosic-Race B. Influence of red clover-derived isoflavones on serum lipid profile in postmenopausal women. J Obstet Gynaecol Res 2009 Dec;35(6):1091-5.

Testai L, Chericoni S, Calderone V, Nencioni G, Nieri P, Morelli I, Martinotti E. Cardiovascular effects of Urtica dioica L. (Urticaceae) roots extracts: in vitro and in vivo pharmacological studies. J Ethnopharmacol 2002 Jun;81(1):105-9.

Thakur CP, Thakur B, Singh S, Sinha PK, Sinha SK. The Ayurvedic medicines Haritaki, Amala and Bahira reduce cholesterol-induced atherosclerosis in rabbits. Int J Cardiol. 1988 Nov;21(2):167-75.

Thathola A, Srivastava S, Singh G. Effect of foxtail millet *(Setaria italica)* supplementation on serum glucose, serum lipids and glycosylated hemoglobin in type 2 diabetics. Diabetologia Croatica 2011;40(1):23-27.

Thayyil AH, Surulivel MKM, Ahmed MF, Ahmed GSS, Sidheeq A, Rasheed A, Ibrahim M. Hypolipidemic activity of *Luffa aegiptiaca* fruits in cholesterol fed hypercholesterolemic rabbits. International Journal of Pharmaceutical Applications 2011;2(1):81-88.

Theerthahalli, Arun Sudheendra, Shenoy, Rekha, Taranalli, Ashok D. Evaluation of saponin rich fraction of trigonella foenum Graecum for antihypertensive activity. Pharmacologyonline 2009;1:1229-1233.

Theobald HE, Goodall AH, Sattar N, Talbot DC, Chowienczyk PJ, Sanders TA. Low-dose docosahexaenoic acid lowers diastolic blood pressure in middle-aged men and women. J Nutr. 2007 Apr;137(4):973-8.

Thirunavukkarasu V, Nandhini ATA, Anuradha CV. Effect of α-Lipoic Acid on Lipid Profile in Rats Fed a High-Fructose Diet. Experimental Diab. Res. 2004;5:195-200.

Tian N, Rose RA, Jordan S, Dwyer TM, Hughson MD, Manning RD Jr. N-Acetylcysteine improves renal dysfunction, ameliorates kidney damage and decreases blood pressure in salt-sensitive hypertension. J Hypertens. 2006 Nov;24(11):2263-70.

Timmers S, Konings E, Bilet L, Houtkooper RH, van de Weijer T, Goossens GH, Hoeks J, van der Krieken S, Ryu D, Kersten S, Moonen-Kornips E, Hesselink MK, Kunz I, Schrauwen-Hinderling VB, Blaak EE, Auwerx J, Schrauwen P. Calorie restriction-like effects of 30 days of resveratrol supplementation on energy metabolism and metabolic profile in obese humans. Cell Metab. 2011 Nov 2;14(5):612-22.

Tinker LF, Schneeman BO, Davis PA, Gallaher DD, Waggoner CR. Consumption of prunes as a source of dietary fiber in men with mild hypercholesterolemia. Am J Clin Nutr 1991 May;53(5):1259-65.

Tiwari S, Singh S, Patwardhan K, Gehlot S, Gambhir IS. Effect of *Centella asiatica* on mild cognitive impairment (MCI) and other common age-related clinical problems. Digest Journal of Nanomaterials and Biostructures 2008 Dec;3(4):215-220.

Toda N, Ayajiki K, Fujioka H, Okamura T. Ginsenoside potentiates NO-mediated neurogenic vasodilation of monkey cerebral arteries. J Ethnopharmacol 2001;76:109-113.

Todorov S, Philianos S, Petkov V, Harvala C, Zamfirova R, Olimpiou H. Experimental pharmacological study of three species from genus Salvia. Acta Physiol Pharmacol Bulg 1984;10(2):13-20.

Toghyani M, Tohidi M, Toghyani M, Gheisari A, Tabeidian SA. Evaluation of yarrow (*Achillea millefolium*) as a natural growth promoter in comparison with a probiotic supplement on performance, humoral immunity and blood metabolites of broiler chicks. Journal of Medicinal Plants Research 2011 Jul. 4;Vol. 5 (13);2748-2754.

Tokede OA, Gaziano JM, Djousse L. Effects of cocoa products/dark chocolate on serum lipids: a meta-analysis. European Journal of Clinical Nutrition 2011;65:879-886.

Tokunaga S, White IR, Frost C, Tanaka K, Kono S, Tokudome S, Akamatsu T, Moriyama T, Zakouji H. Green tea consumption and serum lipids and lipoproteins in a populaton of healthy workers in Japan. Ann Epidemiol 2002 Apr;12(3):157-65.

Tomotake H, Shimaoka I, Kayashita J, Yokoyama F, Nakajoh M, Kato N. Stronger Suppression of Plasma Cholestrol and Enhancement of the Fecal Excretion of Steroids by a Buckwheat Protein Product than by a Soy Protein Isolate in Rats Fed on Cholesterol-free Diet. Biosci. Biotechnol. Biochem 2001.;65 (6):1412-1414.

Tong CC, Choong YK, Mohamed S, Mustapha NM, Umar NA. Efficacy of Ganoderma lucidum on plasma lipids and lipoproteins in rats fed with high cholesterol diet. Nutrition & Food Science 2008;38(3):229-238.

Torres-Duran PV, Ferreira-Hermosillo A, Juarez-Oropeza MA. Antihyperlipemic and antihypertensive effects of *Spirulina maxima* in an open sample of mexican population: a preliminary report. Lipids in Health and Disease 2007;6:33.

Toyoshi T, Kohda T. Antihypertensive Activity of Purple Corn Color in Spontaneously Hypertensive Rats. Foods Food Ingredients J. Jpn. 2004;209(8)

Trinh HN, Quynh NN, Anh TV, Nguyen VP. Hypolipidemic effect of extracts from *Abelmoschus esculentus* L. - malvaceae on tyloxapol-induced hyperlipidemia in mice. 13th Int. Electron. Conf. Synth. Org. Chem. 2009.

Trinidad TP, Mallillin AC, Loyola AS, Sagum RS, Encabo RR. The potential health benefits of legumes as a good source of dietary fibre. British Journal of Nutrition 2010;103:569-574.

Trovato A, Monforte MT, Barbera R, Rossitto A, Galati EM, Forestieri AM. Effects of fruit juices of *Citrus sinensis* L. and *Citrus limon* L. on experimental hypercholesterolemia in the rat. Phytomedicine 1996;2(3):221-227.

Tsi D, Das NP, Tan BK. Effects of aqueous celery (*Apium graveolens*) extract on lipid parameters of rats fed a high fat diet. Planta Med 1995 Feb;61(1):18-21.

Tsi D, Tan BK. Effects of celery extract and 3-N-butylphthalide on lipid levels in genetically hypercholesterolaemic (RICO) rats. Clin Exp Pharmacol Physiol 1996 Mar;23(3):214-7.

Tsi D, Tan BK. The mechanism underlying the hypocholesterolaemic activity of aqueous celery extract, its butanol and aqueous fractions in genetically hypercholesterolaemic RICO rats. Life Sci 2000 Jan 14;66(8);755-67.

Tsuzuki W, Kikuchi Y, Shinohara K, Suzuki T. Fluorometric Assay of Angiotensin I-converting Enzym Inhibitory Activity of Vinegars. Nippon Shokuhin Kogyo Gakkaishi 1992;39(2):188-192.

Tuncer MA, Yamaci B, Sati L, Cayli S, Acar G, Altung T, Demir R. Influence of *Trbulus terrestric* extract on lipid profile and endothelial structure in developing atherosclerotic lesions in the aorta of rabbits on a high-cholesterol diet. Acta hstochemica 2009;111:488-500.

Tuomilehto J, Lindström J, Hyyrynen J, Korpela R, Karhunen ML, Mikkola L, Jauhiainen T, Seppo L, Nissinen A. Effect of ingesting sour milk fermented by *Lactobacillus helveticus* bacteria on blood pressure in subjects with mild hypertension. J. Human Hyperten. 2004;18:795-802.

Twait CM, Slavin JL. Grape Powder Lowers Serum Triglycerides in Postmenopausal Women. The Journal of Applied Research 2007;7(2):196-203.

Uchida S, Ikari N, Ohta H. Inhibitory effects of condensed tannins on angiotensin converting enzyme. Jpn J Pharmacol 1987;43: 242-246.

Ulicná O, Greksák M, Vancová O, Zlatos L, Galbavý S, Bozek P, Nakano M. Hepatoprotective effect of rooibos tea (Aspalathus linearis) on CCI4-induced liver damage in rats. Physiol Res. 2003;52(4):461-6.

Umadevi P, Murugan S, Jennifer Suganthi S, Subakanmani S. Evaluation of antidepressant like activity of *cucurbite pepo* seed extract in rats. International Journal of Current Pharmaceutical Research 2011;3(1):108-113.

Umar A, Imam G, Yimin W, Kerim P, Tohti I, Berké B, Moore N. Antihypertensive effects of Ocimum basilicum L. (OBL) on blood pressure in renovascular hypertensive rats. Hypertension Research 2010 Jul;33:727-730.

Umegaki K, Shinozuka K, Watarai K, Takenaka H, Yoshimura M, Daohua P, Esashi T. *Ginko Biloba* Extract Attenuates The Development Of Hypertension In Deoxycorticosterone Acetate-Salt Hypertensive Rats. Clinical and Experimental Pharmacology and Physiology 2000 Apr;27(4):277-282.

Umeki Y, Hayabuchi H, Hisano M, Kuroda M, Honda M, Ando B, Ohta M, Ikeda M. The Effect of the Dried-Bonito Broth on Blood Pressure, 8-Hydroxydeoxyguanosine (8-OHdG), an Oxidative Stress Marker, and Emotional States in Elderly Subjects. J. Clin. Biochem. Nutr. 2008 Nov;43:175-184.

Ushida Y, Matsui T, Tanaka M, Matsumoto K, Hosoyama H, Mitomi A, Sagesaka Y, Kakuda T. Endothelium-dependent vasorelaxation effect of rutin-free tartary buckwheat extract in isolated rat thoracic aorta. Journal of Nutritional Biochemistry 2008;19:700-707.

Vacha GM, Giorcelli G, Siliprandi N, Corsi M. Favorable effects of L-carnitine treatment on hypertriglyceridemia in hemodialysis patients: decisive role of low levels of high-density lipoproein-cholesterol. Am J Clin Nutr. 1983 Oct;38(4):532-40.

Valcheva-Kuzmanova S, Kuzmanov K, Mihova V, Krasnaliev I, Borisova P, Belcheva A. Antihyperlipidemic effect of Aronia melanocarpa fruit juice in rats fed a high-cholesterol diet. Plant Food Hum Nutr 2007 Mar;62(1):19-24.

Valcheva-Kuzmanova S, Kuzmanov K, Tancheva S, Belcheva A. Hypoglycemic and hypolipidemic effects of Aronia melanocarpa fruit juice in streptozotocin-induced diabetic rats. Methods Find Exp Clin Pharmacol 2007 Mar;29(2):101-5.

Vanhatalo A, Bailay SJ, Blackwell JR, DiMenna FJ, Pavey TG, Wilkerson DP, Benjamin N, Winyard PG, Jones AM. Acute and chronic effects of dietary nitrate supplementation on blood pressure and the physiological responses to moderate-intensity and incremental exercise. Am J Physiol Regul Integr Comp Physiol. 2010 Oct;299(4):1121-31.

Vanitha T, Sumathy H, Sangeetha J, Devaki B, Vijayalakshmi K. Phytochemical analysis of *Allium ascalonicum*. Biomedicine 2009;29(1):22-25.

Varalakshmi B, Thirunethiran Karpagam, Prabha PL, Firdous SJ, Gomathi S. International Journal of Pharmaceutical Research and Development (IJPRD) 2011 Sep;3(7):128-133.

Vasdev S, Mian T, Longerich L, Prabhakaran V, Parai S. N-acetyl cysteine attenuates ethanol induced hypertension in rats. Artery 1995;21(6):312-6.

Vasdev S, Ford CA, Parai S, Longerich L, Gadag V. Dietary alpha-lipoic acid supplementation lowers blood pressure in spontaneously hypertensive rats. J Hypertens 2000 May;18(5):567-73.

Vecera R, Orolin J, Skottová N, Kazdová L, Oliyarnik O, Ulrichová J, Simánek V. The influence of maca (Lepidium meyenii) on antioxidant status, lipid and glucose metabolism in rat. Plant Foods Hum Nutr. 2007 Jun;62(2):59-63.

Venugopal S, Iyer UM. Management of diabetic dyslipidemia with subatmospheric dehydrated barley grass powder. Int J Green Pharm 2010;4:251-6.

Vera R, Sánchez M, Galisteo M, Villar IC, Jimenez R, Zarzuelo A, Pérez-vizcaino F, Duarte J. Chronic administration of genistein improves endothelial dysfunction in spontaneously hypertensive rats: involvement of eNOS, caveolin and calmodulin expression and NADPH oxidase activity. Clinical Science 2007;112:183-191.

Vered Y, Grosskopf I, Palevitch D, Harsat A, Charach G, Weintraub MS, Graff E. The influene of Vicia faba (broad bean) seedlings on urinary sodium excretion. Planta Med. 1997 Jun;63(3):237-40.

Verhoef P, Steenge GR, Boelsma E, van Vliet T, Olthof MR, Katan MB. Dietary serine and cystine attenuate the homocysteine-raising effect of dietary methionine: a randomized crossover trial in humans. Am J Clin Nutr. 2004 Sep;80(3):674-9.

Verma S, Jain V, Katewa SS. Blood pressure lowering, fibrinolysis enhancing and antioxidant activities of Cardamon *(Elettaria cardamomum)*. Indian Journal of Biochemistry & Biophysics 2009 Dec;46:503-506.

Verma SK, Jain V, Verma D, Khamesra R. *Crataegus oxyacantha* – a cardioprotective herb. Journal of Herbal Medicine and Toxicology 2007;1(1):65-71.

Vijayakumar MV, Pandey V, Mishra GC, Bhat MK. Hypolipidemic effect of fenugreel seeds in mediated through inhibition of fat accumulation and upregulation of LDL receptor. Obesity (Silver Spring) 2010 Apr;18(4):667-74.

Vinson JA, Bose P. The effect of a high chromium yeast on the blood glucose control and blood lipids of normal and diabetic human subjects. Nutritional Reports Internationl 1984;30(4)

Vinson JA, Demkosky CA, Navarre DA, Smyda MA. High-Antioxidant Potatoes: Acute in Vivo Antioxidant Source and Hypotensiv Agent in Humans after Supplementation to Hypertensive Subjects. J Agric Food Chem. 2012 Feb 6.

Vishal A, Parveen K, Pooja S, Kannappan N, Kumar S. Diuretic, Laxative and Toxicity Studies of *Viola odorata* Aerial Parts. Pharmacologyonline 2009;1:739-748.

Vittek J. Effect of royal jelly on serum lipids in experimental anmals and humans with atherosclerosis. Experientia 1995 Sep 29;51(9-10):927-35.

Wada K, Nakamura K, Tamai Y, Tsuji M, Sahashi Y, Watanabe K, Ohtsuchi S. Seaweed intake and blood pressure levels in healthy pre-school Japanese children. Nutrition Journal 2011;10:83.

Wagner H. Search for New Plants Constituents with Antiasthmatic and Antihypertonic Activity. Phytomedicines of Europe 1998 Apr 5:691(5):46-61.

Walaszek Z, Szemraj J, Hanausek M, Adams AK, Sherman U. D-Glucaric acid content of various fruits and vegetables and cholesterol-lowering effects of dietary D-Glucarate in the rat. Nutrition Research 1996;16(4):673-681.

Walker AF, Marakis G, Morris AP, Robinson PA. Promising hypotensive effect of hawthorn extract: a randomized double-blind pilot study of mild, essential hypertension. Phytother Res. 2002;16:48-54.

Walker AF, Marakis G, Simpson E. Hypotensive effects of hawthorn for patients with diabetes taking prescription drugs: a randomized controlled trial. Br J Gen Pract. 2006;56:437-443.

Wan WJ, Ma CY, Xiong XA, Wang L, Ding L, Zhang YX, Wang Y. Clinical observation on therapeutic effect of electroacupuncture at Quchi (LI11) for treatment of essential hypertension. Zhongguo Zhen Jiu. 2009 May;29(5):349-52.

Wang J-J, Wang H-Y, Shih C-D. Autonomic Nervous System and Nitric Oxide in Antihypertensive and Cardiac inhibitory Effects Induced by Red Mold Rice in Spontaneously Hypertensive Rats. J. Agric. Food Chem. 2010;58(13):7940-7948.

Waqar MA, Mahmood Y. Anti-Platelet, Anti-Hypercholesterolemic and Anti-Oxidant Effects of Ethanolic Extracts of *Brassica oleracea* in High Fat Diet Provided Rats. World Applied Sciences Journal 2010;8(1):107-112.

Watanabe M, Ayugase J. Effects of buckwheat sprouts on plasma and hepatic parameters in type 2 diabetic db/db mice. J. Food Sci. 2010 Nov – Dec;75(9):294-9.

Watanabe T, Yamada T, Tanaka H, Jiang S, Mazumder TK, Nagai S, Tsuji K. Antihypertensive Effect of y-Aminobutyric Acid-Enriched *Agaricus blazei* on Spontaneously Hypertensive Rats. Nippon Shokuhin Kagaku Kogaku Kaishi 2002;49(3):166-173.

Watanabe T, Kawashita A, Ishi S, Mazumder TK, Nagai S, Tsuji K, Dan T. Antihypertensive Effect of .GAMMA.-Aminobutyric Acid-Enriched Agaricus blazai on Mild Hypertensive Human Subjects. Journal of the Japanese Society for Food Science and Technology 2003;50(4):167-173.

Watanabe T, Arai Y, Mitsui Y, Kusaura T, Okawa W, Kajihara Y, Saito I. The blood pressure-lowering effect and safety of chlorogenic acid from green coffee bean extract in essential hypertension. Clin Exp Hypertens. 2006 Jul;28(5):439-49.

Weck M, Hanefeld M, Leonhardt W, Haller H, Robowsky KD, Noack R, Schmandke H. Field bean protein diet in hypercholesteremia. Nahrung 1983;27(4):327-33.

Weil A, Assmus KD, Neukum-Schmidt A. *Crategeus* special extract WS 1442: Assessment of objective effectiveness in patients with heart failure. Fortschr Med. 1996;114:291-96.

Weil N, Friger M, Press Y, Tal D, Soffer T, Peleg R. The Effect of Acupuncture on Blood Pressure in Hypertensive Patients Treated in Complementary Medicine Clinic. Integrative Medicine Insights 2007;2:1-5.

Wergedahl H, Liaset B, Gudbrandsen OA, Lied E, Espe M, Muna Z, Mørk S, Berge RK. Fish protein hydrolysate reduces plasma total cholesterol, increases the proportion of HDL cholesterol, and lowers acyl-CoA: cholesterol acyltransferase activity in liver of Zucker rats. J Nutr. 2004 Jun;134(6):1320-7.

Whelton SP, Hyre AD, Pedersen B, Yi Y, Whelton PK, He J. Effect of dietary fiber intake on blood pressure: a meta-analysis of randomized, controlled clinical trials. Hypertens 2005 Mar;23(3):475-81.

Wichitsranoi J, Weerapreeyakul N, Boonsiri P, Settasatian C, Settasatian N, Komanasin N, Sirijaichingkul S, Teerajetgul Y, Rangkadilok N, Leelayuwat N. Antihypertensive and antioxidant effects of dietary black sesame meal in pre-hypertensive humans. Nutr J, 2011 Aug 9;10:82.

Wider B, Pittler MH, Thompson-Coon J, Ernst E. Artichoke leaf extract for treating hypercholesterolaemia. Cochrane Database Syst

Rev. 2009 Oct 7;4.

Willi SM, Oexmann MJ, Wright NM, Collop NA, Key Jr LL. The Effects of a High-protein, Low-fat, Ketogenic Diet on Adolescents With Morbid Obesity: Body Composition, Blood Chemistries, and Sleep Abnormalities. Pediatrics 1998 Jan 1;101(1):61-67.

Williams T, Mueller K, Cornwall MW. Effect of acupuncture-point stimulation on diastolic blood pressrure in hypertensive subjects: a preliminary study. Phys Ther. 1991 Jul;71(7):523-9.

Winham DM, Hutchins AM, Johnston CS. Pinto Bean Consumption Reduces Biomarkers for Heart Disease Risk. Journal of the American College of Nutrition 2007;26(3):243-249.

Winther K, Randløv C, Rein E, Mehlsen J. Effects of ginkgo biloba extract on cognitive function and blood pressure in elderly subjects. Current Therapeutic Research 1998 Dec;59(12):881-888.

Witham MD, Nadir MA, Struthers AD. Effect of vitamin D on blood pressure: a systematic review and meta-analysis. J Hypertens 2009 Oct;27(10):1948-54.

Witte S, Anadere I, Walitza E. Improvement of hemorheology with ginkgo biloba extract Decreasing a cardiovascular risk factor. Fortschr Med 1992 May 10;110(13):247-50.

Wójcicki J, Samochowiec L, Juzwiak S, Gonet B, Syrynski W, Barcew-Wiszniewska B, Rozewicka L, Tustanowski S, Ceglecka M, Juzyszyn Z, Mysliwiec Z, Kaldonska M, Górnik W, Kadlubowska D. Ginkgo biloba extract inhibits the development of experimental atherosclerosis in rabbit. Phytomedicine 1994;1:33-38.

Wroblewska M, Juskiewicz J, Wiczkowski W. Physiological properties of beetroot crisps applied in standard and dyslipidaemic diets of rats. Lipids Health Dis 2011 Oct 14;10(1):178.

Wu F, Meng G, Yang L. Preventive effect of Ganoderma lucidum polysaccharides on formation of atherosclerosis in experimental rats. Journal of Nantong University (Medical Sciences) 2008.

Wu L, Noyan Ashraf MH, Facci M, Wang R, Paterson PG, Ferrie A, Juurlink BH. Dietary approach to attenuate oxidative stress, hypertension, and inflammation in the cardiovascular system. Proc Natl Acad Sci USA 2004 May 4;101(18):7094-9.

Wu T, Zhou X, Deg Y, Jing Q, Li M, Yuan L. *In vitro* studies of *Gynura divaricata* (L.) DC extracts as inhibitors of key enzymes relevant for type 2 diabetes and hypertension. Journal of Ethnopharmacology 2011;136:305-308.

Wu YH, Zhu GQ, Lin XY, Oyang L, Su H, Wu B. Effect of needling quchi and taichong points on blood levels of endothelin and angiotension converting enzyme in patients with hypertension. Zhongguo Zhong Xi Yi Jie He Za Zhi 2004 Dec;24(12):1080-3.

Wycherley TP, Noakes M, Clifton PM, Cleanthous X, Keogh JB, Brinkworth GD. A high-protein diet with resistance exercise training improves weight loss and body composition in overweight and obese patients with type 2 diabetes. Diabetes Care 2010 May;33(5):969-76.

Xia W, Sun C, Zhao Y, Wu L. Hypolipidemic and antioxidant activities of sanchi (radix notoginseng) in rats fed with a high fat diet. Phytomedicine 2011 Apr 15;18(6):516-20.

Xia X, Ling W, Ma J, Xia M, Hou M, Wang Q, Zhu H, Tang Z. An anthocyanin-rich extract from black rice enhances atherosclerotic plaque stabiliation in apolipoprotein E-deficient mice. J Nutr. 2006 Aug;136(8):2220-5.

Xie JT, Chang WT, Wang CZ, Mehendale SR, Li J, Ambihaipahar R, Ambihaipahar U, Fong HH, Yuan CS. Curry leaf (Murraya koenigii Spreng.) reduces blood cholesterol and glucose leves in ob/ob mice. Am J Chin Med. 2006;34 (2):279-84.

Xin X, He J, Frontini MG, Ogden LG, Motsamai OI, Whelton PK. Effects of alcohol reduction on blood pressure: a meta-analysis of randomized controlled trials. Hypertension 2001 Nov;38(5):1112-7.

Xiping L, Xianqiong F. Clinical effects of tartary buckwheat on senile hyperlipemia. Current Advances in Buckwheat Research 1995;Vol II:947-950.

Xu GL, Yu SQ, Gong ZN, Zhang SQ. Study of the effect of crocin on rat experimental hyperlipemia and the underlying mechanisms. Zhongguo Zhong Yao Za hi 2005 Mar;30(5):369-72.

Xu H, Xu HE, Ryan D. A study of the comparative effects of hawthorn fruit compound and simvastatin on lowering blood lipid levels. Am J Chin Med 2009;37:903-908.

Xu Q, Zhao Y, Cheng GR. Blood-lipid decreasing action of total saponins of Panax notoginseng (Burk.) F.H. Chen. Zhongguo Zhong Yao Za Zhi 1993 Jun;18(6):367-8.

Xu X, Yu Z, Shuai L, Guo Y, Duan D, Fu P. The effect of kelp on serum lipids of hyperlipidemia in rats. Journal of Food Biochemistry 2011 Dec 30.

Xu YC, Leung SWS, Yeung DKY, Hu LH, Chen GH, Che CM, Man RYK. Structure-activity relationships of flavonoids for vascular relaxation in porcine coronary artery. Phytochemistry 2007;68:1179-1188.

Xu YY, Yang C, Li SN. Effects of genistein on angiotensin-converting enzyme in rats. Life Sci 2006;79(9):828-37.

Xue WL, Li XS, Zhang J, Liu YH, Wang ZL, Zhang RJ. Effect of Trigonella foenum-graecum (fenugreek) extract on blood glucose, blood lipid and hemorheological properties in streptozotocin-induced diabetic rats. Asia Pac J Clin Nutr 2007;16(1):422-6.

Ya-ming F, Min-yuan X, Lu-ya W, Ying Z, Li Z, Hong Y, Peng W, Ping C. The effect of edible black tree fungus (Auricuaria auricula) on experimental atherosclerosis in rabbits. Chinese Medical Journal 1989;102(2):100-105.

Yadav S, Tomar AK, Jithesh O, Khan MA, Yadav RN, Srinivasan A, Singh TP, Yadav S. Purification and Partial Characterization of Low Molecular Weight Vicilin-Like Glycoprotein from the Seeds of Citrullus Ianatus. Protein J. 2011 Oct 12.

Yaghoobi N, Al-Waili N, Ghayour-Mobarhan M, Parizadeh SMR, Abasalti Z, Yaghoobi Z, Yaghoobi F, Esmaeili H, Kazemi-Bajestani SMR, Aghasizadeh R, Saloom KY, Ferns GAA. Natural Honey and Cardiovascular Risk Factors; Effects on Blood Glucose, Cholesterol, Triacylglycerole, CRP, and Body Weight Compared with Sucrose. TheScientificWorldJOURNAL 2008;8:463-469.

Yagnik B, Nilesh K, Rameshvar P, Natavarlal P, Jitendra V, Nurudin J. Antihyperlipidemic and antioxidant activity of *Benincasa cerifera* on high fat diet induced hyperlipidemic rat. Journal of Pharmacy Research 2009;Vol.2.Issue 3.:363-366.

Yahia DA, Madani S, Prost J, Bouchenak M, Belleville J. Fish protein improves blood pressure but alters HDL 2 and HDL 3 composition and tissue lipoprotein lipase activities in spontaneously hypertensive rats. European Journal of Nutrition 2005;44(1):10-17.

Yang, Byung-Keun, Jeong SC, Song CH. Hypolipidemic Effect of Exo- and Endo-Biopolymers Produced from Submerged Mycelial Culture of *Ganoderma lucidum* in Rats. J. Microbiol. Biotechnol. 2002;12(6):872-877.

Yang B, Jeong S, Song C. Hypolipidemic effect of exo- and endo-biopolymers produced from submerged mycelial culture of Ganoderma lucidum in rats. *Journal of Microbiology and Biotechnology* 2002;12(6):872-7.

Yang BK, Kim DH, Jeong SC, Das S, Choi YS, Shin JS, Lee SC, Song CH. Hypoglycemic Effect of a *Lentinus edodes* Exo-polymer Produced from a Submerged Mycelial Culture. Biosci. Biotechnol. Biochem. 2002;66(5):937-942.

Yang TTC, Koo MWL. Hypocholesterolemic effects of chinese tea. Pharmacological Research 1997;35(6).505-512.

Yang X, Yang L, Zheng H. Hypolipidemic and antioxidant effects of mulberry *(Morus alba* L.) fruit in hyperlipidaemia rats. Food and Chemical Toxicology 2010;48:2374-2379.

Yang Y, Zhou L, Gu Y, Zhang Y, Tang J, Li F, Shang W, Jiang B, Yue X, Chen M. Dietary chickpeas reverse visceral adiposity, dyslipidaemia and insulin resistance in rats induced by a chronic high-fat diet. Br J Nutr. 2007 Oct;98(4):720-6.

Yang YC, Lu FH, Wu JS, Wu CH, Chang CJ. The protective effect of habitual tea consumption on hypertension. Arch Intern Med. 2004 Jul 26;164(14):1534-40.

Yam D, Friedman J, Bott-Kanner G, Genin I, Shinitzky M, Klainman E. Omega-3 Fatty Acids Reduce Hyperlipidaemia, Hyperinsulinaemia and Hypertension in Cardiovascular Patients. J Clin Basic Cardiol 2002;5:229.

Yamada T, Oinuma T, Niihashi M, Mitsumata M, Fujioka T, Hasegawa K, Nagaoka H, Itakura H. Effects of Lentinus edodes mycelia on dietary-induced atherosclerotic involvement in rabbit aorta. J Atheroscler Thromb. 2002;9(3):149-56.

Yamagami T, Shibata N, Folkers K. Bioenergetics in clinical medicine. Studies on coenzyme Q10 and essentil hypertension. Res Commun Chem Pathol Pharmacol 1975 Jun;11(2):273-88.

Yamagami T, Shibata N, Folkers K. Bioenergetics in clinical medicine. VIII. Administration of coenzyme Q10 to patients with essential hypertension. Res Commun Chem Pathol Pharmacol 1976 Aug;14(4):721-7.

Yamaguchi T, Chikama A, Mori K, Watanabe T, Shioya Y, Katsuragi Y, Tokimitsu I. Hydroxyhydroquinone-free coffee: a double-blind, randomized controlled dose-response study of blood pressure. Nutr. Metab. Cardiovasc Dis. 2008 Jul;18(6):408-14.

Yamamoto M, Suzuki A, Hase T. Short-Term Effects of Glucosyl Hesperidin and Hesperetin on Blood Pressure and Vascular Endothelial Function in Spontaneously Hypertensive Rats. J Nutr Sci Vitaminol 2008;54:95-98.

Yamamoto Y, Aoyama S, Hamaguchi N, Rhi GS. Antioxidative and Antihypertensive Effects of Welsh Onion on Rats Fed with a High-Fat High-Sucrose Diet. Biosci. Biotechnol. Biochem. 2005;69(7):1311-1317.

Yamamoto Y, Yasuoka A. Welsh Onion Attenuates Hyperlipidemia in Rats Fed on High-Fat High-Sucrose Diet. Biosci. Biotechnol. Biochem. 2010;74(2):402-404.

Yang DH. Effect of electroacupuncture on Quchi (LI11) and Taichong (LR3) on blood pressure variability in young patients with hypertension. Zhongguo Zhen Jiu. 2010 Jul;30(7):547-50.

Yang GY, Wang W. Clinical studies on the treatment of coronary heart disease with Valeriana officinalis var latifolia. Zhongguo Zhong Xi Yi Jie He Za Zhi 1994 Sep;14(9):540-2.

Yannan F, Ruxun H, Yan Z, Jianwen L, Jinru L. A preliminary investigation of Tanakan in the treatment of hypertensive arteriosclerosis and stroke in rats. Chinese Medical Journal 2000;113(5):425-428.

Yao Y, Chen F, Wang M, Wang J, Ren G. Antidiabetic activity of Mung bean extracts in diabetic KK-Ay mice. J Agric Food Chem 2008 Oct 8;56(19):8869-73.

Yazdanparast R, Bahramikia S. Evaluation of the effect of Anethum graveolens L. crude extracts on serum lipids and lipoproteins profiles in hypercholesterolaemic rats. DARU Journal of Pharmaceutical Sciences 2008;16(2):88-94.

Ye XJ, Morimura S, Han LS, Shigematsu T, Kida K. In vitro evaluation of physiological activity of vinegar produced from barley-, sweet potato-, and rice-shochu post-distillation slurry. Biosci Biotechnol Biochem 2004 Mar;68(3):551-6.

Yegnanarayan R, Sangle SA, Sirsikar SS, Mitra DK. Regression of cardiac hypertrophy in hypertensive patients – Comparison of Abana with propranolol. Phytother. Res. 1997;11(3):257.

Yeligar V, Murugesh K, Dash DK, Nayak SS, Maiti BC, Maity TK. Evaluation of Antidiabetic and Antihyperlipidemic Activity of *Luffa tuberosa* (Roxb.) Fruits in Streptozotocin Induced Diabetic Rats. Natural Product Sciences 2007;13(1):17-22.

Yin C, Seo B, Park HJ, Cho M, Jung W, Choue R, Kim C, Park HK, Lee H, Koh H. Acupuncture, a promising adjunctive therapy for essential hypertension: a double-blind, randomized, controlled trial. Neurological Research 2007;29(1):98-103.

Yokogoshi H, Kato Y, Sagesaka YM, Takihara-Matsuura T, Kakuda T, Takeuchi N. Reduction effect of theanine on blood pressure and brain 5-hydroxyindoles in spontaneously hypertensive rats. Biosci Biotechnol Biochem 1995 Apr;59(4):615-8.

Yokozawa T, Kim HY, Kim HJ, Tanaka T, Sugino H, Okubo T, Chu DC, Juneja LR. Amla (Emblia officinalis Gaertn.) attenuates age-related renal dysfuncton by oxidative stress. J Agric Food Chem. 2007 Sep 19;55(19):7744-52.

Yokozawa T, Kim HY, Kim HJ, Okubo T, Chu DC, Juneja LR. Amla (Emblica officinalis Gaertn.) prevents dyslipidaemia and oxidative stress in the ageing process. Br J Nutr. 2007 Jun;97(6):1187-95.

Yoshida H, Yanai H, Ito K, Tomono Y, Koikeda T, Tsukahara H, Tada N. Administration of natural astaxanthin increases serum HDL-cholesterol and adiponectin in subjects with mild hyperlipidemia. Atherosclerosis 2009.

Yu Y-M, Chang W-C, Chang C-T, Hsieh C-L, Tsai CE. Effects of young barley leaf extract and antioxidative vitamins on LDL oxidation and free radical scavenging activities in type 2 diabetes. Diabetes Metab (Paris) 2002;28:107-114.

Yu Y-M, Chang W-C, Liu C-S, Tsai C-M. Effect of Young Barley Leaf Extract and Adlay on Plasma Lipids and LDL Oxidation in Hyperlipidemic Smokers. Biol. Pharm. Bull. 2004;27(6):802-805.

Yuan ZZ, Cheng KM, Huang W, Dilshat, Feng DR. Study on industrialized extraction technology and function of hyperlipidemic regulating of Laminaria japonica polysaccharides. Zhong Yao Cai 2010 Nov;33(11):1795-8.

Yuen KH, Wong JW, Lim AB, Ng BH, Choy WP. Effect of Mixed-Tocotrienols in Hypercholesterolemic Subjects. Functional Foods in Health and Disease 2011;3:106-117.

Zambón D, Sabaté J, Muñoz S, Campero B, Casals E, Merlos M, Laguna JC, Ros E. Substituting walnuts for monounsaturated fat improves the serum lipid profile of hypercholesterolemic men and women. A randomized crossover trial. Ann Intern Med. 2000 Apr 4;132(7):538-46.

Zaoui A, Cherrah Y, Lacaille-Dubois MA, Settaf A, Amarouch H, Hassar M. Diuretic and hypotensive effects of Nigella sativa in the spontaneously hypertensive rat. Therapie. 2000;55(3):379-82.

Zaoui A, Cherrah Y, Alaoui K, Mahassine N, Amarouch H, Hassar M. Effects of Nigella sativa fixed oil on blood homeostasis in rat.

J Ethnopharmacol. 2002 Jan;79(1):23-6.

Zavoral JH, Hannan P, Fields DJ, Hanson MN, Frantz ID, Kuba K, Elmer P, Jacobs DR Jr. The hypolipidemic effect of locust bean gum food products in familial hypercholesterolemic adults and children. Am J Clin Nutr. 1983 Aug;38 (2):285-94.

Zeggwagh NA, Michel JB, Eddouks M. Acute Hypotensive and Diuretic Activities of *Chamaemelum nobile* Aqueous Extract in Normal Rats. American Journal of Pharmacology and Toxicology 2007;2(3):140-145.

Zeggwagh NA, Michel JB, Sulpice T, Eddouks M. Cardiovascular Effect of *Capapris spinosa* Aqueous Extract in Rats. Part II: Furosemide-like Effect of *Capparis spinosa* Aqueous Extract in Normal Rats. American Journal of Pharmacology and Toxicology 2007;2(3):130-134.

Zeggwagh NA, Eddouks M, Michel JB, Sulpice T, Hajji L. Cardiovascular Effect of *Capparis spinosa* Aqueous Extract. Part III: Antihypertensive Effect in Spontaneously Hypertensive Rats. American Journal of Pharmacology and Toxicology 2007;2(3): 111-115.

Zenebe W, Pecháňová O, Andriantsitohaina R. Red Wine Polyphenols Induce Vasorelaxation by Increased Nitric Oxide Bioactivity. Physiol. Res. 2003;52:425-432.

Zeng JF. Clinical study of Semen Raphani in the treatment of hyperlipidemia 38 cases in elder patients. Zhejiang Tradit Chin Med 1995;30:494.

Zern TL, Wood RJ, Greene C, West KL, Liu Y, Aggarwal D, Shachter NS, Fernandez ML. Grape polyphenols exert a cardioprotective effect in pre- and postmenopausal women by lowering plasma lipids and reducing oxidative stress. J Nutr. 2005 Aug;135(8);1911-7.

Zhang J, Marquina N, Oxinos G, Sau A, Ng D. Effect of laser acupoint treatment on blood pressure and body weight – a pilot study. Journal of Chiropractic Medicine 2008;7:134-139.

Zhang J, Ng D, Sau A. Effects of electrical stimulation of acupuncture points on blood pressure. Journal of Chiropractic Medicine 2009;8:9-14.

Zhang Q, Wang GJ, A J, WU D, Zhu LL, MA B, Du Y. Application of GC/MS-based metabonomic profilinf in studying the lipid-regulatig effects of *Ginkgo biloba* extract on diet-induced hyperlipidemia in rats. Acta Pharmacologica Sinica 2009;30:1674-1687.

Zhang W, Wang X, Liu Y, Tian H, Flickinger B, Empire MW, Sun SZ. Dietary flaxseed lignan extract lowers plasma cholesterol and glucose concentrations in hypercholesterolaemic subjects. Br J Nutr. 2008 Jun;99(6):1301-9.

Zhang XF, Tan BK. Effects of an ethanolic extract of Gynura procumbens on serum glucose, cholesterol and triglyceride levels in normal and streptozotocin-induced diabetic rats. Singapore Med J. 2000 Jan;41(1):9-13.

Zhang Y, Li X, Zou D, Liu W, Yang J, Zhu N, Huo L, Wang M, Hong J, Wu P, Ren G, Ning G. Treatment of Type 2 Diabetes and Dyslipidemia with the Natural Plant Alkaloid Berberine. J Clin Endocrinol Meta 2008 Jul;93(7):2559-2565.

Zhang YH, Chen SW, Zhou M, Deng YF. Experimental studies on anti-hypertension effect of Semen Raphani injection. JiLin Tradit Chin Med 1996;41.

Zhang YG, Zhang HG, Zhang GY, Fan JS, Li XH, Liu YH, Li SH, Lian XM, Tang Z. Panax notoginseng saponins attenuate atherosclerosis in rats by regulating the blood lipid profile and an anti-inflammatory action. Clin Exp Pharmacol Physiol 2008 Oct;35(10):1238-44.

Zhao CL, Guo HC, Dong ZY, Zhao Q. Pharmacological and nutritional activities of potato anthocyanins. African Journal of Pharmacy and Pharmacology 2009 Jan;2(10):463-468.

Zhao HL, Sim JS, Shim SH, Ha YW, Kang SS, Kim YS. Antiobese and hypolipidemic effects of platycoding saponins in diet-induced obese rats: evidences for lipase inhibition and calorie intake restriction. International Journal of Obesity 2005;29:983-990.

Zhao HL, Harding SV, Marinangeli CP, Kim YS, Jones PJ. Hypocholesterolemic and anti-obesity effects of saponins from Platycodon grandiflorum in hamsters fed atherogenic diets. J Food Sci. 2008 Oct;73(8):195-200.

Zhao Q, Matsumoto K, Okada H, Ichiki H, Sakakibara I. Anti-hypertensive and anti-stroke effects of *Chrysanthemum* extracts in stroke-prone spontaneously hypertensive rats. J. Trad. Med. 2008;25:143-151.

Zhao Y, Wang J, Ballevre O, Luo H, Zhang W. Antihypertensive effects and mechanisms of chlorogenic acids. Hypertens Res. 2011 Nov 10.

Zheng XX, Xu YL, Li SH, Liu XX, Hui R, Huang XH. Green tea intake lowers fasting serum total and LDL cholesterol in adults: a meta-analysis of 14 randomized controlled trials. Am J Clin Nutr. 2011 Aug;94(2):601-10.

Zhou XZ, Kang L, Tang Y, Li L, Xiong SH. Effect of Valeriana Officinalis Var Latifolia Miq on Heart Rat and Arterial Blood Pressure of Rabbite. Journal of Liaoning University of Traditional Chinese Medicine 2009 Dec.

Zhu W, Chen M, Shou Q, Li Y, Hu F. Biological Activities of Chinese Propolis and Brazilian Propolis on Streptozotocin-Induced Type 1 Diabetes Mellitus in Rats. Evidence-Based Complementary and Alternative Medicine 2011.

Zibadi S, Farid R, Moriguchi S, Lu Y, Foo LY, Tehrani PM, Ulreich JB, Watson RR. Oral administration of purple passion fruit peel extract attenuates blood pressure in female spontaneously hypertensive rats and humans. Nutrition Research 2007;27:408-416.

Zilkens RR, Burke V, Hodgson JM, Barden A, Beilin LJ, Puddey B. Red Wine and Beer Elevate Blood Pressure in Normotensive Men. Hypertension 2005;45:874-879.

Zou Y, Lu Y, Wei D. Hypocholesterolemic effects of a flavonoid-rich extract of Hypericum perforatum L. in rats fed a cholesterol-rich diet. J Agric Food Chem. 2005 Apr 6;53(7):2462-6.

Zulet MA, Martinez JA. Corrective role of chickpea intake on a dietary-induced model of hypercholesterolemia. Plant Foods Hum Nutr. 1995 Oct;48(3):269-77.

Zunft HJ, Lüder W, Harde A, Haber B, Graubaum HJ, Koebnick C, Grünwald J. Carob pulp preparation rich in insoluble fibre lowers total and LDL cholesterol in hypercholesterolemic patients. Eur J Nutr 2003 Oct;42 (5):235-42.